Epidemics and History

Epidemics and History

Disease, Power and Imperialism

SHELDON WATTS

Yale University Press
New Haven and London

First published in paperback 1999

Set in Sabon by Best-set Typesetter Ltd, Hong Kong
Printed in the United States of America

Library of Congress Cataloging-in-Publication Data

Watts, S. J. (Sheldon J.)
Epidemics and history: disease, power, and imperialism/Sheldon Watts.
Includes bibliographical references and index.
ISBN 0-300-07015-2 (hbk.)
ISBN 0-300-08087-5 (pbk.)
1. Epidemics—History. 2. Social medicine. I. Title.
RA649.W27 1997
614.4′9—dc21 97-28168
CIP

A catalogue record for this book is available from the British Library.

10 9 8 7 6 5 4

Contents

Illustrations

Prints courtesy the Wellcome Institute Library, London.

Acknowledgements

This book has been in process for several years. Looking over my notes, I find I gave presentations touching on the social history of plague and cholera at Arts Faculty seminars at the University of Ilorin in 1981–82. I am grateful to my Nigerian colleagues, my Nigerian students and Nigeria in general in helping me develop skills in reflexivity which are a prerequisite for any undertaking of this sort. In England in 1990–91 Professor R. Mansell Prothero of the University of Liverpool had been asked to write a book on human migration and disease, building on his earlier *Migrants and Malaria* (Longmans, 1965). By way of my spouse Susan Watts, his former student, the project passed to me.

For the last six years Roy Porter of the Wellcome Institute for the History of Medicine has been a constant pillar of support and sound advice. He patiently read and commented upon each chapter as it emerged and then read the entire semi-completed work when it was half again as long as it is now. Without Roy's support and encouragement, the book would not have seen the light of day.

Once the project was underway, many scholars were willing to offer advice and bibliographic suggestions. I am grateful to Professor William McNeill (*Plagues and Peoples*) for his comments and suggestions on the Black Death, as well as his earlier suggestion that my *Social History* (1984) might have benefited from a more holistic approach. Professor McNeill was one of the committee members, I was another, in organizing a John Carter Brown Library conference on "America in European Consciousness: An International Conference on the Intellectual Consequences of the Discovery of the New World, 1493–1750," held in Providence, Rhode Island in June 1991. I am grateful to two other committee members, Professors Anthony Pagden and John Elliott, for discussions which helped me develop ideas on the European "Other." Further assisting me in this were discussions I had with David Arnold of the School of Oriental and African Studies during my stay at the Wellcome in the spring of 1993. I am also grateful to Professor Philip Curtin of Johns Hopkins for taking time to comment upon a very early, still unfootnoted draft of "Yellow Fever and Malaria." I am grateful to many scholars for discussions and references: Dr Kenneth Mott (WHO, Geneva) for material on cholera; Professor Barnett Cline of the Department of Tropical Medicine, Tulane University (LA) for important materials on yellow fever; Donald Hopkins (of Global 2000) for up-to-date information on smallpox; Dr Peter Winch of Johns Hopkins for materials on malaria; Dr JoAnne Moran of Georgetown for materials on leprosy; Donald Hiesel (latterly with the UN) for other materials on leprosy; and Dr Elizabeth Sartain (AUC Center of Arabic Studies) for her insights on the Mamluks. Professor Richard Pankhurst (of Addis Ababa) provided me with useful insights into epidemiological contexts in pre-war Ethiopia. Two Ilorin scholars have been particularly supportive, both in running down materials and in prolonged discussion: Dr Ann O'Hear, latterly of Kwara College of Technology, and Dr Hugh Vernon Jackson, one of the last colonial education officers in Ilorin, later Pro-Vice-Chancellor at the University of Botswana at Gaberone, now resident in Cairo. I am extremely grateful as well to Dr Adel Abou Seif (Suez Canal University) for enabling me to visit our local leprosarium and for insightful discussion about epidemic diseases. The staff of several libraries have been most helpful in facilitating research: in the UK, the libraries of the Wellcome Institute for the History of Medicine, the School of Tropical Medicine, the University of London (Senate House), the School of Oriental and African Studies, and the Institute of Historical Research; in the US, Northwestern University, Evanston, and the University of Minnesota at Duluth; in Egypt, the American University in Cairo and the Mubarak Library. A Wellcome Institute for the History of Medicine research grant (038042/Z/93/Z) in 1993 enabled me to meet a wide range of scholars and to enjoy a solid block of library research time. Two anonymous readers for Yale University Press provided me with insights into a variety of topics and mindsets; some of these are reflected in the final version of this book. At the Press itself, Robert Baldock has always been most helpful.

Finally, my gratitude to my spouse companion for half of my life. Susan has been involved with the project from its very inception, and has always been most generous with her time, with Conradian and all other forms of support, reading and commenting upon each draft chapter as it emerged. Without her, the project would never have been conceived, nurtured and brought to final completion.

Cairo / Ilorin / Lokoja
1 January 1997

Introduction

> Cairo and Plague! During the whole time of my stay, the plague was so master of the city, and stared so plain in every street and every alley, that I can't now affect to dissociate the two ideas. . . . The orientals, however, have more quiet fortitude than Europeans under afflictions of this sort. . . .[In the cities of the dead], tents were pitched, and *swings hung for the amusement of children*—a ghastly holiday! but the Mahometans take a pride . . . in following their ancient customs undisturbed by the shadow of death.
>
> Alexander Kinglake, *Eothen*, 1835[1]

Living and writing in largely Islamic Cairo 160 years after the author of *Eothen* observed it in time of plague, I am struck by the continuing integrity of Egyptian culture when confronted with life-threatening crises. I am also aware that the sort of cultural imperialism trumpeted by Kinglake is far from dead. For instance, one of the quality London newspapers recently available on Cairene streets revealed that a United Nations panel on climatic change estimated the cash value of each individual in the Third World at only one-fifteenth that of persons in Western Europe or America.[2]

One of the first questions to be asked of a study in comparative history concerned with power relations and the impact of epidemic diseases is about the role played by university-trained medical doctors; have they always performed the same functions as they do today? The short answer is a firm "no". Until the early twentieth century and the "medicalization" of the West, most sick Europeans not of high or middling status relied on their family for basic health care. If the situation worsened, they might call in healers from the village and perhaps supplement this by cures recommended by wandering pedlars. Aside from financial costs and status considerations, one reason why ordinary Europeans so seldom had recourse to medical doctors was the perception that they were unable to cure any serious illness.

Following guidelines laid down by Galen (131–*c.* 201 CE) and Avicenna (in Arabic, Ibn Sina) (d. 1037), doctors themselves saw their task as providing clients with special individualized techniques for preventing ill health. When a client who had been acting on a medically prescribed regimen was

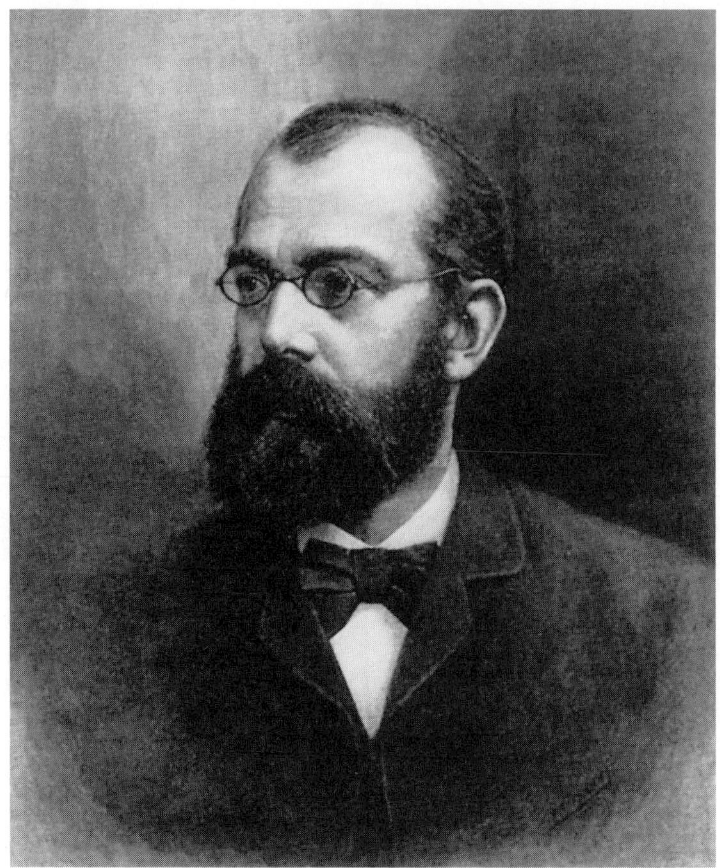

1. Professor Robert Koch. Engraving by P. Naumann for the *Illustrated London News*, 29 November 1890.

actually struck by a serious sickness, the doctor's function was to give the impression of *caring*, through placebos, bathings, bleedings, and dietary recommendations. He (before the nineteenth century, a woman doctor would have been a contradiction in terms) knew full well that he could not actually *cure* the illness.[3]

For our purposes, modern medicine begins with the work of the Prussian medical scientist Robert Koch (1843–1910). Koch discovered the tiny living organism (vibrio) that causes cholera while in Alexandria (Egypt) in 1883 and confirmed his finding in Calcutta (Bengal) in 1884; he had discovered the causal agent of tuberculosis two years earlier.[4] Yet it was some time before Koch's radical ideas won general acceptance and came to influence therapeutics. Doctors trained in the "scientific truths" of the Great Tradition held that most diseases were caused by miasmas, undisciplined life-styles, and anything other than tiny *living* organisms. Confronted with Koch's ideas, they were unwilling to give up what they had always believed. Only with their retirement did younger men trained in the new paradigm finally come to the fore.[5]

The transitional years (1880s–1930s) that led to the full medicalization of the West (lay people's acceptance of medical doctors as their first line of defense against disease) coincided with the great age of European and North American imperialism; the two phenomena were not unrelated. Coming out of the scramble for Africa, the scramble for China, and the conquest of Spain's old empire in the Caribbean and Pacific by the USA was the new discipline of Tropical Medicine. From its very onset tropical medicine was thus an "instrument of empire" intended to enable the white "races" to live in, or at the very least to exploit, all areas of the globe. Justifying this new role were the "truths" concocted by Herbert Spencer and later incorporated into popularizations of Charles Darwin's seminal works on evolution. As generally understood, the Social Darwinistic message was that Europeans were at the very summit of the evolutionary chain and that they should, by right, dominate all other humankind.[6]

Yet as we know, the only thing new about these assertions was the scientism used to support them; as an actual phenomenon European imperialism dates back some five hundred years. Europe's first moves toward world domination were undertaken by the Portuguese and the Spanish in the fifteenth century, followed in the next two hundred years by the Dutch, French and English. Then in the mid-seventeenth century, emerging from what had already become a true global economy touching all habitable continents except Australia were the beginnings of mass consumerism. This phenomenon was part of a larger scheme, *Development*, which was managed by agents living in the financial capitals of Europe: Genoa, Lisbon and Antwerp and later Amsterdam and London.

Regarded for our purposes as a principal motor force of the early modern and modern world, Development was capable of taking on a multiplicity of forms. Most required four elements: (1) fertile land, seeds, forests, mineral and other *raw materials* that could be converted into products (some of them entirely new) which consumers could be enticed to buy; (2) the *laborers* who did the actual converting and who might or might not double as consumers, depending on what their owners or employers permitted; (3) the *credit* and credit facilities needed to meet the costs of bringing together on one site the raw materials and the labor needed to convert it into a saleable product and then to take it to whichever market would provide the highest profit; and (4) the *consumers* who, by handing over cash, promissory notes or verbal promises to pay, converted the finished product into gold or silver, the species on which the pre-1930s European credit system rested. Until the final quarter of the nineteenth century (when high-tech industry finally prevailed), the actual nature of finished products—whether completely manufactured by hand, by machine, or by a combination of both—was immaterial. What did matter was that the European agents of Development kept its processes turning over and brought under its influence more and more of the world's people.[7]

Among the unintended consequences of Development was the creation of disease networks which—like the trading network first put in place by the Portuguese—spanned the world. Before Columbus's fateful crossing of the Atlantic in 1492, none of the epidemic diseases treated in this book—bubonic plague, leprosy, smallpox, cholera, malaria, yellow fever or venereal syphilis (as opposed to yaws) had existed in the New World. This happy condition has been seen as the result of two sets of happenings. The first was the migration of proto-Asian peoples overland across what is now the Bering Straits some 40,000 years ago; rising seas closed this route 30,000 years later. These incoming settlers formed the genetic core of the population of the pre-Columbian New World. Second, occurring in the Old World *after* the emigrants had departed, was the evolution of modern diseases.[8]

Theory—based on Europeans' idea that their own past establishes rules applicable always and everywhere—holds that in order to evolve, the types of epidemic disease we deal with here required sizeable populations of settled people. In the Old World, settled agriculture (as opposed to root-gathering and hunting) began between 10,000 BCE (in Asia) and 9,000 BCE (in Egypt and the Fertile Crescent). This chronology fits nicely with time schedules positing the evolution and appearance of Old World diseases. The theory however does not explain why (except for TB) these failed to develop in the New World. In the western hemisphere, in existence from around 500 BCE, principally in Meso-America, were large market towns and populous cities (many with over 50,000 inhabitants).

The evolution of microscopic organisms capable of causing epidemic diseases on the Eurasian land mass several thousand years *after* Native Americans' ancestors left meant that the latter's descendants had no occasion or need to develop immunities against them. The consequences of this were catastrophic, particularly in the case of smallpox. Beginning only twelve years after the death of Columbus himself, in any New World region invaded by infective Europeans, within a generation or so nine out of ten Native Americans would be carried off by smallpox, or other lethal illnesses which seemed like it, before they had time to have children of their own.

But for the Development agents in Europe who were determined to reap maximum profit from mines of gold and silver in the New World, the destruction of Native Americans was no great loss. Thanks to Portuguese naval technology (soon surpassed by that of the Dutch and English) and to Portuguese bases in Africa and Asia, it was relatively easy to import *African* slaves to work the *American* mines. Thus within a few short decades of European contact, the holocaust of smallpox (together with measles and typhus) combined with white greed and other human behaviors to transform the ethnic composition of the New World completely.[9]

In any polity, whether in Europe itself, or in a non-European-ruled region being transformed by Development, or in a proper European colony, an epidemic impacted on the power relationship between the dominant few and the dominated many. Obviously, it was the rulers who determined the official response to the disease threat (sometimes in consultation with medical doctors). Though epidemiological contexts differed, very often the elite would claim that the disease targeted one particular set of people while leaving others alone. Arrived at through a complex of cultural filters, this perception was part of what I term the disease Construct (as in Construct leprosy, or Construct yellow fever). In establishing official responses, this Construct determined what—if anything—should be done in an attempt to limit disease transmission.[10]

Very often, ordinary people found that the policies put in force during an epidemic—the quick burial of corpses in lime in mass graves, confiscation of the property of the dead, closure of markets, establishment of quarantines—posed far greater threats to their world of lived experience and expectation than the disease itself. Yet the privileged few could never understand why their own ideas (taken to be exemplary of the wisdom of the learned Great Tradition) should not be taken as the universal norm. With the coming of the Enlightenment in France, England and Scotland, the divergence of elite and popular attitudes became wider still.[11]

In the following six chapters, I place each epidemic disease in two different cultural settings, one European and the other Non-Western. Contextualization in time, space and culture means that I have set myself a rather different task than William McNeill assigned himself twenty years ago; essentially what McNeill did was to assess the impact of epidemic diseases on humankind in general.[12] Working chronologically, I begin with a study of the bubonic plague in West Europe and in the Cairo-based Mamluk Middle Eastern empire, both hit by the illness in 1347. In Europe it disappeared in the 1690s/1720s but lingered in the Middle East until the 1840s. In the West, centuries after the plague had disappeared it remained the quintessential scourge against which later crises tended to be compared.[13] Yet, horrendous as Europe's experiences were, at least the plague did not open it to conquest by aliens in the way that smallpox later did the Americas.

The second chapter, on leprosy, begins in the Middle Ages in Europe with an examination of the growth of the potent Construct, the "leper" as stigmatized being, then proceeds to case studies of the way this Construct was applied in the colonized world in the nineteenth century. Beginning with Hawai'i and India, I move on to South Africa, Nigeria, the Philippines and Malaysia. The chapter ends with a note of warning: though there is now an effective cure for leprosy if applied in time, the medieval Christian Construct remains. People prone to accept current western wisdom about Construct lepers seldom seek medical care early enough to prevent the irreversible loss of fingers and toes.

Chapter 3 deals with smallpox in the Americas and in Europe. The fourth chapter examines the hidden plague, venereal syphilis, in Europe and in the Americas after *c.* 1493. The chapter ends with a discussion of the ways in which the proud civilization that was China confronted Construct syphilis.

Cholera in India and in Great Britain is the subject of the fifth chapter. During the years of British rule, *c.* 1786–1947, cholera claimed the lives of upwards of 28 million people. Before the British arrived, it is unlikely that it had ever been a major threat to the subcontinent as a whole. Cholera thus may be seen as the quintessential disease of colonialism. Within the British Isles, where the disease first struck in 1831, cholera and Construct cholera (in this instance a Construct not related to the colonial experience) are seen as one of the several anvils on which the still inchoate middle class beat down their social enemies, the communitarian artisans and craftsmen, who in older understandings were the true people of England.

Malaria and yellow fever in the Atlantic world (Africa, the Caribbean, mainland America) are treated in the penultimate chapter. In the evolution of these diseases, Development (involving the involuntary migration of millions of potential laborers from East to West) is again found to be a principal motor force. As with leprosy in the nineteenth century, disease Constructs were important in shaping dominant peoples' attitudes. Construct yellow fever held that black Africans were immune to the disease. This mischievous understanding was taken to demonstrate that the Christian God had specially created them to serve as slaves in North, Meso- and South America. In Africa and Liverpool in the 1890s, British medical personnel further marginalized blacks by creating a malaria Construct.

This harsh vision of the uses of epidemic disease in the past leads in the "Afterword" to a brief discussion of the situation at the time this book went to press. I take as my point of departure the fact that, building on the insights of Robert Koch, modern doctors and technicians have finally achieved the capacity to control all of the epidemic diseases discussed in this study. In the case of malaria, today still a major killer, it can be argued that failure to control it is due to socio-intellectual-economic barriers rather than to technical ignorance *per se*. With the overcoming of similar barriers, smallpox was abolished from the face of the earth in 1977.[14]

Though scientific knowledge advances year by year, medical personnel remain part of larger social systems and cannot avoid sharing their underlying values. So it is that in the economically advanced North and in certain urban enclaves in the tropics, key groupings of people have agendas for personal gain that do not give high priority to the control of infectious diseases now found mainly in the South. Yet *ordinary* people of the sort Alexander Kinglake observed in Cairene cemeteries in 1835 and I see on Cairo's streets every day have time and again shown their willingness to accept the equal worth and dignity of each of their fellow human beings. In such people lie the seeds of a more humane future.[15]

1 The Human Response to Plague in Western Europe and the Middle East, 1347 to 1844

Introduction

In the summer of 1347 rats and fleas infected with bubonic plague boarded Genoese merchant ships at Caffa on the Black Sea. Later that year some of these ships passed through the Dardanelles, touched down at Messina (Sicily) and then sailed to Pisa, Genoa and Marseilles: other Genoese ships sailed directly from Caffa to the mouths of the Nile in Egypt. Within a few months pestilence of a form unknown to contemporaries began killing men, women and children on both sides of the Mediterranean. As 1348 wore on, the plague began striking populations along the Atlantic and Baltic coasts. Then, travelling up rivers, along paths and across fields, it reached Europeans living deep in the interior.

Though reliable information is scarce, it would seem that during the five years (1347–51) the Black Death was darting about, mortality varied from an eighth to two-thirds of a region's population. Overall it may have killed three Europeans out of every ten, leaving some 24 million dead. This remains the worst epidemic disease disaster in Europe since the collapse of the Roman Empire.[1]

Also appallingly high was the casualty rate in the Muslim Middle East: between a quarter and a third of the population died. Writing in 1349, Ibn Khatimah, a medical writer from Andalusia (Muslim southern Spain), testified that:

> This is an example of the wonderful deeds and power of God, because never before has a catastrophe of such extent and duration occurred. No satisfactory reports have been given about it, because the disease is new. . . . God only knows when it will leave the earth.[2]

In the years after 1351, bubonic plague continued to make sporadic appearances, sparing neither lands to the north nor to the south of the Mediterranean. Though no category of person was immune, it seemed that on every second or third visitation the plague targeted a region's pregnant women and young children. The net effect was to prune back the sprouts of population growth by killing young people before they were old enough to have children of their own. In the case of ill-favored Florence, generally taken to be the birthplace of the Renaissance, after being hit by plague eight times between 1348 and 1427 the city was left with little more than a third of its pre-plague population of 100,000.[3]

Then for reasons that remain unclear, after around 1450 mortality rates in Christendom began to diverge from those found in the Muslim Middle East; in the latter region pestilence continued to be a frequent population-slashing visitor until the 1840s. By way of contrast, in a Europe that was still overwhelmingly rural, except for localized outbreaks such as those which hit north Italian *urban* centers in 1575–76, 1630–31 and 1656, the ability of plague to significantly reduce the numbers of humans of reproductive age ended in the mid-fifteenth century. Thereafter, outbreaks of plague became increasingly random, missing whole regions for decades. This pattern allowed the population gradually to recover and then to forge beyond its 1347 proportions.[4]

Within this framework, beginning with Western Europe, I will explore the reasons why elites did not respond to the plague as a *sui generis* disease crisis requiring a special response until around 1450; only then did well-born north Italians create plague-specific policies based on what I will call the Ideology of Order.[5] After these policies were introduced in the most politically pliable provinces of Europe (Tuscany, Liguria, Lombardy, Venetia) there was a time lag of 200 years before they were given general continental application. As used after 1660, quarantine and the other standard control techniques probably were the agencies that forced pestilence into retreat, though not all experts agree on this.[6] Be this as it may, it is abundantly clear that the new policies severely strained traditional ideas about the roles appropriate to rulers and those who were ruled. As will be seen, within Europe the creation of plague controls greatly strengthened both the image and the reality of elite authority.

Turning then to the Cairo-based Mamluk Empire and the Ottoman Turkish regime that succeeded it in 1517, I will investigate why no interventionist policy was developed until Muhammad Ali became Viceroy of Egypt in 1805. By that time Egypt's population stood at a mere 3 million, less than a third of what it had been before the onset of plague in 1347.

In this chapter, I do not intend to enter into the debate about the role which urban and rural depopulation, caused by the Black Death and succeeding pestilences, played in the long-term fortunes of the various regions of West Europe and the Middle East. It should be pointed out however that these debates have led to the unsensational discovery that a sudden decrease in human numbers is only *one* of the variables that can decisively tilt the balance between an old established, flourishing economic region (such as northern Italy) and regions such as England and the Netherlands from which new-style entrepreneurial opportunists emerged. With regard to Italy, the Cambridge historian S. R. Epstein has recently compared the fortunes of Sicily and Tuscany. He suggests that though initial plague mortalities may have weakened the importance of both regions' long-distance trade in luxury goods (of concern only to elites), of more lasting importance was the impetus sudden population decline gave to the development of regional markets for non-luxury goods, and with it the growth in the proportion of local people who depended on market transactions for their livelihoods rather than on subsistence agriculture. Within each region, what counted most was the institutional framework and mindset of the governing classes. In a loosely articulated setting where competition between rival rule-givers left large areas of ordinary people's lives unpoliced (the situation in Sicily), peasants and artisans who survived the plague had room to work out strategies for long-term family betterment. Able to control their spending patterns and family size, they could produce the specialized goods for sale on regional markets which gave them the disposable income they needed to became market-orientated consumers. In contrast, in Renaissance Florence and its *contado* (hinterland) where the pre-plague institutional framework was authoritarian and efficient, and remained so after the population hemorrhages of 1348–1450, tax burdens and labor requirements imposed on ordinary people prevented them from rising above the poverty level.[7] Here then in two regions hit by the same mass killer disease, differing patterns of elite behavior resulted in quite different consequences.

Shifting Attitudes towards Disease

Anthony Molho has recently written of the need for a language "with which to express . . . the alienness of late medieval Italian culture."[8] In that alien past, literate elites confronted with the Black Death tended to interpret it in ways that matched their ideas of what a disease disaster was *supposed* to entail based on readings of ancient Greco-Roman authors.[9] One example of the hold the Ancients had is the entry made by Agnolo di Tura in the chronicles of Siena:

> The mortality began in Siena in May [1348]. It was horrible and cruel. . . . And it is not possible for human tongue to tell of the horror. . . . Father abandoned child, wife, husband. . . . None there were who for money or friendship would bury the dead. . . . And in many places in Siena huge pits were dug and the multitude of the dead were piled within them. . . . And I, Agnolo di Tura . . . buried my five children with my own hands. And there were those so poorly covered with earth that the dogs dug them up and gnawed their bodies throughout the city. And there were none who wept for any death, for everyone expected to die.[10]

Deeply moving though this description is, parallels in wording and phraseology suggest that it may owe more to di Tura's awareness of what the ancient historian Thucydides had written about a disease disaster said to have occurred in Athens in 427 BCE than it did to lived experience in 1348 CE.

When plague re-emerged in 1347 (an earlier, all but forgotten, pandemic had raged from 541 to 775 CE), the Judeo-Christian notion prevailing among the learned held that humans were a special kind of being; they alone had souls, they alone had a contractual relationship with their creator God. In Renaissance Florence, added to this scripturally based construct was the Neoplatonic philosophy of pagan origin (derived from the writings of Plotinus of Asyut, Egypt, d. 270 CE) that again came into fashion in the early fifteenth century. In this sanitized Christian form, Neoplatonic theory posited that all living things were linked in a Great Chain of Being. In this chain, noble humankind came next after the angels, archangels and the glorious company of heaven and was separated by many links from lowly rats. This concept, together with the idea that humankind was of unique interest to the God who controlled the stars, impeded recognition of a possible link between humans and rats in such matters as plague transmission.[11]

Learned people's prejudice against empirical observation—regarded as a practice typical of peasants, craftsmen and other disreputable types—also formed a barrier to untrammelled observation of what was essentially a new phenomenon. Thus in the north Italian town of Busto Arsizio in 1630 it was reported that there was "a great quantity of rats . . . one could count them by the hundreds in every house . . . they were so hungry that they gnawed at doors and windows." But such were the mindsets then in existence that this sort of behavior by rats was regarded as a discrete happening, unconnected with plague. In fairness, it should be noted that the considerable time lag between the death of the first plague-stricken rats, the movement of rat fleas from dead rat to live human, the biting process, the two- to six-day incubation period within the victim, followed by the death of the first plague-stricken human, then by the deaths of whole groupings of people, also made it difficult to conceptualize any connection between rat behavior and the plague.[12]

The trail which eventually led to the unravelling of the mysteries of the causal agents and transmission patterns of the bubonic plague—in its third pandemic form (1890–1945) and by analogy in its 1347–1844 form as well—began with the seventeenth-century scientific revolution.[13] One consequence of this intellectual revolution was the creation of an alternative vision which dethroned humankind from its central place in the great scheme of the universe. Two hundred and fifty years down the road some of the constructs that emerged from seventeenth-century seeds of doubt began to make an impact on medical thinking: combining doubts and empirical observation of the real world the germ theory at last came into being.

Working independently, in 1876 and 1877, Robert Koch and Louis Pasteur discovered that anthrax—a disease of cattle and horses which can jump species and attack humans—was caused by a micro-organism too small to be seen with the naked eye but large enough to be detected by a high-powered microscope. The two medical doctors who, working independently of each other, first applied this insight to bubonic plague were the Japanese doctor Shiba Saburo Kitasato (who was with Koch in Berlin between 1886 and 1891) and Dr Alexander Yersin, a Swiss student of Louis Pasteur and Emile Roux. While in Hong Kong during the plague of 1894 both men found that the bacillus now known as *Yersinia pestis* was present in the tissues of plague-dead rats and of plague-dead humans. Two years later, in Bombay, Dr Paul Lewis Simond of France established that the link between rats and humankind was the rat flea *Xenopsylla cheopis.* Though a hundred other flea species could also transmit plague, *Xenopsylla cheopis* is now thought to be the principal vector of the plague in its bubonic form.[14]

Once infected with the plague bacillus, the rat flea is unable to digest its food—rat's blood—and becomes voraciously hungry. After the rat dies of plague, the flea looks desperately around for food and if a human host is available moves there. However, because one human being cannot transfer *bubonic* plague directly to another, the unseen force governing the bacillus *Yersinia pestis* regards humans as a cul-de-sac. While waiting for a new animal host, a displaced rat flea might hibernate for up to fifty days in grain (for making bread, for most people the staff of life) or in soft white things, such as woollen cloth. Since both grain and cloth were important items of trade, their transport was one of the ways in which humans spread the plague.[15]

The name of the plague in its bubonic form came from the name of the swellings (buboes) of a human's lymph glands in the groin, under the arms and in the upper neck below the ears. Late fourteenth- and fifteenth-century autopsies recorded swellings the size of eggs or grapefruit. Some victims who had no external buboes reportedly died of internal swellings of tissues near vital organs. Mortality rates for bubonic plague ranged from 30 percent to 80 percent depending on when in the outbreak infection occurred; the bacillus was usually most lethal in the first months after it arrived. Yet in 1347–48 this lethal phase continued in both summer and winter. At Avignon the plague broke out in January 1348 and according to eyewitness Dr Guy de Chauliac continued for seven months. However after the mid-fifteenth century the usual pattern was that the plague confined its slaughter to the summer months then, with the coming of cooler weather, gradually lost strength. In Constantinople it followed much the same pattern. In contrast, according to early nineteenth-century accounts from Egypt, in Alexandria plague usually peaked in July and ended in October. Further south at Asyut, following the migration of rats from harvest fields along the Nile to human habitations between August and December—the most favorable month for fleas to breed—it was not until January that quantities of humans began to die of plague.[16]

Bubonic plague was no respecter of persons. High-status people in the wrong place at the wrong time were as likely to be struck dead as were half-starved vagrants or peasants. Moreover, there was no long-term immunity: those who recovered from a bout in one year might be carried off by the disease in the next. Perhaps this was why Europeans who witnessed outbreaks of what may have been plague in sixteenth-century Meso-America did not see death by plague as ethnically selective.[17]

In addition to bubonic plague narrowly defined, there were two variants of the disease, both dependent on the presence in the first victim's body of the bubonic form. In one form, the vector was the human flea, *Pulex irritans*. If an infected human flea changed hosts and bit another human, transferring the bacillus directly into the bloodstream, death within a few hours was almost certain. In pre-nineteenth-century Europe where two or three people slept in the same bed, it was not difficult for human fleas to move from person to person. The third form of the disease was pneumonic plague, a secondary infection in the lungs brought on by the presence of the bubonic form in the first victim. In this case the disease was contagious (spread from one human directly to another) and could be transferred by droplets exhaled by the victim while breathing or coughing up blood. The incubation period for pneumonic plague was from one to six days, and the death rate close to 100 percent.[18] Some historians hold that the loss of a third of the population when plague swept Europe in 1347–51 was caused by a combination of bubonic and pneumonic forms of the disease. It seems likely that combined forms were sometimes also at work in Egypt.

In West Europe two sorts of rat seem to have been involved, the black rat, *Rattus rattus*, and one of the several varieties of field or country rat. Though the outer reaches of the territory of a clan of country rats might overlap with the territory of sedentary black rats, country rats did not usually come into direct contact with human beings. In contrast, *Rattus rattus* preferred to establish its burrow near the grain reserves of humans or in their houses. These rats willingly boarded ships and settled down in the saddle-bags of overland travellers. In the mid-1340s, it was probably black rats accompanying merchants on the Silk Road from central Asia to the East–West trade center near Lake Balkhash in Kazakhstan and then on to the Black Sea that brought plague to Caffa in the Crimea. From Caffa plague-bearing black rats were transported by sea to Messina where they had no difficulty in climbing down hempen ropes and finding their way ashore.

Once on land (as in Messina), the black rat liked to establish burrows near human habitations. Because human and rat dietary preferences were similar, black rats established burrows near supplies of grain or flour; bakers and millers were frequently the first local victims of a plague. After burrows of black rats were infected by infective fleas, diseased and dying rats might rush to the surface as they did in 1630 in Busto Arsizio ("one could count them by the hundreds in every house").[19] In upper Egypt where most *fellahin*

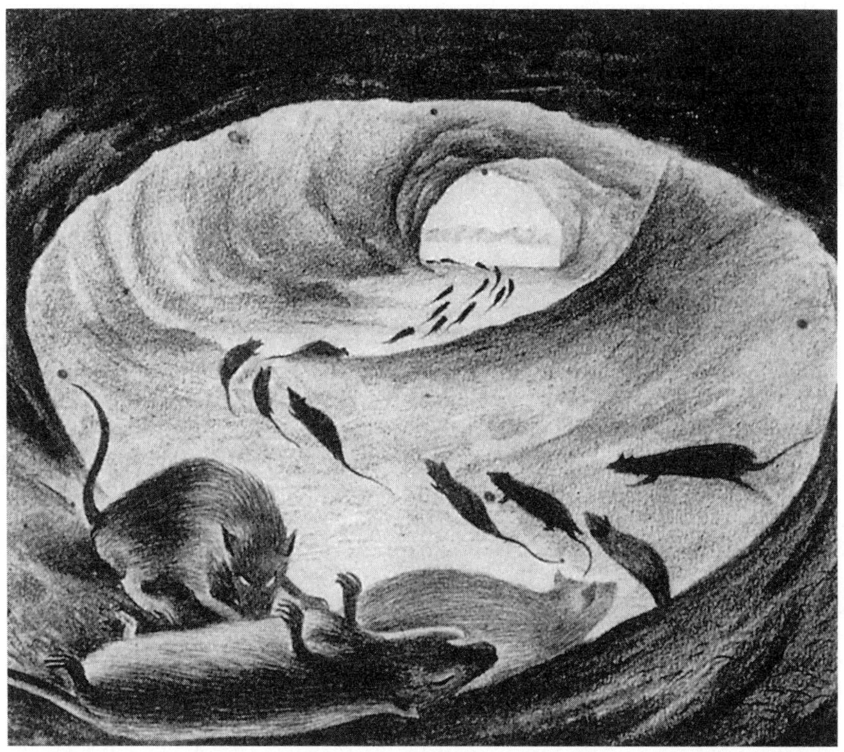

2. Rats Roaming the Sewers. Drawing, 1940s, by A. L. Tarter.

built pigeon lofts on the roofs of their houses in the 1940s and probably also did so earlier, a fortnight before people in the rooms below began dying of plague, dead rats (while living attracted to the eggs laid by pigeons) dropped from the rafters. Ironically, in *fellahin* wisdom it was held that any house on which pigeons voluntarily nested would escape from plague.[20]

Our knowledge of patterns of disease transmission among rats and fleas in Europe during the second pandemic is admittedly scanty. It may be that near every sea port or market town where they were introduced, plague-bearing fleas from black rats managed to find their way to the burrows of country rats. Feeding on their blood, infected fleas moved inland on the backs of their rodent hosts, field by field. Coming to the edge of a human settlement the fleas might desert a dying country rat and feast for a time on black rats, the near companions of humankind. Fortunately (from the human perspective), the country rats in an infected burrow tended to die off in six to ten years; infected burrows of black rats died off in an even shorter time. This pattern meant that there were no permanent reservoirs of epizootic infection in Europe or in Egypt in historic times: once a territory of country rats became plague free, the region itself remained free until a fresh source of the bacillus was introduced on human transport from disease reservoirs in central Asia. It was this accident of nature (which no one at the time knew anything about) that enabled the quarantine controls put in force by Italian administrators in the 1450s and given general application in Western Europe after the 1660s, to be effective.[21]

Professional Paradigms: Continuities and Change

During the first century of plague, magistrates of Europe's semi-autonomous towns either made no official response to an outbreak, or if required to do something, introduced controls of the type used when dealing with disease crises in general. The rationale behind this was simple. Even in the most advanced parts of the West—the trading cities of northern Italy and the Iberian peninsula—magistrates had only recently (in the 1290s) come to regard public health as a legitimate concern.[22]

As part of their new interest in health as *publica utilitas*, urban Italian rulers had accepted recently reinterpreted medical teaching about the six Non-Naturals the Ancients (such as Hippocrates and Galen) had thought caused disease. For our purposes the most important of these was what medieval people called "climate," which translates into socio-physical surroundings, including air. Fourteenth-century experts thought that contaminated air in the form of a *miasma* (from the Greek word for "defiled") caused disease. Another Non-Natural was the category type "afflictions of the soul" which translates as mental depression or melancholia. Using a tool of logic (argument by analogy) which medieval schoolmen often applied to the writings of ancient pagans (such as Aristotle and Plato) to bring them into line with Christian revelation, "afflictions of the soul" came to mean ill health caused by contamination of the space of the *civitas* (city or city state).[23] Using another tool of scholastic logic, it was held that the whole of a community might be targeted by the arrows of God (in the form of a miasma) to demonstrate His wrath against a defiling few.[24]

Building on these learned understandings, before 1347 (and the coming of plague) whenever an up-and-coming north Italian or Aragonese town was racked by influenza, strange fever or other disease crisis, authority trotted out the emergency rules. Following this sanitary regime, the heaps of offal which butchers left rotting in front of their shops, the scraps and liquids that leather-workers pushed out into the streets, the human excrement that people tossed out their front doors, and all other smelly things were collected and bundled out of town. If the disease crisis was unusually serious (a subjective understanding which was not constant over time), prostitutes and other morally contaminating people would also be driven from the city.

In Tuscan towns in the forefront of secular civic thought such as Florence and Siena, the outbreak of plague in 1347–48 was greeted with these recently devised responses to disease. Orders were given that streets be swept clean and that smelly rubbish and rotting cadavers be promptly buried. Then, using elements of the even older crisis response maintained by Christian priests, representatives of the moral community were ordered to join penitential processions to propitiate the angry deity. And since the crisis was seen as especially grave, anyone who followed an irregular life-style seen as offensive to God was banished.[25]

In Florence in 1348, to oversee these activities a temporary pre-plague-type Board of Health was set up. However, during later visitations (before 1450) no health boards were created because there were not enough magistrates left in town to staff them. Alerted by their own private warning systems, most members of the 500 leading Florentine families removed themselves to places known to be free of the plague. Here and elsewhere in Europe, the dictate "flee early, flee far, return late" became the propertied person's standard response to a rumor of plague.[26]

Yet in their rush to save themselves by flight, Florentine magistrates worried that the common people left behind would seize control of the city; this fear was perhaps justified. In the summer of 1378 when factional disputes temporarily immobilized the Florentine elite, rebellious wool-workers won control of the government and remained in power for several months. In later years, men of magisterial rank were terrified lest something like this happen again. It nearly did during the plague of 1383. On 22 July, the anniversary of the Ciompi rising of '78, Florentine artisans stormed around the city yelling rebel slogans. Fortunately for the on-going cultural Renaissance, they were captured, tortured and decapitated. Then, according to the chronicler, Marchionne Stefani:

> many laws were passed that no citizens could leave because of the said plague. For they feared that the *minuti* [the vulgar] would not leave, and would rise, and the malcontents would unite with them. . . . [But] it was impossible to keep [the citizens in the city] . . . for it is always so that large and powerful beasts jump and break fences.[27]

More than seventy years were to pass before the Florentine oligarchy developed a policy which, under the guise of controlling the spread of plague, would cow the common people.

Before 1450, in the absence of plague-specific responses by magistrates, two professional groupings—the Christian clergy and university-trained medical doctors—took the lead in explaining what caused plague epidemics. Of the two, the clergy were the more numerous, reflecting the fact that by 1347–48 the Christian faith was well established among the 10 percent of the European population who lived in towns with populations of 2,000 or more. The remaining 90 percent lived in small villages or scattered settlements where they might or might not have access to the services of a cleric. If they did, this cleric was usually a semi-literate man of peasant birth.[28]

Among the 10 percent of the population who were both urban and fully Christian (and who tended to despise peasant country bumpkins), the first response to news that the Black Death had broken out in the port cities of Italy was that the scourge had been sent by an angry deity. Led by their priests, some thought this required that non-conformists be rooted out. Though the choice of victims was not everywhere the same, along the River Rhine, the main internal north–south route of European trade and communications, genocidal violence was directed against the Jews. Like most reactions to plague, this response was a re-enactment of what had gone before, in this case the ethnic cleansings of the 1090s in the lead up to the First Crusade.

As in the past, in the 1340s Jews were suspect because they were descendants of the people thought to have crucified Christ at Calvary. Forbidden in many polities to cultivate land as peasants, Jews tended to be urban folk who sometimes dabbled in lending money and in selling medical drugs. Moreover, unlike most Christian youth, Jewish boys were trained in literacy at an early age. Among other skills this training provided, Jews' knowledge of Hebrew and other Middle Eastern languages gave them access to ancient medical knowledge. In many of the mainland polities in which Jews were still found (the Plantagenets had driven them out of England in 1291), a high proportion of learned medical practitioners were Jewish; doubtless some medical irregulars were of the same persuasion. In any case, because of who they were by repute and because of the distinctive clothes the Fourth Lateran Council (1215) required they wear, Jews were a highly visible minority, easily targeted in time of crisis.[29]

In exemplary fashion, 900 Jews were burned alive at Strasbourg on St Valentine's Day 1349 before the plague actually came near. Only later that spring did the arrows of pestilence rain down on the tight-packed medieval town and its preachers. To his credit, the then Pope, Clement VI, secure in sealed-off rooms in his palace at Avignon in southern France (where he worried about the demons trapped in steel-framed mirrors), condemned the slaughter for, as he noted, the plague struck down Christians and Jews alike.[30]

In addition to supporting attacks on Jews, another clerical response to plague was the staging of outdoor processions. The purpose here was to demonstrate that rival local vendetta groups had put aside their hatred to join in an act of communal solidarity pleasing to God. Therapeutic in intent, long processions of close-packed people were also nicely suited to the movement of fleas. In Paris in 1466, the reliquaries of saints Crépin and Crépinien were carried at the head of a solemn procession witnessed by thousands as it wound its way past the twin-towered cathedral of Notre Dame through the plague-infested Île de la Cité. Though cause and effect can

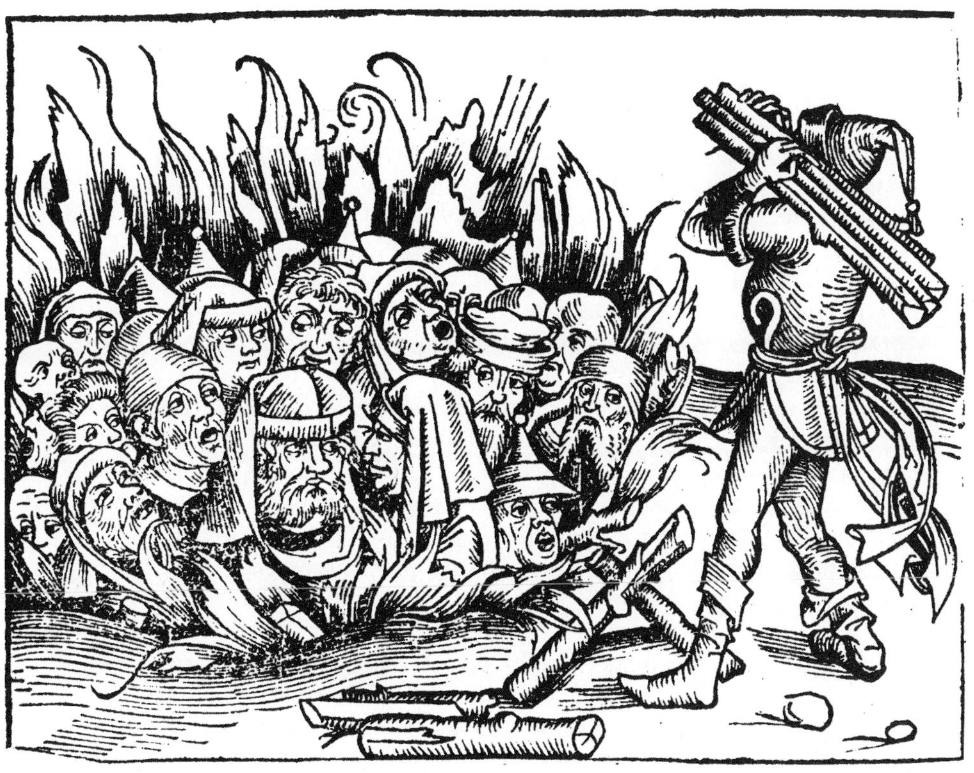

3. Jews being burnt in time of plague. Woodcut by Hartmann Schedel, 1493.

only be conjectured, within a short time the plague redoubled its violence within the city walls and moved out into the suburbs.[31]

In Italy, after *secular* magistrates hit upon the idea that crowds of people spread plague by contagion and that processions might not be a good thing, clerics addressed themselves to this problem as well. Preaching before the Doge of Venice on Christmas Day 1497, a Franciscan Observant warned:

> Gentlemen you are closing the churches for fear of the plague, and you are wise to do so. But if God wishes it, it will not suffice to close the churches. It will need a remedy for the causes of the plague, which are the horrendous sins which are committed, the blaspheming of God and the saints, the schools of sodomy, the infinite usury contracts made at Rialto. . . . And worse, when some gentleman comes to this city you show him the nunneries, not nunneries but public brothels. Most Serene Prince, I know that you know all this better than me. Take action, take action and you will deal with the plague.[32]

As late as 1570, Charles Borromeo, Archbishop of Milan, one of the architects of revitalized Catholicism, was still insisting it was essential to cool the wrath of God by penitential processions. The matter did not end there. During the Mantuan War which brought French and Spanish armies deep into Italy in 1630, Pope Urban VIII excommunicated the Florentine sanitary commission for banning processions.

Supported in this way by the successors of St Peter, priests in rural parishes continued to uphold old notions about appeasing the wrath of God. In 1631, Father Dragoni, the priest of Monte Lupo, ignored bans sent out from Florence duchy headquarters and defiantly led his parishioners in procession, heedless of the consequences this might have for their plague-prone bodies. Subsequently, scores of them died.[33]

University-trained physicians also had a role in formulating responses to the plague. Thus in 1348, King Philip VI of France consulted with the medical teaching faculty at Paris about disease causation. The Sorbonne masters concluded that plague had come into being with the conjunction of the planets Saturn, Jupiter and Mars on 24 March 1345. They further explained that this unusual planetary event had led to the heating of the air, which as a miasma evidenced itself in the buboes of plague.[34]

Astrology, for most modern health provisioners an alien country, was part of a larger paradigm of medicine which fourteenth-century experts inherited from the Greeks. Here the great master was Galen of Pergamon (d. 201 CE), often introduced to Latin readers through a translation of an Arabic introduction, Johannitius' *Isgoge*. Galen's own voluminous works incorporated writings by an even older authority, "Hippocrates" (a collection of medical writers on the island of Cos in the fifth century BCE). In addition to Galen, students in training at one of the four leading universities—Padua, Bologna, Montpellier, Paris—also studied Aristotle, known to pre-moderns simply as the Philosopher.[35]

In a seminal essay, H. J. Cook has provided a framework for understanding the paradigm within which learned medical men worked between the fourteenth and the seventeenth centuries.[36] As Cook explains, within a university, convention allotted the title *physician* to scholars who concerned themselves with *physics*. Physics was the study of the natural world and was part of the larger discourse known as *natural philosophy* which was based largely on the works of Aristotle.

In the minuscule world of the literate, rootedness in Aristotle was essential since it earned physicians the right to wear the "long gowns of learning" and to be "grave councilors worthy of respect, whether in church or civil society." Even so, they had less authority than did the five-star intellectuals of the day, theologians and jurists.[37] Important for their status, physicians' knowledge of ancient scribal wisdom was in fact the only skill which clearly set them apart from "empirics," the rival health provisioners who greatly outnumbered them. Though a few empirics may have been university dropouts, most acquired their skills in curing by learning informally from senior empirics, by observing the success of one medicine and the failure of another, and by making mental notes. Proper medical doctors regarded empirics as low-status hacks.[38] Writing during London's experience of plague between 1603 and 1611, an English physician named Eleazar Dunk trumpeted the superiority of his own kind:

> the name of an Empirike is derived from the Greek word which signifieth experience; and by an Empirike is, as you know, understood a Practitioner in Physicke, that hath no knowledge in Philosophy, Logicke, or Grammar; but fetcheth all his skill from bare and naked experience. Ignorance then is the difference whereby these men are distinguished from other Physicians.[39]

Proper physicians learned from Galen that disease was caused by an imbalance in the four humors (bodily juices) which corresponded to the four elements from which all matter is formed: fire, earth, air, and water, and to the four qualities, hot, cold, dry and moist. In the case of bubonic plague, which in the absence of other ideas physicians regarded as a fever, Galenic orthodoxy held that the disease manifested itself by an increase in the hotness of the heart which in time suffocated that vital organ.[40] Medical doctors also held that the connecting link between the macrocosm (earth and the celestial spheres) and the microcosm (individual human beings) was air. As every respectable physician knew (ignoring ideas post-1450s magistrates on boards of health had about the spread of disease through contact between one person and another—contagion), it was bad air that caused plague.

Part and parcel of the learned medical paradigm was the generalized concept of disease. According to Vivian Nutton:

> A disease did not have an existence in its own right, but as a deviation from the normal within the patient. . . . always . . . taking into account "the peculiar nature of each individual". The nature of disease was to be found in [each] man's temperament, the structure of his parts, his physiological and psychological dynamism, and could be defined very much in terms of impeded function.[41]

As Nutton suggests, practicing physicians regarded their *primary* social function as tending the health of patients who were able to control their own diet, environment and other Non-Naturals. This *caring* function would involve close study of the life-style of the client, leading to the establishment of an appropriate regimen for him to follow. Because this was a lengthy and necessarily costly process, prized patients included men who controlled landed estates (lay and clerical princes and aristocrats), as well as the rich bankers and merchants who formed the upper strata of the bourgeoisie. Though many of the towns in the Crown of Aragon and in northern Italy and, after 1436, in the German Empire hired physicians to attend to the needs of the poor, this assignment was regarded as irrelevant to a proper professional career in medicine.[42] As described by an Italian physician in 1576, the urban poor were a "sickly looking people full to overflowing with the coarsest and filthiest humors."[43] Typically, the practitioner who served as town doctor in Florence in the thirty years before the plague first broke out was Magistro Jacopo de Urbe, "bonesetter."[44]

In the mid-sixteenth century, a credible explanation for the inability of learned medical men to cure disease was given by a Dr Varchii. As he put it:

> Medicine has its rules and principles and they are true and well established. . . . If anything goes wrong, it is not the art which is at fault. The physician may have blundered or the ailment is such that it does not yield to treatment, or, as so often is the case, the patients are blamable because they do not do what is prescribed, or the apothecaries are at fault.[45]

Drawing on his knowledge of two centuries of European history, Cardinal Gastaldi, minister of health for Rome during the plague epidemic of 1656–57, sourly noted that: "Practical experience shows that the remedies used by medical doctors are useless and sometimes noxious."[46]

In post-Kochian retrospect it seems doubtful that pre-modern university-trained physicians contributed much to the control of plague. Yet this may not have been the way recruits to the medical profession understood the situation. For whatever reason—personal status enhancement or sense of duty—in the half-century after the Black Death swept away a third of Europe's population, student recruitment in university faculties of medicine remained at nearly the same level as it had been in the first four decades of the fourteenth century.[47]

Among ordinary unlettered people (95 percent of the population of the West) who knew little of the medical theory taught in universities, demons or wandering souls were often seen as the causal agents of disease and death. For example, in late fourteenth- and fifteenth-century rural Luxembourg and the Massif Central, cultivators held that the supernatural forces that controlled human and animal health were ambivalent beings which could work either for good or for ill. In this understanding (which avoided the Manichean tendencies of Christianity with its polarity of the evil Devil and the benevolent God), the way in which supernatural forces acted depended on the balance between harmony and disharmony within the village, and on the control of contact with strangers. Peasants of this sort—who put a premium on isolation and wore leather instead of flea-bearing wool—stood a good chance of escaping the plague until some tithe-collecting priest or wandering pedlar brought it in.[48]

Several examples of peasants who violently refused to have anything to do with strangers coming from plague-infested towns have been recovered from the archives. In 1628, after Lyon, the second city in France, was hit by plague, its rich bourgeoisie fled to their country estates as rich people were wont to do. But when the populace attempted to leave Lyon in their turn, stone-throwing peasants forced them back. In the next year peasants in Provence threatened to bombard Digne rather than let refugees from that plague-threatened town invade their *pays*.[49] Based on a rationale derived from their own mental worlds, these peasants had hit upon an eminently sound plague-control technique: the curtailment of human movement. Yet it is to the rather different mental world of Italy's urban elites and later of the European elite as a whole that we must turn to find the insights which eventually enabled them to conquer the plague.

The Invention of Controls

In northern and central Italy, during this era the part of Europe where most innovative thinking arose, elite ideas underwent a transformation around 1439–50.[50] To still new notions of health as *publica utilitas* were added intellectual stimuli brought in from Ottoman-threatened Byzantium. Confronted by the advance of the Ottoman Turks, in 1439 the Byzantine Emperor came to Florence to request military aid. None was forthcoming; Constantinople fell in 1453. However, several leading Byzantine scholars stayed in Florence, greatly increasing the number of people in the West who could translate ancient medical works from Greek and Arabic into Latin.[51]

Leading on from this was the clutch of ideas known as civic humanism. Among other things, civic humanism held that society was analogous in its organization to a living organism and that the oligarchs at the top of the hierarchy owed paternalistic oversight to the lower orders, the artisan wage earners of the town and peasant cultivators of the *contado*. In their turn the lower orders owed their rulers deference and obedience.[52]

No sooner had these ideas gelled than they were put in jeopardy as the population slowly began to recover to pre-plague levels. Sons and daughters of peasants, finding no land to farm or other ways to make a living in their villages, flocked to the cities to find work. Once there, some of them took to petty theft, prostitution or begging. Earlier (when they had been comparatively few in number) seen as exemplars of Christ, the immigrant poor were now viewed as potential criminals who might band together to overturn the social order.[53]

This feeling was reflected in the new depth of contempt with which the poor were coming to be regarded by the privileged few and by the extension of the category "the poor" to include most working people. Under the new dispensation it was commonly held that "butchers, meat sellers, innkeepers, bakers, grocers" and other persons who earned their daily bread by manual labor—which is to say more than two-thirds of the population of any Italian city—were "squalid, public or sordid people."[54] These sordid people obviously had to be kept in place by the gibbet, the whip, the galleys and other condign punishment which only by a distortion of language could be termed instruments of benevolent paternalism.

Once these harsh ideas were in place (Carmichael and Henderson see it as happening in Florence during the plague crisis of 1448), it required only a short imaginative leap to conclude that the collective "poor" were carriers of disease, and that plague itself was contagious, spread from person to person.[55] Empirical observation of the way the plague behaved after the mid-fifteenth century (when it had moved into its random patchy phase) seemed to confirm this argument. By force of circumstance, many poor people lived in flea-infested environments, in wood and thatch slums on the urban fringe. Rich people on the other hand, who lived in the city center in stone-built houses and were able to flee to country estates as soon as plague neared, were far less likely to come into contact with infected rats and fleas. There was also the issue of raw power: magistrates were not above warning low-status health inspectors that suspicious deaths of poor people were to be marked down as "death by plague." Perhaps for this reason surveys showing the place of residence of "plague victims" during moderately virulent plagues in mid-fifteenth-century Florence and in London after 1532 always demonstrated that the poor were at far greater risk than the wealthy.[56]

Emerging from this complex of perceptions was an Ideology of Order which during epidemic crises justified intervention into the lives of ordinary people. First created in Florence and its sister city states by humanist scholars, jurists and health magistrates (who were usually *not* university-trained physicians), the order ideology gradually spread to France and Spain; decades later it took root in remote northern kingdoms such as Sweden and England. Put into effect only once or twice in the lifetime of every adult (outbreaks of plague by then having entered their random phase), interventionist policies were a clear demonstration that authority was able to disrupt the everyday lives of subject peoples at its whim. What was not demonstrated, however, was that the policies actually blocked the spread of plague.[57] In Florence, a city with control measures as authoritarian as those anywhere, outbreaks of plague occurred in 1497–98, in each year between 1522 and 1528, again in 1530 and 1531, and once again in 1630, 1631 and 1633. Whether as a republic or as the capital of a Medici duchy (after 1527), Florence did not regain its pre-plague level of population until the nineteenth-century.

In a nutshell, full-blown Italian plague control consisted of five elements: (1) rigorous policing of human movement from plague-infested regions to those still plague free by the use of marine or land quarantine; (2) compulsory burial of the plague dead in special pits and the destruction of their personal possessions; (3) isolation of people sick with plague in pesthouses and the shutting up of their families in their own houses or in temporary

30. Cerusico, Medico, e Confes.ri sporchi. 31. Carrette, e Profumatori sporchi, che pr
le robbe, che mandano allo spurgo. 35. Carretoni, che portano uia le dette rob

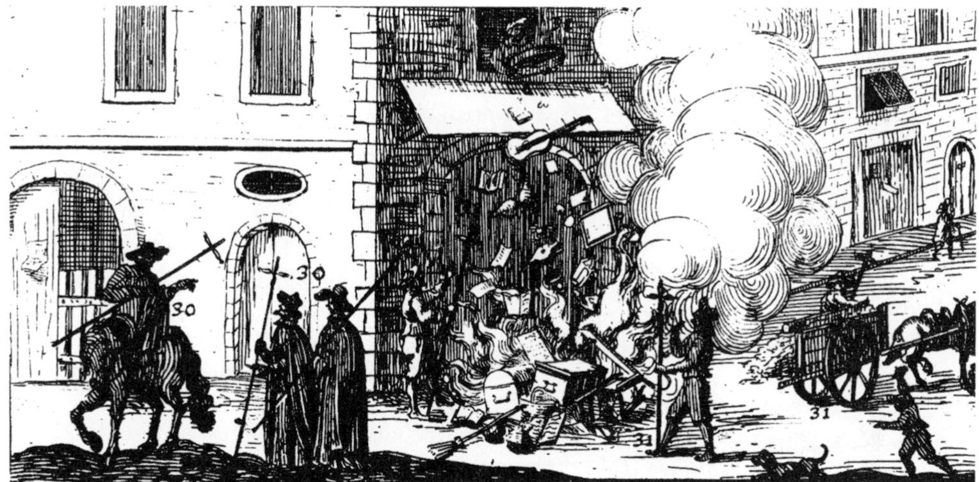

4. Burning plague-infected possessions, Rome, 1656.

cabins far from built-up areas; (4) assumption of responsibility by the local unit of taxation to provide free medical service and food to people placed in isolation; (5) provision of subsistence to those whose livelihoods had been wrecked by the closure of markets and who had no food reserves to fall back on.

From this listing two points emerge. Under pretext of blocking the plague, what Andrea Zorzi terms "the project of control and of social mediation" touched the lives of subject peoples to an extent hitherto unknown.[58] Among the casualties was the old idea that rich and poor should join together in religious processions, festivals such as Carnival, and in well-heeled people's rites of passage. There was also the problem of funding; in most polities, families of noble blood were exempt from direct taxation. This meant that an elite's capacity to extract from ordinary taxpayers the great sums needed to enforce controls was itself a test of the new Ideology of Order. With wry humor a Palermo health official chose as his motto during the plague of 1576, "Gold, Fire, the Gallows": gold to pay the costs, fire to burn suspect goods, and the gallows to hang poor men who disputed the authority of the Board of Health.[59]

In the heavily governed Italian city states where power relationships among the great families had been regularized by 1450, the new controls were applied relatively easily. Here the threat of plague strengthened order-conscious bureaucrats' sense of collective responsibility. Thus in Milan when the ruling duke was assassinated during the plague of 1476 the health magistracy carried out plague-control measures as efficiently as if the duke had still been alive. In contrast, in Transalpine Europe, before kings or territorial rulers could apply interventionist policies to the common people, they first had to establish effective control over lesser members of their own caste. After 1517 centralization required that kings tame the passions stirred up by the reformations in religion and convert semi-autonomous provincial magnates into fawning courtiers. So it was not until the mid-sixteenth century that plague controls tentatively began to be applied in some of the cities in the German Empire and in the Spanish kingdoms. In the Hexagon of France, no sooner had centralization begun than rival elites tore society apart in thirty years of religious war (ending only in 1598). In England, the oldest coherently organized dynastic state in Europe, nation-wide plague regulations were not established until 1578.[60]

Everywhere they *were* imposed, plague regulations met with a muted or overtly hostile response from the populace. Evidence from Sweden, England and elsewhere suggests that people were terrified by the plague for the first week or so after it arrived, but that they then grew accustomed to its depredations and, when left alone, attempted to go about their ordinary affairs. If social breakdown did occur, it was more likely to be caused by the enforcement of a plague code than by the disease itself.

In a famous passage, Jean Delumeau sketched out what householders took to be appropriate behavior:

> Ordinarily, sickness and its rites cemented the unity of the patient and those whose surrounded him; and death even more followed a familiar funerary liturgy; the death watch around the corpse, the burial and entombment. The tears, the words in a low voice, the recalling of memories, the furnishing of the death chamber, the prayers, the final cortège, the presence of family and friends; as many of the elements which constitute a rite of passage as are appropriate for order and propriety. But in time of epidemic [all proprieties are abandoned] and the social personality of the dead person is abolished.[61]

Delumeau found that ordinary people bitterly resented the magisterial banning of funerals and funeral processions at which the living honored the dead and accepted the fact of their passing. Commenting on the popular response to such measures in London in 1603, a member of the elite noted that "the poorer sort, yea women with young children, will flock to burials, and (which is worse) stand (of purpose) over open graves where sundry are buried together, that (forsooth) all the world may see that they fear not the Plague."[62]

Also at odds with fundamental values was the requirement that plague dead be salted down with lime and buried in mass graves. In the popular mind, denial of burial in a churchyard was appropriate only for animals and social pariahs—suicides and apostates who had renounced God. Rather than allow their dead to suffer this fate, traditionalists in post-Reformation Sweden (a particularly well Christianized country) resorted to stratagems which included keeping bodies at home until, perhaps in the dead of night, they could be properly buried. One secret graveyard digger was Per Månsson in Småland province. After surreptitiously burying his own plague-dead wife and children near his parish church in 1730–31, Månsson offered his services to families of other victims: his only slip was to ask that he be paid in cash, not as a neighbor, but as an entrepreneur. Warned by local authorities that he was violating a state law (of which they themselves disapproved), Månsson continued his secret burials until he was jailed and flogged. Elsewhere in the Swedish kingdom it was without thought of private gain that communities attempted to maintain their traditions. In the province of Blekinge in 1710 riotous parishioners disinterred an entire plague cemetery (which they termed a "wolf-pit") on the hill outside the country town and brought the dead back to the parish church for proper burial. In incidents such as these, the local *Volk* directly challenged the authority of the Swedish state—which at Poltava (1709) had just lost a major war to Russia.[63]

For simple people, the regulation that the clothing and bedding of plague victims be burned, and household possessions be washed down with lime (ostensibly to prevent contagion), also cut deeply into customary norms. In late fifteenth-century Turin, anti-plague measures went a step further: houses suspected of harboring plague were burnt to the ground. In a court case heard in 1461, the heirs of a burnt-out owner claimed that they still had not been compensated for their parents' loss. Most poor people would not have the cash needed to bribe court attendants to undertake a lawsuit of this sort.[64]

In Florence in 1630–31, many of the cases tried before the special court enforcing plague regulations (the Public Health Magistracy) concerned what duchy officials regarded as theft, but what ordinary people regarded as the normal recycling of dead people's goods. One particularly contentious matter was the disposition of deceased people's best suits of clothes. Earlier, the practice had been to hand these over to the gravedigger to ensure that he give special attention to the dead person. Before 1348 this custom had been written into the rules of the gravedigger's guild affiliate: now the Duchy claimed possession. Rights to other forms of property were at issue in a case involving a baker named Salvatore Tortorelli in 1630–31. After the death of his childless brother-in-law, Tortorelli had secretly entered the dead man's house to remove jewels that had been part of the dowry of the widow, his sister. Tortorelli claimed that if he had left them lying around, they would have been pocketed by the duchy household decontamination squad. This argument did not wash with the Health Magistracy: Tortorelli was imprisoned and tortured. While his arms were being wrenched out of their sockets, he shouted that whatever the State might claim, the jewels he had taken were part of his family's patrimony and by right belonged to them.[65]

In addition to putting the inheritance patterns of ordinary people in peril, plague regulations closed normal venues of neighborhood sociability: cock-fighting and bull-baiting rings, houses of prostitution, alehouses and taverns. Most self-employed married masters, unmarried apprentices and journeymen lived in the building in which they worked. For them, taverns and the like were neutral centers of sociability where they exchanged news, found jobs, and decided how to enforce traditional moral codes governing the behavior of wives and young unmarried women. Their closure threatened the very cement which held neighborhoods together.

Also oppressive was the enforcement of plague regulations which deprived people of ways of making a living. For humble folk who survived by hawking fish or second-hand clothes on street corners or in the town market and had no reserves to fall back on, the closure of meeting places meant destitution. Dire too was the situation facing wage laborers who were dependent upon manufacturers who closed down operations in time of quarantine, throwing employees out of work. If only a few household heads were affected, neighbors might be able to help out at meal times. However, in a not untypical urban situation where more than a third of the workforce was in the textile or similar industry, the closure of workshops when rich owners fled threatened to wreck whole neighborhoods. Charitable donations, usually late to arrive and small in scale, might save the unemployed from starving but would not be enough to prevent them falling prey to typhus (the famine disease *par excellence*). Once dead from typhus or pneumonia, heads of household and family members might suffer the further indignity of being added on the gravediggers' lists to the toll chalked up to "plague," thus confirming the elite conceit that there was a direct correlation between poverty and pestilence.[66]

Great merchants dependent on the exchange of goods in regional, interregional or international networks worried that suspension of commerce as a result of quarantine might allow outside rivals to usurp their markets. Thus they were notoriously slow to accept that quarantine was needed.[67] Following this rationale, in 1629 Venetian oligarchs ignored warnings that plague was nearby and claimed that a cordon sanitaire was unnecessary. The short-term consequences were grave enough. Plague moved unhindered from Mantua and Milan to enter Venice in 1629. It remained until the autumn of 1631 and became the most serious disease disaster Venice suffered in the seventeenth century. Though rural in-migration from Terra Firma enabled it to recover its pre-plague size within a generation, other consequences proved irreversible. While Venice was closed down and its plague-dead leadership was being replenished from youthful entries in its Golden Book (which listed the families from which council members were chosen), Dutch and English entrepreneurs moved into its traditional marketing territories around the Adriatic and eastern Mediterranean. Once in possession they stayed. Shorn of its major markets and burdened with leaders suffering from sclerosis (young in body but old in mind), Venice soon found itself only a regional power with no economic clout. From this it was but a short step to becoming a museum city.[68]

In the Italian city states, and after 1578 in England, where governments imposed household isolation on the entire family of plague victims, the new authoritarianism required that doors of afflicted houses be boarded up; necessary foodstuffs were put in baskets lowered from windows on ropes. In England in 1604 anyone thought to have the plague who was found out on the streets could legally be hanged. During the plague of 1630–33, in Florence, artisan families devised ways to circumvent household isolation. When a family member showed plague symptoms, men of working age slipped off to the shop where co-workers provided them with raw materials and food: womenfolk and children were left at home to tend the plague sick. Several instances of families following this strategy came to the attention of the special sanitary court—with its firm, summary justice—when spiteful neighbors informed the police that things were not as they should be in the boarded-up house next door. In Milan, the boarding up of houses in 1468 was apparently done at the request of medical doctors motivated by personal gain; for a sum of money slipped to the plague doctor, long-standing neighborhood feuds could thus be resolved.[69]

A policy sometimes used in Milan and Venice was to cart off suspect co-residential groups to specially constructed wood and straw shacks far from other habitations. But whether locked up in these shacks or in their habitations in town (as in London), it was likely that caged-up people, who had been innocent of plague when confined, would be killed either by plague spread by desperate fleas or by typhus, pneumonia or starvation. Writing of the situation in the English kingdom after boarding up entire families had become the norm, Paul Slack found that "between one-third and two-thirds of all burials during an epidemic of plague occurred in families which had three or more deaths."[70]

Another institutional device much favored by the Ideology of Order was the establishment of purpose-built pesthouses. Such institutions cost a great deal, with the result that there was often a time lag between the initiation of a building campaign and actual opening. For example, in Genoa the Great Council commissioned a pesthouse in 1467; sixty years passed before the building was finally completed and in operation. In the interim, plague hit the city in 1499, 1501 and in the three years 1524–26. Once a pest hospital was set up—in most parts of Europe not until the early seventeenth century—essential services were provided by municipally funded medical doctors or barber-surgeons required by their contracts to provide treatment to the poor free of charge; the results were predictable.

Typical perhaps were conditions in the pesthouse in Bologna where according to Cardinal Spada: "Here you are overwhelmed by intolerable smells . . . you cannot walk but among corpses. . . . This is the faithful replica of hell since here is no order and only horror prevails."[71] In Venetian pesthouses, medical personnel wore masks and heavy protective clothing to protect them from the miasma allegedly rising from the sick. As depicted in paintings and engravings from the period, pesthouse practitioners looked like actors in a grotesque festival of death.

In Milan during the plague of 1630 and in Genoa in 1656, extraordinarily high death rates (70 percent of the Genoese population) can probably be attributed to the policy of carting off suspects to pesthouses to die of starvation, typhus and plague. After the holocaust of 1656 the director of the Genoese lazar house asked: "If no measures had been taken to rid the city of the epidemic, would Genoa have suffered greater losses?"[72] Nothing came of this musing. Confronted with the coercive power of authority and their own internalized habits of obedience, ordinary people could do little to prevent removal.

If there *was* resistance, it was likely to be led by women, often widows, who felt that pest hospitals deprived them of one of their natural roles: nursing the living and laying out the dead. In the England of King Charles I, women in Salisbury in 1627 and in Colchester in 1631 burned down pest hospitals. This assertion of traditional values demonstrates the resilience of popular culture when confronted with the Ideology of Order. Similarly in Florence under its Grand Dukes, women who as wives, daughters or sisters of the sick were trapped inside boarded-up houses shouted defiance from the windows; with their encouragement, riotous youths threatened officials. In the Via Porcia district in 1633, a 200-strong crowd put Jacopo Sassi, food distributor to the confined, into such "great danger and fear" that he resigned.[73]

Yet the terrifying threat of pest hospitals or household isolation did not obtain everywhere. In the Netherlands where groups of gentlemen of the corporate sort painted by Rembrandt were accustomed to use "opportune force for minimum risk" to create a trading empire which spanned the globe, people were encouraged to visit plague-afflicted neighbors to help them through the last painful hours of life. Plague victims able to walk could leave their houses to take the breeze so long as they carried a wand symbolizing sickness; family members living with them were encouraged to come to church to share in the consolations of religion. Here then, despite the triumph of aggressive forms of capitalism applied to non-Dutch peoples overseas, customary values prevailed. In the Netherlands plague mortality was never exceptionally high.[74]

In more authoritarian lands, in addition to isolating plague victims, another technique was isolation of an entire town. The first known cordon sanitaire predated the humanists' Ideology of Order by seventy-five years. In 1374, Bernardo Visconti, tyrant of Milan, regarded by his contemporaries as exceptionally cruel, ordered the town of Reggio nell'Emilia 150 kilometres south of Milan to be sealed off by troops. This precaution notwithstanding, the plague made its way to Milan, seemingly disproving the effectiveness of cordons sanitaires.[75] Yet with the triumph of authoritarianism, the Milanese measure earlier thought ineffective was adopted lock, stock and barrel by

Milan's one-time republican rival, Florence, now under its Grand Dukes. Managed by its Board of Health, during plague alerts it became standard Florentine practice to employ squads of soldiers to deal with subordinate towns in the *contado*; people who slipped away from a plague-ridden place were tracked down and shot. Following another Milanese precedent, the Florentine board demanded that people planning to travel between one town and the next first secure a health passport from their place of origin. In France while Marie de Medici, the widowed queen of Henry IV enjoyed power at court, the health passport system was brought in from her native Florence.[76]

Throughout Europe, by the second decade of the seventeenth century perceptive members of directing elites began to realize that in some mysterious way plague was kept at bay if plague regulations were enforced throughout a large territory. Yet before they were able to persuade themselves that they should put aside mutual animosities in the interest of creating a *continental-wide* network of social controls and order, a revolution in attitudes was required.

There is no general agreement as to what brought this revolution to pass. Theodore Rabb gave pride of place to the revulsion felt by elites to events in the Thirty Years War (1618–48). In the course of this gruelling conflict which left between a fifth and a third of the population of the German lands dead, Europe hovered on the brink of moral anarchy. Troops under the command of King Gustavus Adolphus of Sweden and his like systematically raped, murdered and plundered civilians in north, central and southern Germany. In regions peripheral to the war, mercenaries slaughtered civilians just for the fun of it. Appalled by this collapse of civilized values, after the Peace of Westphalia (1648) European monarchs reorganized their military by creating standing professional armies funded by peasant taxpayers. They thus rid themselves of the need to employ mercenaries swept up from the overpopulated Alpine cantons and other rude corners of Christendom. Rulers, moreover, insisted that their troops obey newly established rules of war; battles were to be fought well away from urban places and in no circumstances was plundering or murdering of civilians permitted. A new concept of international order was in the making.[77]

Then too, in mid-century a new balance was established between regional aristocracies and the prince. In France the king (Louis XIV) who as a youth had been chased from his capital by revolting nobles and judges (the Fronde of 1648–52), was able within a few years of his return to Paris to bring all French aristocrats to heel. Triumphant over their magnates, centralizing monarchs, patterning themselves on the French, built up efficient fiscal-military states. In Spain and Spanish Italy, in Sweden, Denmark and England aristocrats recognized that they had more to gain by working in alliance with this State than they could achieve by revolt. The same thing happened in the constituent parts of the still fragmented, proto-federalist German Empire (much troubled by plague between 1675 and 1683).[78]

In the decades after 1648, the willingness of Europe's elites to settle differences by compromise was paralleled by the rise of political economists, a new breed of experts who argued that a nation's strength depended upon the wealth-generating capacities of its inhabitants. In addition to full employment in homeland industries, national well-being would, they claimed, be enhanced by the establishment of food-provisioning networks in time of dearth. Converting theory to practice, agents of state mercantilism organized famine and disaster relief programs, paid for by taxes exacted by growing armies of revenue collectors.

The growth of interventionist agencies gave aristocrats hope that people of their sort could solve every problem, if they worked together. One of their first priorities was the eradication of plague, beginning with the rigorous control of land routes between plague-free and afflicted regions. Typical were the measures put into force in June 1679 by the government of Spain to protect Madrid from the plague then raging in the south. Ignoring the old notion that plague was caused by a miasma (Madrid was said to be the most smelly capital in Europe), officials sealed off land routes running north from Andalusia with two cordons of troops and kept Madrid plague free. After this scare pestilence never returned to the city.[79]

As we saw earlier, in the natural order of things plague-infected burrows of country rats died off in six to ten years: once a region was clean it remained so until reinfected by companionable black rats and their infective fleas brought in from an affected region. As it happens, Italian port cities had been using quarantine ever since 1450. The problem was it didn't seem to work, presumably because small sloops bearing rats, fleas and high-value goods from the Levant came ashore in isolated coves in defiance of local government regulations. All this changed in the late seventeenth century.

Borne up by their optimism that international cooperation could overcome problems that earlier defeated the efforts of individual cities, territorial governments began to coordinate control measures. Building on perceptions that plague originated in the Levant or North Africa, early warning systems based on European consuls and travellers alerted home authorities of the whereabouts of plague and smugglers; news-sheets regularly reported disease conditions in Ottoman lands. Ships from suspect ports were forced into quarantine for three or four weeks.[80]

The combination of quarantine on incoming ships and land-based controls gradually forced plague to retreat. It was last seen in Scotland in 1647, in England in 1668, in the Low Countries in 1670, in west Germany and Switzerland in 1679, in Spain in 1711, and in northern and central Italy in 1714. Into a nearly clean France, plague was reintroduced from the Levant in 1720 by the ship *Le Grand Saint Antoine* whose skipper had bribed the Marseille port authorities to avoid quarantine. After a campaign costly in lives (100,000 dead) and taxpayers' dues, plague was contained to that Mediterranean city and its *pays* and thereafter effectively disappeared from the West.[81]

In the Habsburg lands (south-central Europe) the plague was last seen in 1716, though it long continued in neighboring Balkan territories ruled by the Ottoman Sultan. Still in the dark about why cordons sanitaires and quarantine were effective, after the Peace of Belgrade ended a Habsburg–Ottoman war in 1739, the Habsburgs created a plague-control zone which covered about half of the provinces of Slavonia and Croatia and provided jobs for around 4,000 troops; similar military zones were set up in Transylvania and south of the Danube. All along the Military Frontier, sentry posts backed up by mobile patrols had orders to shoot unauthorized travellers. People coming from Ottoman lands had to submit to groin and armpit strip-searches and a quarantine which might last forty-eight days. Trade goods were fumigated. In the case of suspect raw wool the practice was to put it in a warehouse where low-status people were made to sleep; if they developed plague symptoms they were shot and the wool was burned.[82]

Habsburg plague policies imposed hardship on Balkan people with extended family on both sides of the line: they waved and signalled to each other but because of the forty-eight-day quarantine period seldom met. Habsburg policies also hampered Bulgarian and Greek merchant-capitalists on the Ottoman side whose dependent artisan workers made up cloth for sale in Christian Europe: in earlier years cloth and grain had been major exports. Now, with the prolonged Habsburg quarantine, in the time it took to travel the 1,300 kilometers between Istanbul and Vienna one could sail from an Atlantic port to the colonized New World. Alexander Kinglake, after going through the hassle of quarantine himself, was perhaps right to claim that the Muslim and Austrian lands "are as much asunder as though there were fifty broad provinces that lay in the path between them."[83]

It was not simply a matter of time and space. As Daniel Panzac pointed out, the application of Austrian controls further deepened the ideological rift between the Christian West (which saw itself as plague free and civilized) and the Muslim Middle East (seen as disease ridden and primitive). In this spirit, readers of a British medical journal were reminded in 1799: "No nation was ever long engaged in a war with the Turks without taking the plague."[84]

Responses to Plague in the Middle East

When bubonic plague re-emerged in the Middle East in 1347, the western Islamic world was under the control of the Mamluk military regime.[85] Centered in the Citadel in Cairo, the Mamluk Empire extended south beyond Aswan and north to Palestine and Syria. Among its settled people, the first plague outbreak resulted in catastrophic loss of human life, perhaps a third of the population. In Cairo, with an estimated pre-plague population of half a million (the world's largest or second largest city), between October

1347 and January 1349 some 200,000 people were carried off. On the caravan route linking Cairo and Bilbeis in the south-eastern Nile Delta, there were said to be corpses everywhere along the way. In the far north at Alexandria, with the death or flight of thousands of workers, the production of silk, fine cotton and other high-quality cloth collapsed. Hrbek rightly claims that the Black Death and the famine which followed it were "the greatest catastrophe to befall Egypt during the whole Muslim period."[86]

Inseparable from the plague itself were localized famines that followed the visitation. Though documentary evidence is sparse, it would seem that famines were often caused by the flight of peasant cultivators to Cairo, Damascus or other large cities where they hoped to find food. Peasants also went in search of wonder-working urban exorcists thought to be effective against the jinn which carried the plague; in the language of the people "the stinging of the jinn" was a euphemism for the pestilence. Many *fellaheen* also sought freedom from oppressive landlords and once they had joined an urban workforce did not return to their natal villages. Because much of the arable land depended upon irrigation, the flight of able-bodied men and women disrupted agricultural regimes in whole regions: unless attended to, heavy reeds grew up, blocking ditches and canals.[87]

In peripheral regions of the empire where absentee landlords were unwilling to invest in land reclamation or to coerce settlers to come in, following the plague great sections of productive land fell out of use. In Upper Egypt and Nubia the situation was complicated by the successful revolt of a Bedouin faction against central authority and their disruption of trade routes. Thus at Luxor, of the 24,000 *feddans* of arable land under crops before 1347, only 1,000 were still being cultivated in 1389.[88] There was extensive depopulation in northern Syria where a century after the Black Death hundreds of village sites lay abandoned. Yet, rather than entire village groupings being exterminated by plague, it would appear that many cultivators who had survived had moved south to take up farms in the Nile Delta and then stayed on.[89]

In this agricultural heartland of Egypt, plague and famine had wrought their usual havoc in 1347–49. Yet within seven or eight years, most of the Delta's 2,300 villages were again producing the wheat and other foodstuffs needed to feed Cairo. And within the capital itself, craft-work, buying, selling and other everyday activities had resumed in reassertion of the continuity which was the special Egyptian way.

To assess the consequences of the Black Death and later visitations of plague on the Mamluk lands we must examine the web of relationships among particular social groupings. In a nutshell, we will find that between 1347 and 1805 human responses did not change in any appreciable way because no group had any compelling reason to alter accustomed behavioral patterns. This was true for the *fellaheen* who had always been at the bottom of the social heap as well as for the various power-brokers who had authority over other people's lives.

During the long centuries when plague was present, in theory each *fellah* head of household had hereditary use-rights to his land under the watchful eye of the village headman, the *shaykh al-balad.* This headman was the single link between the village and the world outside. When Mamluk government was strong, village headmen recruited the corvée labor needed to construct new irrigation canals and ditches. The *fellaheen* resented these corvée requirements as well as the oppressively heavy taxes collected by the headmen on wheat, poultry, fruit trees and other products. Though when confronted by alien forces coming from the outside, villagers would stand together as a moral whole, in ordinary times they tended to divide into feud-prone extended family groupings. Any headman worth his salt knew how to manipulate the two or three factions in the village for his own profit.[90]

In addition to these human forces, Egyptian peasants had to worry about when the Nile would flood and how high the waters would rise. Only a full-scale inundation would bring soil-enhancing silt to all their parcels of land; several years of low water or no inundation at all (as in 1374) would result in famine (as in 1375–76). Famine might also follow if the village lands were invaded by grain-devouring locusts or rats. Such crises had a long history. While in exile in Egypt during the years that included the reign of Akhenaten (*c.* 1379 BCE) the Hebrews had coined the phrase the "ten plagues of Egypt" as a catch-all term to cover disasters caused by locusts, rats, floods, dearth and disease.

Three thousand years later, after 1347 CE, Nile Valley peasants had to sort out how to respond to the particular problems caused by the pestilence of bubonic (perhaps aided by pneumonic) plague. The alternatives were to sit it out and hope for the best or to give up farming and flee to Cairo or Alexandria to become unskilled wage laborers.

Standing outside the troubled world of settled peasants were the nomadic Bedouin. Living in deserts a few miles beyond the cultivated banks of the Nile (95 percent of the land of Egypt was desert), the Bedouin had for centuries avoided contact with settled people they knew were suffering from strange diseases. In 1347–48, from listening posts they maintained in market towns, they learned of the bubonic disease crisis and acted accordingly. Travelling at camel speed, the Bedouin retreated further into the deserts and both then and during later outbreaks of pestilence outdistanced the movement of the disease. Soon after 1348, the life-preserving behavior of the nomads was favorably commented upon by Ibn al-Khatib, a Muslim scholar on his way across north Africa to Andalusia.[91] Yet because of the fierce antipathy between settled *fellaheen* and nomads (in current colloquial Arabic, the word Bedouin translates roughly into "filthy savage"), Nile Valley peasants were unwilling to learn anything from semi-pagan nomads.[92] Instead, whenever the plague raged, they tended to flee to the cities to add to the number of potential urban victims.

The long-term effects of the contrasting behavior of settled people and nomads were of some consequence. At a time when the population of Egypt was in decline (perhaps 8 million in 1346 moving steadily downwards to perhaps 3 million in 1805), the nomadic population remained more or less constant (at best a few hundred thousand). In peripheral regions, such as the far south, the middle Nile Valley, and in areas bordering the Delta, in times of weak Mamluk government (the situation after 1399) charismatic Bedouin chieftains were able to establish semi-autonomous regimes of their own. Emboldened by their own strength, in the fifteenth century and again in the eighteenth, eastern desert nomads attacked isolated Coptic monasteries (St Paul's and St Anthony's), slaughtering the monks and burning their libraries. Yet so long as nomadic tribesmen paid something in tribute, Mamluk central authority generally left them alone.

Bearing in mind our concern to identify the reasons why no group (other than nomads) even contemplated the idea that plague might actually be controlled by human agency, let us turn to the decision-makers at the summit of fourteenth- and fifteenth-century Middle Eastern society, the Mamluks. These rulers were a self-recruiting military elite in which, in stark contrast to European aristocratic and knightly landholders, sons did not inherit their fathers' status. Among Mamluks, the usual practice was to recruit each generation afresh from fair-skinned non-Islamic Turkish or Circassian nomadic families living on the southern steppes of Russia, north of the Black Sea.[93] At a time when Italians regarded slaves (generally black Africans) as household ornaments unfit for serious responsibility, in the Mamluk world almost everyone recruited for high-status jobs was originally a slave.

Once enslaved in their western Asiatic homelands and cut off from further ties with their kinsmen, young Circassian or Turkish nomads were loaded on ships at Black Sea ports and carried through the Dardanelles to the Egyptian port of Dumyat (Damietta). From there they were brought to the barracks in the Citadel in Cairo. Within that great fortress (built by Saladin), recruits who were destined for service under the Sultan (Royal Mamluks) or under a leading emir were superficially instructed by eunuchs (men who had sacrificed their testicles to their careers) in the truths of the Muslim faith. At the more practical level recruits were trained in horsemanship and the use of lance and bow and arrow. After cavalry training was completed, a recruit was manumitted to become a Mamluk, formally joined in service in the invincible army and sent to live in the household of a graded commander of cavalry; one of these commanders held the office of Sultan.

It was the Mamluk cavalry which in 1250 had captured the saintly King Louis IX of France and wrecked the Sixth Crusade. It was again the Mamluk cavalry which had forced the pagan Mongols to retreat to their central Asian homeland in 1258 after they sacked and destroyed Baghdad, the then chief city of the Islamic world. At a time when the warriors of Christendom were notoriously unable to work for a common cause (Acre, the key crusader fortress, fell to the Mamluks under Sultan al Ashraf Khalil in 1291), it is not unlikely that these Mamluk victories over Mongols saved central Europe from ruin. And in the era of plague, immediately after 1400, Mamluk cavalry again saved the West by defeating a fresh wave of Mongol invaders led by Tamberlane (Timur Lang) and persuading him that his future lay in China, rather than in the Middle East or in Christendom.

Ever victorious and convinced that their military tactics were flawless, in other areas of human concern the Mamluks were ill-prepared to innovate. Most of them were functionally illiterate (an attribute they shared with most aristocrats north of the Alps before 1550) and were thus cut off from stray new ideas that might have come their way through written sources. Mamluks were isolated in other ways as well. While on active service, they were not commonly allowed to marry or encouraged to have much to do with indigenous Cairenes other than those they encountered on visits to female or male brothels in the town. Though they provided inspiration for the web of fabulous stories which became *The Thousand and One Nights* (the *Arabian Nights*), few Mamluks bothered to learn Arabic as spoken by the majority of Cairenes, or in its classical form, the language in which Allah had communicated the contents of the Holy Qur'ān to the Prophet Muhammad. Few learned Coptic, the language of the Christian minority, which in the fourteenth century was being gradually phased out as the language of daily use. Among themselves the Mamluks spoke a Turkish dialect that was unintelligible to the general Egyptian population.[94]

To support their households, Mamluk magnates were assigned blocks of land, *iqta*, by the central Army Board; deeds of possession were then registered in the central Chancery. Mamluk *iqta* estates were usually scattered about in Upper and Lower Egypt and Syria and reassigned every five years to prevent an individual Mamluk from building up a local power base of retainers of the sort found among fief-holding magnates and nobles in pre-bureaucratic Europe. On the death or retirement of a Mamluk his lands were returned to the Army Board for reassignment. From what has been said so far, it is clear that the members of the Mamluk oligarchy had practically nothing in common with the indigenous people whom their local agents so thoroughly exploited.[95]

In time of plague, the alien Mamluks of course had to make individual decisions about how to cope. In 1347–48, led by the eleven-year-old Sultan, many Mamluks fled Cairo to plague-free villages north of the city. Yet in later years, most decided that it was best to stay in the Citadel to defend their interests against Mamluk rivals. Staying put, however, was perhaps not a good idea; contemporaries noted abnormally high plague mortality among fortress inmates. Overall, Mamluk numbers dropped from 10,000 in 1346 to only 5–6,000 at the time of the Turkish invasion in 1517. Even so, this force was fifteen times the size of the company the crusaders left behind to hold the Holy Land after its conquest by the First Crusade. Perhaps one consequence of falling Mamluk numbers was that this drained their morale. Yet Mamluk proneness to plague meant that they had no reason to assume that there was a link between poverty, moral turpitude, and the spread of plague. This humane attitude contrasted sharply with the situation in northern Italy after 1450.[96]

At a time when Italian humanists and princes were creating the cultural phenomenon known as the Renaissance, the Mamluk regime fell into intellectual decay.[97] Convinced of the continuing invincibility of the cavalry that had earlier defended the Middle East from Mongols and Christians, sixteenth-century Mamluks failed to notice that their Ottoman Turkish rivals had recovered from their defeat at the hands of Tamberlane (1402) and were making effective use of infantry armed with hand guns and cannon. At a great battle north of Cairo in January 1517 the Turks defeated the Mamluk cavalry. Thereafter the Ottoman Sultan in Istanbul (the Byzantine capital captured by the Turks in 1453) ruled Egypt through local deputies. Yet behind the screen on which were played out the transient movements of actors' shadows, few things in Egypt actually changed. Under the Ottoman Sultans, the Mamluks stayed on as *de facto* rulers until those who survived the Battle of the Nile (1798) against the young French general, Napoleon, were gunned down at the Citadel by the Ottoman Viceroy in 1811.

As it existed before 1517 and after, Mamluk power was buttressed by a highly centralized state bureaucracy. Because the curriculum at Al Azhar University (founded in 927 CE) was intended to produce Muslim theologians and jurists rather than civil servants, the bureaucracy was staffed largely by native-born Coptic Christians literate in Arabic, assisted by a few Jews.[98] As members of a religious minority in the service of an alien elite, Coptic bureaucrats knew that their survival depended on their skill in bringing tax receipts into the Sultan's central treasuries even during an era when plague, famine and disasters were drastically cutting the size of the taxable population. In 1423 on the initiative of Copts in the central treasury, a state monopoly of the sale of cane sugar was created. This was followed in 1429 by the creation of a monopoly on the sale of spices to European agents cooped up in *funduq* (walled compounds) in Alexandria. These supplemental revenues helped to keep the Mamluk regime in being and lessened Mamluk rulers' need to worry about the well-being of plague-threatened peasant populations.[99]

As city-dwellers banned from holding landed estates in rural areas, Coptic bureaucrats were vaguely aware of the slow decline of fifteenth-century Cairo's population (in-migration notwithstanding) and with it the decay of the urban tax base. To find out more precisely what was going on, in time of plague counts were made of the number of victims' coffins leaving the city gates; other counts were made of the plague dead for whom special prayers were said at Friday mosque. Aside from this, bureaucracy took no notice of recurring bouts of pestilence and never contemplated establishing health boards on the Florentine model.[100]

Below the Mamluk civil service—and in personal wealth sometimes exceeding them—were the great merchants and bankers of Cairo, Alexandria and Qus, the city in southern Egypt which controlled the shortest route from the Nile to the Red Sea. The most famous of these were the Karimi merchant clan; some Karimi were Jewish, others regarded it as politic to be Muslim.[101] So long as their Mamluk masters controlled access to the Red Sea at Aden, these merchants had naval contact with the great spice-trade treasures of India, Ceylon, Indonesia and China. Within Egypt, merchants' primary concern was that receipts and bills of exchange came in regularly. After Sultan Barsbay created a state monopoly of the spice trade in 1423, many merchant clans simply moved to India and carried on business from there. Historians now realize that it was this migration rather than Portuguese discovery of a new route to Asia via the Cape of Good Hope in 1498 that contributed most to the decay of Mamluk tax revenue from long-distance trade.[102]

The principal customers for the Asian spices in which merchants dealt were the Mamluk elite of Cairo and the Genoese traders in Alexandria who serviced well-born people in Europe; there was no demand for these luxury goods among rural *fellaheen*. Presumably for this reason, these non-consumers were beyond the pale of merchants' concern. Similarly absent from mercantile minds was a willingness to try out Italian-style maritime or land-based quarantines which would halt the flow of shipping. In any case, Mamluk masters delegated no political power to Egyptian merchants in the cities where their warehouses and principal residences were found. Untroubled by requirements of service on a board of health (in the style of a German, French or English burgher in an early modern town), in time of plague merchants simply barricaded themselves into well-provisioned houses and waited the crisis out.

Within the cellular framework of extended families and corporate groupings that was urban Cairo, craft production was controlled by guilds.[103] There were guilds for wood-workers, metal-workers and food processors and for the makers of fine cottons and silks for elites, for rough cloth for workers and peasants; there were also guilds for prostitutes and pick-pockets. Each guild was headed by an official appointed by the regime who saw to it that taxes assessed by the central bureaucracy were regularly paid. Since all categories of people, moral or immoral, were tax-rendering subjects, in the tolerant world of Mamluk and later Ottoman Egypt there was no need to stigmatize any social group as carriers of plague. Lacking indigenous scapegoats (other than the spectral jinn found in peasant culture), there was no room for the development of the idea that human movement should be restricted to block the plague.

In looking at Egyptian reactions to pestilence, some historians stress the apparently unchanging nature of the official Islamic religious response; this interpretation oversimplifies a complex reality.[104] To begin with (ignoring the pagan residuum), it was not until the fifteenth century that the majority of people outside of the Delta and Cairo considered themselves to be Muslims at all. Egypt had been among the first provinces of the Roman Empire in which Christianity became the religion of the people. This was achieved by the mid-300s, some years before Augustine of Hippo (d. 430) created the construct "original sin" that thereafter distinguished western followers of the cult from other Christians. After the Arab invasion of 640, welcomed by Copts as a way to free Egypt from the tentacles of the Byzantine (Greek Orthodox) Church, Copts co-existed with Muslims. For its part, Islam recognized the right of other peoples of the book (Jews and Christians) to their own forms of religion so long as they did not proselytize Muslims. Co-existence continued during the Mamluk period. However, at times of special crisis when, for example, Genoese and Venetians were raiding the Egyptian coasts (they burned down Alexandria in 1356), many Copts found it convenient to have a family member convert to Islam.[105] New-made Muslims were unlikely to challenge established teachings about the appropriate responses to plague.

Until the re-emergence of bubonic plague, the practice among Copts was for one of their sons to become a monk; monasteries like those of St Anthony in the Eastern Desert and in Wadi Natrun in the desert west of the Nile were true bastions of the faith. However, because monastic building plans were so nicely suited to the dietary needs of flea-bearing rats (a flour mill was generally located near the monks' living quarters), these communities were particularly hard hit by plague: the monastic records of Wadi Natrun fall silent after 1346. According to a contemporary report, of the hundred monasteries tucked away in desert Egypt in 1346, only seven were functioning around 1450.[106] In the Coptic vision there was no doubt that plague was sent by God; human intervention was futile.

The small Jewish community in Egypt also failed to come up with an alternative interpretation of the meaning of plague. Jews were especially numerous in Alexandria (where they had lived on and off since Roman times) and in Old Cairo near Fustat. Many of them engaged in the spice trade with India. Others were medical doctors trained in the Yünäni (Greco-Arabic) tradition that accepted Galenic ideas about miasmas and humors. Like their colleagues in the West, in Egypt Jewish doctors often served as personal physicians to great men at court. Because it was necessary to have eight household heads in attendance to establish a synagogue (a number seldom found in peasant villages), most Jews were city-dwellers who knew nothing of the plague-prone world of rural people.[107]

For somewhat different reasons, after 1347–49 Islamic theologians and jurists learned in the law (subjects taught at Al-Azhar university and at *madrasa* in Cairo) did not alter the basic interpretation of the response to plague worked out around 870. As Lawrence Conrad has recently shown, in the lifetime of the Prophet Muhammad (*c.* 570–632) during the first pandemic of bubonic plague (541–775), the disease became a byword for a horrifying presence before which all humans were powerless. During those early years of Islam in and around Mecca and Medina, nomadic Arabs who were still pagan held that plague was caused by demon jinn working on their own, unbidden by any higher authority. To Muslims this was a heretical explanation which denied the unchallengeable power of God. Accordingly, the Prophet's followers undertook to turn the pagan argument on its head so that it would conform to the requirements both of theology and of popular understanding. This took time: Conrad suggests that the completed formulation did not emerge until around 870.[108]

As incorporated into the Sayings of the Prophet (*hadith*) remembered after 870, plague was an instrument of Allah the Merciful, the all-powerful God: this reading ensured that it was not seen as caused by non-God-directed demons. And recognizing that two of the Prophet's companions had died of plague, the *hadith* also asserted that the death of a Believer by plague provided immediate access to paradise; in this the plague-dead joined Muslims martyred for the faith or killed in a jihad. On the other hand, it was held that pagans, infidels and other non-believers struck down by plague would proceed immediately to hell. In further recognition of plague as an instrument of the All-Powerful, the *hadith* advised Muslims that "If you hear that the plague is in a country, do not enter it, but if it appears in the country you are in, do not leave and do not flee that country."[109]

Taken together, these teachings make it clear that there was no need for family members to flee the household if one of their number were carried off by plague or to search for scapegoat humans. What Allah wills happens; in time of plague people should carry on their lives as if nothing unusual were going on. A commentary on this was written by Ibn Hagar al-Asqalāni, a Cairo *imam* who lived through the plagues of 1417, 1429–30 and 1444 and died in 1449. Inspired (Dols suggests) by this *imam*, after 1437 in time of plague it became customary to read out the appropriate *hadith* to the assembled faithful at Friday prayers at Al-Azhar.[110]

In Mamluk and Ottoman times, Al-Azhar scholars learned in theology and in the law issued formulations to guide medical attitudes to disease. Yet in practice, medical pluralism prevailed; each social grouping had several traditions to choose from. J. P. Berkey cites the case of a teaching *madrasa* known as the Jawhariyya founded in 1430 to instruct students in forms of law appropriate to Islamic identity. Incorporated into its deed of endowment was the command that room be found for a special pearl which, when immersed in water poured into a silver dish, cured a urinary disease. As a practical demonstration of cultural pluralism, the endowment ordered the *madrasa* to ensure that the common people always have access to the curing waters this pearl produced.[111]

Somewhat similar was the medical pluralism found at the Mamluk court. Here a hypothetical emir might place a sick, kin-less, slave-soldier in the care of a Jewish physician in the Greco-Arabic (Yünäni) tradition. If suffering from a (non-plague) fever, the slave might be treated following the medical tradition used by fourteenth-century Jewish and Gentile physicians in princely courts in the West, which is to say, the relevant sections of Ibn Sina's *Canon*. Alternatively, our hypothetical emir and his fair-skinned slave might turn to a Sufi, a person with healing powers which he had obtained from his contact—through reading, prayer and meditation—with the spirit of life and regeneration. Or the emir might turn to a practitioner of what was known as the Prophet's Medicine. Under a nomenclature that conferred authenticity, this included pagan Pharaonic, pagan nomadic, settled Arabic and other ancient ideas about how to prevent and to cure disease. Included in its wisdom was the proverb that every disease had its cure *except plague*, madness and old age.[112] For the urban poor, a less costly option was a magical amulet guaranteed to keep away the evil eye which struck down individual people or the jinn of plague which struck communities.

As in the Christian West in the early sixteenth century, in the Muslim world the heartbeat of orthodoxy was stronger in the great cities than in the countryside. Thus in Cairo during the terrible plague visitation in 1695–96, among people of middling rank the decencies expected of believers were scrupulously maintained. Expanding the Islamic doctrine of good works, family, friends and neighbors regularly visited plague-afflicted people and assisted in their feeding and bathing.Caring family members tidied up the dead, placed them in coffins and brought them to the grave accompanied by large processions of mourners. According to the chronicler, Garbarti, "Many rich men, emirs, great merchants and others, joined in this charitable work and assisted personally with the burial of a great number of plague dead" in the Eastern and Southern Cemeteries.[113] In doing what they did, believers accepted that the visitation had been sent by Allah the Merciful to open to the faithful one of the 360 doorways of Paradise.

The situation in rural areas may have been different. Here among unacculturated *fellaheen*, plague continued to be seen as a visitation by dart-throwing jinn, best responded to by flight to Cairo where there was a chronic labor shortage.[114] In eastern Anatolia in the Ottoman heartland, during the plague of 1720 many villagers took to the hills; after the crisis some stayed in their new-found settlements. Travelling opposite Egypt on the Red Sea coast in 1816 John Lewis Burckhardt was told by fleeing people that "the plague is a blessing which Allah has sent to the world to call the virtuous to paradise; we believe we have yet to achieve this state of grace and so we are withdrawing ourselves until another time."[115]

In Egypt, in determining how to cope with plague, each extended family, peasant community or self-contained urban neighborhood seems first to have looked at how their forebears had done things. Finding no precedents for intervention, no interventions were made. And so the plague continued. Somewhere in Egypt in at least sixteen of the fifty years between 1750 and 1800 great numbers of people died of the disease. Then, early in the nineteenth century, a new alien ruler arrived on the scene. Unlike his predecessors, when confronted by plague, Muhammad Ali proved himself willing to take forceful action.

The son of a Macedonian soldier/merchant, Muhammad Ali had served in the Ottoman army and may have picked up some ideas about plague control from Turkish medics; in such matters the Turks were half a century in advance of the Egyptians.[116] In 1801, while still a dashing young man he was sent to Egypt as second-in-command of an Albanian contingent to clean out the remnants of Napoleon Bonaparte's army (which had been hit by plague earlier in Syria). In 1805 Muhammad Ali Pasha became Viceroy and *de facto* ruler of Egypt under the Ottoman Sultan.

Inasmuch as one man could, Muhammad Ali transformed Egypt and the Syrian province his army occupied after 1805. As heir of the power of the Mamluks, within the settled lands his word was law. To rid himself of intrigues, in March 1811 he invited 470 Mamluks to dinner at the Citadel and gunned them down as they left. At his command, Sufi teachers established colonies in Upper Egypt and Nubia and used Muslim converts to expand the area of arable land. Beyond Egypt, military campaigns brought Sinai and Syrian nomads into his system as taxpaying subjects. Further afield, his sons commanded armies that defeated a fundamentalist sect in control of the holy cities of Mecca and Medina and, in 1816, established the Pasha as the protector of orthodox Sunni Muslims within the Ottoman Empire. All this was done with an army which at maximum strength numbered 200,000 men and a naval establishment of 30 ships based on the new-built arsenal at Alexandria.

Muhammad Ali intended to modernize Egypt so that it could compete on equal terms with its European trading partners—principally England and France—as well as expand its already considerable trade in the Middle East.[117] Had he succeeded, Egypt would have been the first non-European country to come successfully to terms with the modern world of advanced capitalism and imperialism. If the Pasha failed in the end, it was not through any fault of his own, but because the European states (wherein reigned the liberal values, *laissez-faire* and possessive individualism) had vastly superior resources of manpower, advanced technology and advanced credit finance. They also had vastly superior access to raw materials and markets. In contrast to Britain's 20 million people and France's 34 million, Muhammad Ali's Egypt consisted of only 3 million mostly illiterate people, heirs to 450 years of periodic exposure to bubonic plague, living on an area of arable land smaller than the Netherlands.[118]

Never daunted by statistics, Muhammad Ali established a command economy in part funded between 1809 and 1814 by the export of wheat to the British forces under Wellington, which were driving Napoleon's armies out of Portugal and Spain. Then building on fifteenth-century Mamluk precedents, the Pasha established state monopolies in cotton, linen and manufactured goods; he also created a monopoly on Egyptian trade with

Europe and Anatolia and built up the navy to enforce it. After 1838, overriding existing use-rights, he resumed (Pharaonic) state control of all arable land and established a new landholding class, largely of Turkish or Circassian descent, which became the basis of the aristocracy until it was undermined by Gamal Nasser in the 1950s. To make these state agencies work, and to harness the energies of the whole of the Egyptian population to the task of producing cotton, grain and other goods for export to the Middle East and Europe, Muhammad Ali devised an Ideology of Order based on Pharaonic precedents touched up with what his Italian and French advisers told him were ideas current in Europe. In its application, it worked in much the same way as did the full-blown Italian system.

Many of Muhammad Ali's state-building activities ruffled the feathers of liberals in Europe. With perhaps unconscious irony, P. J. Cain and A. G. Hopkins (1993) summed up the British position:

> this emerging complementarity [raw cotton from Egypt, in exchange for cotton goods from Manchester] could not disguise the fact that Mohammed Ali was a centralising autocrat who favoured state monopolies and protectionism, and had expansionist ambitions of his own, whereas Britain was treading a path toward free trade and minimal government, and needed to create obedient and pacific satellites.[119]

In 1827 at Navarino Bay a combined Franco-British fleet sank the navy Muhammad Ali had sent to help his Ottoman Sultan master discipline the rebelling Greeks.[120] In 1830 French and British consuls in Cairo teamed up to ensure that the Pasha did not help his co-religionists in Algeria drive newly arrived French settlers back into the sea.

Indicative of mid-nineteenth-century non-governmental attitudes towards the Pasha's Egyptian subjects and their medical practices were the comments of the British back-packer, Richard Burton. Briefly in Cairo while preparing to slip illegally into Mecca, Burton found himself in need of money. As he reported:

> From my youth I have always been a dabbler in medical and mystical study. . . . Moreover the practice of physic is comparatively easy amongst dwellers in warm latitudes, uncivilized peoples, where there is not that complication of maladies which troubles more polished nations . . . so . . . I therefore considered myself as well qualified [to practice medicine in Cairo] as if I had taken out a *buono per l'estero* diploma at Padua . . . I request the reader not to set me down as a mere charlatan; medicine in the East is so essentially united with superstitious practices, that he who would pass for an expert practitioner, must necessarily represent himself an "adept".[121]

This was written nearly forty years before Robert Koch of Prussia brought modern medicine into being, finally justifying the assumption that western medicine was itself more than a "mix of superstitious practices."

As an enlightened despot, Muhammad Ali recognized that all members of society, to be productive, needed access to modern health care. To this end, he created the first state-supported rural health scheme in the Mediterranean world; no similar scheme would be found in liberal Britain until the coming of socialism in 1945. To achieve universal rural health coverage, the Pasha brought in European medical advisers in the clinical tradition, headed by Dr A. B. Clot. In 1827 Clot and Muhammad Ali established the first western-style teaching hospital in Egypt, the Kasr el Ainy Hospital; instruction was in Arabic. Students were recruited from Al-Azhar where they had been studying law and theology; these programs were just as appropriate for students of medicine as was the program in Classics at Oxford to which the *crème de la crème* of the British medical profession was exposed. By 1830, *graduates* from Kasr el Ainy—Dr Clot refused to let them call themselves medical doctors—were out in the field staffing rural clinics.[122] Four years later Egypt was hit by the first of two harsh bouts of plague; it is to these we now turn.

By 1834 Muhammad Ali was already committed to an Ideology of Order in time of disease crisis. In 1812, learning that plague was in Istanbul, the chief city of his political master and leading trading partner, he imposed a naval quarantine on Turkish ships; the plague did not enter Egypt. Later, to deal with the problem of men and goods coming in from plague-ridden Levantine ports, he established a pesthouse and warehouse in Damietta. Ironically, his chief medical adviser Dr Clot, being a miasma man, derided the contagion theory on which these programs was based. However in 1830s Egypt, as in baroque Italy, the opinions of medical men were easily overridden by the mandates of the Prince.

Despite quarantine precautions taken in 1834, the plague entered Egyptian Mediterranean ports in great force in the following year. During early months, while only outlying regions near Alexandria were affected, Muhammad Ali imposed a cordon sanitaire around the city. When plague broke through, he used tough measures much like those used in Genoa in 1656. Police and soldiers imprisoned plague victims in pesthouses and burned their personal effects. As in Europe, status considerations held; middling or high-ranking Alexandrians who had a family member suspected of being sick got off with household isolation. In contrast, whole families of poorer people in the same plight were rounded up at night and carted out to quarantine stations on the edge of town. Heads of households failing to report a family member dead of plague were summarily shot.[123]

What particularly offended Alexandria's Muslims about Muhammad Ali's Ideology of Order was that Christian infidels (Western doctors) seemed to be commanding Muslim medics to do things which were against the law of God. Seen as gross examples of defilement were the autopsies conducted by medical personnel on the nude dead which were then buried in lime. To stop the rounding up of suspects (who, it was rumored, might be converted into "plague" dead for clinical observation) groups of Muslims barred the way of soldiers who were taking people away under cover of darkness. The results were predictable: a score of people shot dead, whole neighborhoods cowed and the further rounding up of plague victims and their families. Faced with the failure of neighborhood solidarities, some families took measures of their own. Burrowing away secretly at night they buried their plague dead in courtyards, or left the corpse on some distant street where it could not be recognized and thus bring punishment to the family.

Yet in the end, the application of the Ideology of Order was futile. Once pestilence was well established among the rat, flea and human population all the way between Alexandria and Luxor, there was nothing that Muhammad Ali could do but wait for it to run its course. By the time the visitation ended in October 1837 some 75,000 Cairenes and 125,000 other Egyptians were dead. Total mortality was equal to the size of the entire army, roughly 7 percent of the Egyptian population.[124]

For a small non-western nation struggling to emerge on terms of equality with the liberal imperial powers of Europe, this loss was a staggering blow. It was the first of many. In 1838, under the siren call of Free Trade (ancestor of GATT), Lord Palmerston forced the Ottoman Sultan and his Viceroy in Egypt to allow British agents to buy cotton direct from producers; this destroyed the Egyptian state monopoly of a vital export and income generator. Three years later liberal Europe forced the Egyptians to withdraw from Syria (since 1250 an integral part of the Mamluk Empire). Deprived of his tax base in Syria and of revenues from state monopolies in Egypt, by the mid-1840s Muhammad Ali was unable to prevent European usurers from winning control of the money markets of Egypt. It seemed that his dream of establishing an Egypt under nominal Ottoman suzerainty, independent of the West, was rapidly becoming an illusion.[125]

So too, if western ideologues had their way, would the Pasha's main line of defense against fresh imports of plague from abroad. Determined to end the "barbarism and self-sufficiency" of a non-European state which put up barriers to Free Trade, British diplomats worked to prevent the establishment of further quarantines on shipping.[126] Writing in 1839, the British ambassador to the Sublime Port, Lord Ponsonby, made clear his contempt of Orientals' policies of inspecting and impounding ships and warehouses. In his lordship's words:

> This power will occasion a serious inroad upon one great and precious principle and right created by our capitulation, that is the inviolability of the domicile of a Frank [a British person]; and it will probably occasion robbery, perhaps murders, and certainly infinite distress and misery to the sick. . . . therefore I am adverse to these measures.[127]

Despite the setbacks Europe's imperialists inflicted on Muhammad Ali, when plague broke out in northern Egypt in 1841 he again took up the fight. This time, his foreign plague doctors were accompanied by battalions of troops and, as a concession to the gender differences of plague victims, women curers. Confronted with this support system, local people stiffened their backs, determined not to cooperate. Typically, in the Delta province of Gharbiyya, 300 village headmen met the provincial governor in February 1841 and assured him that their dependent peasants were plague free. This was patently false; a few days later it was learned that 650 people, nearly half the inhabitants of one of these villages, had already died of the disease. In another plague-swept village, survivors lynched the soldiers Muhammad Ali sent in and for several hours prevented reinforcing troops from even rescuing their corpses. Elsewhere however, the shock-troops of the Ideology of Order successfully maintained control.[128]

As perfected by Dr Masserano and other medical hirelings in the Delta in 1841, plague measures were enforced with brutal thoroughness. In any suspect village, living victims and family members were separated from healthy peasants and placed in isolation; the entire village was surrounded with a cordon sanitaire manned by soldiers instructed to shoot to kill. Within the village, clothes and housing belonging to the plague dead were burnt. All other peasants were rounded up, segregated by sex and, in crude violation of Muslim ideas about the impropriety of public nudity, made to take an all-over *spoglio*, a bath in full view of medical attendants (hence the need of a woman curer to supervise the washing of females). The *spoglio* completed (nobody then knew that the fleas which might carry the plague were thus banished), the peasants were given clean clothes and kept for several days under medical supervision.[129]

Backed by rigorous control of shipping coming in from suspect Mediterranean ports, this time Muhammad Ali's plague measures appeared to work to wondrous effect. The plague slowed down (the last localized outbreak was in October 1844), then petered out. Thereafter Egypt became plague free and would remain so for three generations. Standing before the Pasha's tomb in his mosque in the Citadel today, visitors may be excused for thinking they hear a sigh issuing forth which, translated from the Arabic says: "But at least I won the victory over plague." Augmenting the Pasha's boast is the modern understanding that quarantines, working in phase with the dying off of afflicted populations of rats, might indeed free sizeable regions from the Great Scourge.

2 Dark Hidden Meanings: Leprosy and Lepers in the Medieval West and in the Tropical World under the European Imperium

Introduction

In 1885 Henry Wright, archdeacon in the Church of England at Grantham, warned that "loathsome" leprosy, long thought to be extinct among civilized beings, was in India "eat[ing] into the nerve-tissues of [England's] people." Looking to the near future when he thought many of his nation would be settled in India, Wright predicted that travel back and forth would bring the terrible disease to England's own "closely packed population." To head off this "Imperial Danger," Wright pleaded for Christian commitment to the despised "Lazar in his rags," who like the lepers known to Jesus "invites us to hasten and help him."[1]

Six years later, coming from within the medical profession rather than the clergy, was a book-length survey of the affliction Archdeacon Wright had in mind. In *Leprosy* (1891), Dr George Thin confirmed that "modern nerve leprosy" was the same disease for which prescriptive behavior was laid down in Leviticus chapter XIII verses 44–46. Here the operative words were "now whosoever shall be defiled with the leprosy and is separated by the judgement of the priest . . . shall dwell alone without the camp."[2] Like others with career interests in this disease—such as Health Officer Acworth in British-occupied Bombay—Dr Thin believed that medieval regimes had literally followed the Old Testament injunction to capture and confine lepers and that this policy had led to the disappearance of leprosy in Europe by the end of the sixteenth century. Instancing modern ideas about civil rights, Thin boasted that "the drastic measures by which the people of England freed themselves from the plague of leprosy are hardly likely to be repeated in any country governed by a civilized power."[3]

Yet at the very time Dr Thin was writing, coinciding with the rise of the penny-cheap press, an aggressively civilized United States of America was rigorously segregating lepers in Hawai'i in the mid-Pacific. In Britain, media-led sympathy for Father Damien de Veuster, the Belgian Roman Catholic missionary priest who martyred himself for Hawaiian lepers in 1889, led to the establishment of the National Leprosy Fund with the Prince of Wales as honorary chairman.[4] Following this, the first World Leprosy Congress was held in 1897 in Berlin, the city where sub-Saharan Africa had recently been portioned out to the colonial powers. Not surprisingly, leprosy professionals at the congress voted overwhelmingly for the segregation of lepers world-wide.

Against this background I will open this chapter by looking at the leprosy situation in medieval Europe. Following in the footsteps of two quintessential late Victorian medical men, Charles Creighton and Jonathan Hutchinson, I argue that the time has come to reject *orthodox* nineteenth-century historical accounts of medieval leprosy of the sort exemplified by Wright and Thin and, in our own time, Foucault. As I as see it, depending on context, medieval "leprosy" lay somewhere along a spectrum ranging from:

leprosy as *moral* impurity moving on to leprosy as imagined disease (a Construct, but in official perceptions, requiring *no* police action);
leprosy as the full Construct and call to action by accusers and magistrates: this led to the imprisonment of "lepers" in lazar houses;
leprosy as Hansen's disease, i.e., clinically true leprosy.

Unlike Mary Douglas, I assume that at least a few sufferers from Hansen's disease were found among the "lepers" dealt with in late eleventh-, twelfth, and thirteenth-century northern Europe. I also assume that as Construct (delusion), leprosy was for a time an epidemic threat. Building on the findings of Hutchinson and Creighton, I will then argue that medieval responses to "leprosy" were actually a heterogeneous hodgepodge which left most "lepers" wandering about at will.[5]

After looking at medieval accusers and victims of "leprosy" I will pinpoint those elements Victorian orthodoxy chose for its usable history of leprosy. Emerging from this was the scripturally based Construct summed up by Dr George Thin. In this version, as applied to the tropical colonial world, particular stress was laid on the transference of identity which transformed a normal colonialized person into a dehumanized leper.[6] From the 1860s on, application of this Christian paradigm formed a basis of policy in Hawai'i, South Africa, Malaysia and the Philippines.

Elsewhere, especially in India, colonial administrators regarded the Hawaiian model as the ideal towards which they might like to aim, all other things being equal. In practice however, many of them recognized that local cultural attitudes to the colonial intruders would make it impolitic to intervene in ordinary people's lives on the scale the Hawaiian model required. There was also the always touchy issue of finance. Who was to pay for any campaign of mass leper incarceration? Accordingly, in India and in other areas which looked to its government's policies as models, instead of following the Hawaiian paradigm to its logical conclusion, colonial administrators resorted to face-saving tokenism. Yet even the confinement of a tiny number of lepers was usually accompanied by loud scoffing at indigenous peoples' medical ideas. This had important long-term consequences. One of

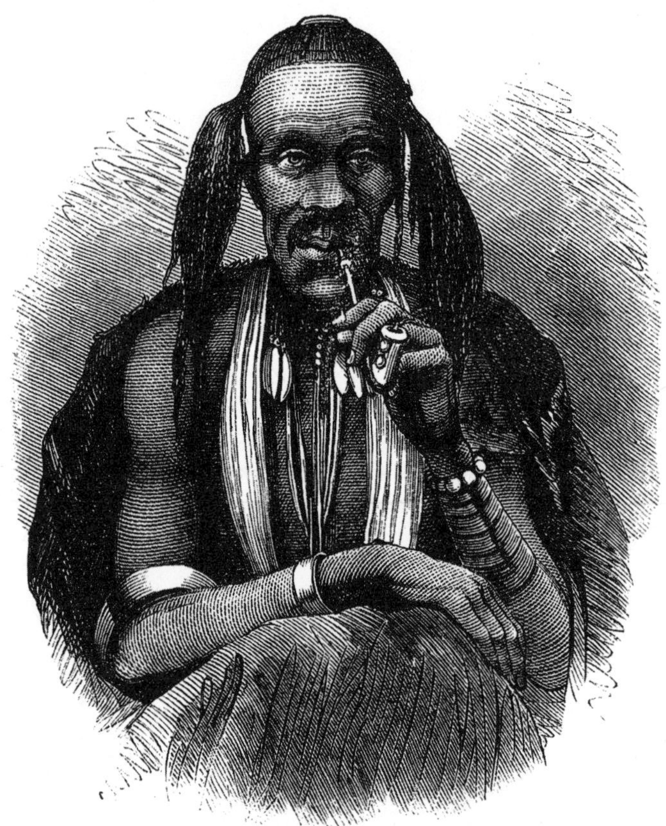

5. The "Other": a "Kaffir Witch-Doctor", from the *Illustrated London News*, 10 December 1864.

the little-known secrets of nineteenth-century imperialism was that trivial interventions, often seen by the colonialists as mere window dressing for the benefit of some special interest group back home, were seen by the imperialized peoples themselves as massive interference. However, this understanding often escaped the notice even of long-serving colonial officers who prided themselves on their knowledge of local conditions and local languages.[7]

Among late nineteenth-century westerners worried about "Imperial Dangers," it was thought that leprosy was a hereditary, contagious, incurable disease that condemned once normal people to years of living as shrivelled wrecks with collapsed noses, claw-like stumps for hands and feet, stinking flesh and breath, and raucous voice. Even more degrading was the stigma attached to the disease. Among the historically informed, opinion held that leprosy was God's punishment for dark, hidden thoughts, words and deeds, usually involving disgusting forms of sex. Lepers needed moral uplift even more than they needed medical care. Inspired by this notion, most of the work among lepers in India and Africa was carried out by missionaries, missionary doctors, and religiously motivated volunteers from European homelands. These people formed a powerful interest group which colonial administrators ignored at their peril.

Ironically, in view of the small input laboratory-based science actually made to the control of its spread until very recently, leprosy was one of the first human illnesses for which the bacteria causal agent (*Mycobacterium leprae*) was discovered. Armauer Hansen of Norway made the breakthrough in 1873, nine years before Robert Koch of Prussia located the causal agent of tuberculosis; it is now known that the two disease agents are closely allied. Yet despite this head start, Hansen's disease was one of the last of the infectious diseases in this book for which something resembling a full cure was devised. The first seemingly satisfactory curative drug—dapsone—was discovered in the early 1940s, but because many patients developed resistance, it had to be replaced in the 1980s by a multi-drug treatment. This new therapy halts the degenerative processes (cures the disease) but is only *fully* effective for cases caught in time; lost nerves can never be restored.[8]

In the modern understanding, Hansen's disease is a spectrum of types ranging from highly destructive lepromatous leprosy to tuberculoid leprosy.[9] In the 1920s, clinical technology revealed that lepromatous leprosy went through three stages. During its early stage when it was at its most infective, it caused little visible tissue damage. Only during its third and final stage when the victim was no longer infective (and had thus become a "burnt-out case") did the leper acquire the collapsed nose, claw-like remains of feet and hands and other gruesome evidence of lepromatous leprosy.[10]

Globally, during the "Imperial Danger" scare, leprosy was most commonly found in the tropics. Yet in those regions it was unclear why so few—perhaps 5 percent—of the people who came into contact with an infective leper developed the illness. One of the barriers to problem resolution was the seven- to ten-year interval between contact and first disease symptoms; leprosy was seldom an illness of young children. If, as now thought, most members of a population exposed to *Mycobacterium leprae* had immune systems able to resist the bacteria, this did not explain why the residual 5 percent were susceptible. Among the possibilities suggested by early twentieth-century experts were "predisposing diseases" such as syphilis, gonorrhea and malaria. Other predisposing causes which one or another expert added to the list were physical weakness brought on by malnutrition, living in squalor with a large family in tight quarters, living near peat-bogs, or eating contaminated fish. In the antebellum American South, plantation doctors tended to regard leprosy as yet another disease of black people.[11]

During the 1920s, there was uncertainty about how leprosy was spread. The argument that it was airborne, broadcast through nasal discharge, ran against the counter-argument that during this era of "Imperial Danger" immigrants known to be carriers of leprosy living in Paris and other large cities did not trigger epidemics. Similarly, it was pointed out that the 170 leprous Norwegians who had emigrated to Minnesota and Wisconsin in North America after the Civil War had failed to set off epidemics, or indeed to produce children who became lepers. Back in Europe, aside from the odd case, leprosy was confined to sparsely settled rural places such as coastal Brittany, the Pyrenees and coastal Norway.[12]

Over the centuries very few lepers have written accounts of what the disease (imagined or real) personally meant to them. Aware of this informational gap, I thought I should visit my local leprosarium at Abou Zaabal on the outskirts of Cairo.[13] Once there I saw several dozen blind, claw-handed, skeletal human wrecks, victims of Hansen's disease, who matched any description of physical horror I found in written sources; French Catholic nuns were in attendance. By coincidence, it had been in the Egyptian southwest, in Dakhlah Oasis, that the first skeletal remains of a leper were found (from the second century BCE). Literary evidence, however, suggests that the disease was first found in India around 600 BCE.[14]

Leprosy in the European Middle Ages: Background

The relatively recent discovery of twenty to thirty leprosy-damaged skeletons belonging to people who lived in Roman Britain and Gaul, and beyond the frontiers of the Roman Empire in Hungary and the Nordic lands, conclusively proves that leprosy was not introduced into Europe during the era of the Crusades as many Orientalists thought, but that it had been there much earlier.[15] What probably happened was that sufferers from Hansen's disease had been in the entourages of Roman conquerors such as Julius Caesar (who was in Gaul 58–49 BCE). They in turn probably picked up leprosy in Roman-ruled lands in the Levant: the disease seems to have appeared in that region soon after Alexander the Great's attacks on India in 327 BCE.[16]

Moving to the seventh and eighth centuries of the current era brings us to Lombard precedents for the mixing of accusations of religious heresy and leprosy which would be typical of the situation half a millennium later, in the high Middle Ages. Coming south after 550 these Germanic *Volk*, the last tribal group to settle in Italy, were adherents of the Arian interpretation of Christianity (named after Arius of Alexandria) which claimed that Jesus was *of similar* substance to God the Father. Once settled in and around Pavia and Milan, the Lombard minority found themselves living among a conquered underclass who followed Athanasius (also of Alexandria) in claiming that this was not so, and that Jesus the Son was *of one* substance with God the Father. For believers, these differences were of critical importance.

Hemmed in by a populace who followed the creed of Athanasius and the authority of the Bishop of Rome, the Lombard king Rothari spoke of the adult male Lombard population as "the most fortunate army." Presumably he was thinking in terms of the "purity" of insiders like himself and the "danger" posed by outsiders.[17] Living in these strained circumstances, in 635 Rothari incorporated into a law code a chapter prescribing action in case of leprosy:

> If anyone is affected with leprosy and the truth of the matter is recognized by the judge or by the people and the leper is expelled from the *civitas* or from the house so that he lives alone, he shall not have the right to alienate his property or to give it to anyone because on the day he is expelled from the home it is as if he had died. Nevertheless, while he lives, he should be nourished on the income from that which remains.[18]

Though the meaning of leprosy (as disease, as Construct, or both) within Lombard society remains opaque, in determining the tone of Lombard relationships with neighboring Frankish Gaul while it was ruled by King Pepin meanings became transparently clear. The Franks had became the armed protectors of the papacy against the Lombards in 753–54. After Pepin brought the Lombards to heel, he accepted the Pope's warning that dynastic ties cemented by marriage between himself or his son and a Lombard princess would introduce hereditary leprosy into the Frankish royal line; it seems that popes were already infatuated with the tainting qualities of leprosy. Thereafter following the papal lead, it became *de rigueur* for Franks to claim that Lombards were "perfidious and fetid, amongst whom it is certain that the race of lepers took their origins."[19]

During the long era between the collapse of Rome and the birth in the tenth to eleventh centuries of a set of societies recognizable in retrospect as "Europe," medical doctors in the classical learned tradition lived almost exclusively in the urbanized *eastern* half of the old empire, either in the Christian core centered on Constantinople or in the Islamic world centered on Baghdad and Cairo; in both regions the heartbeat of urban life continued to be strong.[20] In stark contrast, in the post-Roman West (proto-Europe), by the end of the fifth century internal social decay had destroyed all but the most rudimentary forms of town life and with it the sort of patronage/clientage networks learned physicians required. Worse was to follow. After the death of the peripatetic Frankish king/emperor, Charlemagne (Pepin's son) in 814, the West was overrun by rural terrorists, at first predominantly outsiders—Vikings, Magyars, Saracens—then by locally born raiders.

In the west Frankish lands in the late tenth century and in the eastern (Germanic) lands in the late eleventh, casual lawlessness gave way to the systematic exploitation of cultivators by the holders of rude fortresses (castellans) and resident warriors (later known as knights); many of these thugs were ostensibly in the employ of great territorial lords.[21] Writing in 1127, Peter the Venerable, Abbot of the great Benedictine abbey at Cluny in Burgundy, noted that it was common practice for lords and under-officers arbitrarily to beat, plunder and torture peasants who had been unable to take refuge in flight. Victimized by armed predators year after year, most peasants capitulated to an oppressor; in order to regularize exactions they became his serfs.[22]

During these centuries of terror and disintegration in the Christian West, health provisioning lay almost entirely with village curers, sorcerers, magicians, wandering spirits and wonder-working protector saints.[23] When in the eleventh century elements of learned medicine finally reappeared in the form of written texts, they necessarily came in from outside. Before 1236, one source was the Andalusian city of (Muslim) Cordoba with its library of 400,000 books in Arabic, Hebrew, Greek and Latin which, before they were burned in that year by conquering Christians, probably contained much of the wisdom of the Ancients.[24] Another lay in the manuscripts brought into monastic libraries in coastal Italy from scriptoria in the Levant. Among these imported sources were ancient writings on leprosy. But in establishing which medical interpretation would henceforth become standard in the West, much depended on the accidents of chance.

As Michael Dols, Mirko Grmek and others have pointed out, the first extant description of proper leprosy was for a long time lost or ignored. Written in the first century CE by the Alexandrian physician, Aretaeus of Cappadocia, it is one of the great "might-have-beens" of medical history. Like the imperial masters he mentioned, Nero and Vespasian, Aretaeus believed in the traditional pantheon of Roman gods, none of whom connected sickness with private moral behavior. This neutral ethical position permitted Aretaeus to regard Hansen's disease as merely a disease of the body. However, he did point out that because of the physical disfigurement it caused, true leprosy frightened many people: "for this reason there are those who abandon their most cherished relatives in the desert and the mountains . . . even if [they are] one's own son, father, or brother."[25]

Between the seventh and the eleventh centuries medically informed Muslim authors drew on other late antique writers to present more or less clinically correct descriptions of Hansen's disease. This held that *judhäm*, *bahq*, or *baras* (Arabic words for various forms of clinical leprosy) was one of the hazards of life to be endured; it was not seen as a moral category or as a punishment sent from on high.[26] However, because of the near absence of open-minded Christian scholars literate in Arabic in apposite times and places, it would not be from these medical and medical/literary sources that instrumental people in the West would find the insights they needed to coin functional meanings for "leprosy." Instead they used sources that were heavily influenced by *priestly* interpretations of Judaic-Christian scriptures.

This brings us to the point in the emerging western mind at which Old Testament ideas and words associated with skin problems, deadened nerve ends, collapsing bones and ritual conditions of impurity come to the fore. According to the practices prescribed in Leviticus chapter XIII verses 44–46, Hebrews accused of having scaly skin were to be examined by a priest. If the skin condition and its associated white spots continued, they were judged to have offended the Hebrew God and had to withdraw from the tents and camp of the healthy *until* such time as the skin and/or ritual condition (*zara'at*) cleared. This presumably is the meaning of the sentence from Leviticus: "All *the time that* he is a leper . . . he shall dwell alone without the camp." In a perceptive comment in 1906, J. Hutchinson, earlier president of the Royal College of Physicians, pointed out that:

> [the Old Testament] scriptural record makes no mention of the paralysis, the loss of sensation and the helpless crippling which attend the true disease, but speaks of it as if it affected the skin only, and had its consummation in whiteness.

Hutchinson drew on the insights of Armauer Hansen (1873) and others in holding that Hansen's disease was incurable by human agency and that most self-cured lepers would be in the third phase of the disease—without fingers, toes or nose. In this deformed state they would probably better fit Aretaeus of Cappadocia's category of human wrecks before whom sons, fathers or brothers fled in terror than any category of cleansed, ritually pure folk fit to be welcomed back to their camp by kinsmen and priests. This leads us to accept Hutchinson's conclusion that the disease category *zara'at* which had existed in Palestine at the time Hebrews were reciting Leviticus around their campfires and altars was not what any modern physician would accept as leprosy.[27]

Archaeology also cast doubt on the connection between Hansen's disease and whatever it was that the prescription in Leviticus was all about. Archaeologists who have exhumed several hundred skeletons from Palestine from the sixth and fifth centuries BCE, when Leviticus was entering Jewish oral tradition, have discovered no human remains with evidence of true leprosy. Though this negative evidence might at any time be countered by a large find of ancient leprous remains, the current archaeological presumption is that true leprosy was not found in Palestine when Leviticus was being composed.[28]

Our next certain knowledge of developments in the making of "lepers" through priestly agency comes from a period 200 years closer to our own time, the third century BCE. Working in Alexandria for the benefit of bilingual offspring who in everyday conversation were more at ease with Greek than with Hebrew, Jewish scholars created a Greek translation of the Old Testament (the Septuagint). When they came to Leviticus, they translated the Hebrew *zara'at* (ritual impurity) into the Greek word *lepra*. Four hundred years later, in the first century CE, Josephus, a Jewish literary man and Roman collaborator also living in Alexandria, again used the Greek *lepra* when recounting (in order to refute) a 300-year-old anti-Semitic myth about Jews being driven out of ancient Egypt because they were lepers.[29] The next major contributor to the making of "lepers" was St Jerome (d. 419 CE), the compiler of the Latin Bible standard throughout the Middle Ages (the Vulgate), who we are assured was comfortable with Hebrew and didn't need Greek cribs. However, in Latinizing Leviticus's *zara'at*, Jerome used the same word—*lepra*—that the compilers of the Septuagint and Josephus had earlier employed.

Five hundred years later, monk Constantinus Africanus (*c.* 1020–87) at Monte Cassino (north of Naples) consolidated the translation of the Arabic-language medical texts which would become part of the standard literature available to physicians in the Latin-reading West. Using whatever cribs lay at hand, he employed the word—*lepra*—to denote true leprosy rather than a Latinized version of the Arabic word, *judhäm*. As a Christian who had sworn to obey the rules of the Benedictine order, Constantinus was obviously prepared to accept that whatever word St Jerome had chosen for purposes of translation was necessarily closer to fundamental Christian truth than any word used by Muslim scholars. As a result of this decision, the way was clear for literate people in the eleventh-century West to suppress morally neutral Classical World and Arabic meanings.[30] On this foundation would be built the conviction that leprosy was God's punishment for sin and that lepers must be driven out of the camp.

The Great Leper Hunt, c. *1090 to 1363*

In his 1987 study of the Great Hunt which lasted from *c.* 1090 to 1363, R. I. Moore cautioned that: "The whole question of how lepers were identified and their diagnosis confirmed is of central importance, and our ignorance of it is still almost total." More recently (1991), Mary Douglas suggested that the leper hunt was not concerned with a physical disease at all, but that accusations were merely a ploy to put inconvenient people out of the way.[31]

To move the argument forward, we can begin with the observation that among late eleventh-century brokers of power, Leviticus continued to be a talismanic force, just as it had been in the time of Pepin. As we know, according to that ancient Hebrew text, responsibility for judging lepers rested with priest, magistrate and "people". How this was interpreted during the early days of the hunt is unknown since no trial evidence seems to have survived. However, mid-fourteenth-century evidence from around Calais shows that by then "the people" had taken the form of juries. We don't know how these particular jurors were chosen, but in the analogous case of fourteenth-century England jurors were chosen because they were local men of good moral standing who knew the background of the disputants. In deciding innocence or guilt, jurors' concern was with the "repute" of the accused and how he or she meshed with networks of kinsfolk, friends and patrons who might be prepared to even out scores in a feud.[32] Set against this customary usage, one could hardly expect an impartial "diagnosis" for leprosy: indeed to do so would be anachronistic.

This still does not bring us closer to answering Moore's question about who "identified" lepers during the Great Hunt. As posed, the question does not distinguish between accuser and magistrate judge. Yet in any hypothesis which might be suggested, the sort of people defined as the new clerkly literati of the late eleventh and twelfth centuries would probably find a place. Moore suggests that these clerks (men in holy orders, necessarily literate in Latin) were being employed in proto-bureaucracies by centralizing territorial magnates and that they were leading agents in the "formulation of a persecuting society." In any leprosy trial set in motion by an accuser and conducted before "priest," "magistrate" and "people," a new-style clerk could presumably act in any capacity required by his magnate employer.

For religio-political authorities *circa* 1090 who hit upon the leprosy Construct as a felicitous way of ridding themselves of troublemakers, the last people they wanted meddling about were medically informed experts. There was little danger of this. In the 1090s even medical generalists were rare birds; Salerno, for long the sole medical school in the West, was only then beginning to feel its way forward.[33] There was also the matter of personal safety; in the French Hexagon and its satellites where religio-political hierarchies were determined to use the leprosy Construct as a tool of social control, medical doctors who valued their lives probably kept quietly out of the way. As Danielle Jacquart and Claude Thomasset tactfully put it: "especially in the case of leprosy . . . medicine offered a nosological conceptualization in conformity with the *demands* of the sacred and its textual tradition."[34]

In the pages that follow, having established the rationale for the beginning of the Great Hunt, I will then examine why after the mid-fourteenth century hegemonic authority lost interest in the leprosy Construct as an agency of social control. As will be seen, one reason was that it came to focus instead on the targets Carlo Ginzburg has so ably described: Jews, heretics and witches.[35] Once this shift in targeting was underway, two changes in leprosy processes occurred. One was a judicial innovation, the summoning of *medically competent* experts from *outside* the community to judge the truth or error of an accusation. Secondly, with the opening of a new market for up-to-date medical information, Guy de Chauliac (personal physician to Pope Clement VI at Avignon in 1348) put into circulation manuscript copies of his *La Grande Chirvrgie* (1363). Among its other features, this vernacular text contained a listing of the distinctive marks and signs of leprosy.[36] Equipped with this updated tool and called upon to use it at trials, medical doctors played an integral part in the process of identifying true lepers. Now that these humanitarians were at last in a position to influence decisions, it is little wonder that after the 1360s the number of certified lepers began its precipitous decline.[37]

Yet even during the era of transition (away from lepers towards more modern forms of social deviant), the role of learned physician did not remain unchallenged. In Valencia in the Crown of Aragon in 1318, a medical doctor who used a proto-guide to pronounce a person called Bernat Cubells free of leprosy was overridden by the local justiciar who had sentenced Cubells to confinement in the first place and whose will prevailed in the end.[38] Some decades later in the Rhineland town of Haguenau, barber-surgeons who had been on the local leprosy detection jury for years—and grown accustomed to pocketing fees—claimed that they knew far better how to identify a leper than did the bearded university medical men who had come in from Heidelberg, Speyer and Metz. In the barber-surgeons' complaint was a throwaway comment that one of the alien doctors was a Jew.[39]

Now that I have suggested a relationship between the Great Hunt (1090–1363) and the Great Void—the near absence of medical doctors at leprosy trials before *c.* 1363 (or slightly earlier in the Crown of Aragon)—we can return to the main issue, the use of Construct leprosy as a tool of social control during the high Middle Ages. Let us begin with the well-known but nonetheless extraordinary statistical fact that between 1090/1120 and 1240/60 several *thousand* lazar houses (leprosaria) were opened in West Europe. According to one account:

> there were 43 in the diocese of Paris alone . . . the two largest were in the immediate vicinity of Paris: Saint-Germain and Saint Lazare . . . England and Scotland alone had opened 220 lazar houses for a million and a half inhabitants in the twelfth century.[40]

Taken at face value, this sudden explosion in the number of asylums for lepers would seem to indicate that disease incidence had increased precipitously. Using the figures listed for England, there would have been 1.4 leprosaria for every thousand people; with an average of 10 inmates each, this would have worked out at a truly incredible 14 lepers per thousand.[41]

Historians who are unwilling to attribute this "leprosy" epidemic to a collective delusion similar to the seventeenth-century fantasy about the ability of old ladies to interfere with the workings of the weather through witchcraft, generally attribute the "rise of the number of lepers" (itself a fallacious concept) to changes in the physical and economic environment. This explanation is based on the orthodox historical understanding that in the late tenth and eleventh centuries the West finally broke through its post-Roman pattern of civil, economic and demographic decline. Using new tools and mindsets, forests were cut down, and wolves, werewolves and Green Men were forced into retreat. Along the banks of inland rivers and along the Atlantic, Baltic and Mediterranean coasts, market centers were refurbished or created anew. Some towns numbered 500 people, other giants contained 10,000 or 20,000 souls all needing foodstuffs produced by agriculturalists in rural hinterlands. Pushed along everywhere by the demands of urban–rural exchange, and in a handful of cities by long-distance trade in luxury goods with Cairo and other Muslim centers, Europe's old-style gift-economy based on the exchange of gold, jewels and spices among warrior elites gave way to a more broadly based economy which depended on the exchange of goods for money or letters of credit—the Arab model. As an unintended consequence of what was Europe's first brush with development, population began to grow. And added to the threat of too many mouths and too little food was the moral threat posed by sharper differentiation between *the few* who grew very wealthy (territorial lords, high-ranking clerics and great merchants), and *the many* who remained downtrodden and poor.[42]

Following elementary rules of logic, in newly vibrant Europe the number of lepers in each locality should have been roughly proportional to the density of its population. Yet as things worked out, leprosy did not bulk large in the records of the two most highly urbanized regions—northern and central Italy, and the Low Countries. Looking at the matter from a slightly different perspective, and supporting my contention that epidemic "leprosy" was a mindset rather than a physical disease, was the high prevalence of "leprosy" and leprosaria in the aggressive new cultural heartland of West Europe, the Hexagon of France, and its cultural satellite across the channel. (England had acquired that status with the Norman Conquest of 1066.)

In looking for dramatic change in the Hexagon, historians give pride of place to the Gregorian reform movement underway after 1050. As R. W. Southern explained, driven by the impetus of reform, the features which distinguished most aspects of medieval religious life were put in place in a few short years.[43] As part of this exercise, reforming clergy deliberately set themselves apart from ordinary secular rulers who in Pope Gregory VII's graphic phrase of 1081, had "raised themselves above their fellows by pride, plunder, treachery, [and] murder."[44] To further differentiate themselves from the laity, Gregorian clerics argued that God regarded contemplators of pure thought as infinitely superior to brute copulating humankind and, for their part, vowed to remain forever chaste.

Having established their own links with God as spirit, clerical reformers extended their claims to *imperium* by asserting control over lay sexuality. Between 1159 and 1181 Pope Alexander III (earlier known as Master Roland, the jurist who was a frequent table companion of the French king Louis VII) set down some basic rules. Marriage between lay man and lay woman was to be monogamous, non-incestuous, indissoluble, witnessed by a priest, and contracted only with the consent of both parties. None of this of course applied to celebate clerics.[45]

Also as part of the Gregorian effort to control, to categorize and to separate out, reformers attacked the lax practices of the great Benedictine monastery at Cluny on the eastern fringes of the Hexagon. According to Robert Arbrissel of Brittany (*c.* 1055–1117), Cluniac monks had been corrupted by their quest for gold, silver and jewels to adorn their altars and had allowed the work of Christian charity to lapse.[46] Seeing nothing at Cluny of spiritual worth, Robert looked to the fourth-century hermetic monasteries of St Anthony's and St Paul's in Egypt's Eastern Desert for inspiration. In his "New Egypt" model of authentic Christian society, Arbrissel paid special heed to the poor of Christ, the lepers such as those Jesus had healed on his way to Calvary, who in their modern form still offered Christians an opportunity to practice charity.[47]

Robert Arbrissel's vision of lepers as an essential element in Christian charity culminated in the good works of St Francis of Assisi (d. 1226). When not in Egypt trying to convert Muslims or working among the poor in Italy, St Francis was found among the lepers. As he put it:

> While I was in sin it seemed to me too bitter to look at lepers. But the Lord himself led me among them and I showed pity to them. And when I left them that which had seemed so bitter to me was turned into happiness of body and soul.[48]

St Francis's successor as missionary in Egypt and as foot-washer of lepers was St Louis IX of France (captured by the Mamluks in 1250). Louis's biographer and friend, Jean de Joinville, was often troubled by the king's physical contact with lepers, but was warned off with the words: "For you ought to know that there is no leprosy as ugly as the leprosy of being in mortal sin, because the soul that is in mortal sin is like the devil."[49]

In this sentence are found the ambiguities central to Construct leprosy. Though a leper could be seen as a representative of Christ offering opportunities for Christian charity, the leper was also seen as a sin-curst being who, following the precepts of Leviticus, must be cast out of the community of the faithful. Further linkage between leprosy and sin is found in words written in the third or fourth decade of the twelfth century by Richard of the Abbey of St Victor, not far from the famed lazar houses of Paris. According to this monk:

> fornicators, concubines, the incestuous, adulterers, the avaricious, usurers, false witnesses, perjurers, those likewise who . . . look upon a woman concupiscently . . . all, I say, such as these, who through guilt are cut off from God, all are judged to be leprous by the priests (who know and protect the law of God) and are separated from the company of the faithful, if not physically, nevertheless spiritually.[50]

In a seminal paper published in 1970 Zachary Gussow and George Tracy reminded readers that the universalizing notion that humans everywhere regarded leprosy as a stigmatizing disease was itself a cultural construct formed by the hegemonic few in the West. In contrast, most other people tended to regard leprosy as a disease like any other.[51] This insight, intended to relate to the modern colonized world, applies with equal force to rural medieval Europe. There, in the vast tracts where the influence of the universalizing institutional Church (foster parent of the later Enlightenment) remained weak until the sixteenth century, cunning women, healers, wizards and other oracles of oral culture maintained traditional values. These values held that disease was brought into the village by morally ambivalent forces from outside and that leprosy was but one disease among many. Unfortunately, this idea was a peasant artifact, alien to the mental world of the aggressive elites who, in the eleventh century, were constructing a new Europe using, among other tools, Construct leprosy.

Tying together loose strands in the Construct were pronouncements made at the Third Lateran Council in 1179. For lepers, the results of any council summoned by Pope Alexander III (formerly Master Roland) were perhaps a foregone conclusion. A few years earlier this pontiff had launched the fiery encyclical *Cor nostrum* against a royal leper known to be insensitive to pins pricking his skin, Baldwin IV, ruler of the crusader kingdom of Jerusalem. Alexander had warned that under the rule of a king who, since he was a leper, was clearly immoral and out of favor with God, Jerusalem would fall to its Muslim enemies. Two years after Baldwin IV died, Jerusalem duly fell.[52]

At the Third Lateran Council, under Pope Alexander III's direction, prelates considered the evils of male homosexuality (guilty clerics were to be excommunicated) and the threat posed by the Cathar heresy in the uplands of southern France (convicted heretics to be burnt at the stake), then turned their attention to "lepers." The assembled fathers took it for granted that authorities in Europe's provinces already knew that lepers threatened the morals of the common people and that they had segregated them in special housing. They also recognized that those confined in leprosaria were unable to attend religious services in ordinary churches or to bury their dead in consecrated ground. To make good these deficiencies, Canon 23 established that confined lepers be allowed to have a special chapel and a burial ground in their leprosarium and that the foodstuffs grown in its garden be exempt from payment of the tithe.[53]

Building on the Canon 23 assumption that it was spiritually useful for lepers to have their own chapels staffed by priests, one interpretation of the foundation of several thousand new leprosaria between 1090 and 1260 (seven for the city of Toulouse with its 20,000 people) was that these institutions provided jobs for thousands of priests who otherwise would have no altars before which to perform their sacred rites. In a no-nonsense way in his *History of Epidemics in Britain*, Creighton pioneered this interpretation as early as 1891.[54] Yet, in light of Marcus Bull's (1993) historically informed study of knightly piety in the age of the First Crusade, the rage for founding leprosaria can perhaps be given a more authentic gloss.

The new interpretation builds on the understanding that knightly arms-bearers greatly respected pious monks of the New Egypt variety. At the same time, as laymen deprived of the special status that the Church claimed God had allotted to men in holy orders, knightly arms-bearers felt overwhelmed by the weight of their personal sins. They were also troubled by the plight of members of their lineage who had preceded them in death and whose sin-stained souls were presumed to be lingering in the half-way station between hell and heaven. Many of these ancestors were of the sort who had risen to positions of authority through "pride, plunder, treachery and murder," as Pope Gregory had averred in 1081. Though the Church had already provided propertied laymen with outlets through which they could work for salvation for themselves and their ancestors, many knightly arms-bearers craved for more.[55] By creating the delusion that Europe was awash with "lepers" who had to be confined in purpose-built leprosaria, a market-oriented Church created an exciting new form of Good Works.

As early as 1135, Waleran, Count of Meulan, in Normandy, made it clear that the funding of a leper hospital was an act as full of merit on St Peter's scales as the act of donating fiscal rights to a monastery of the conventional sort. The count himself was founder of the Leper Hospital of St Gilles at Pont-Audermer. Bernard of Clairvaux, statesman and intellectual giant of the New Egypt variety, made the same point: to found a leprosarium was a substantial act of merit which might alter the fate of dead kinsmen. Bernard's observations were made while he was visiting the leprosarium at Grand-Beaulieu at Chartres not long after the Bishop of Chartres had complained that his own under-officers (laymen) were exacting ransoms and torturing hapless peasants.[56]

Detailed local research has shown that founders of leprosaria could be divided into several categories. In Normandy, local knights seem to have dominated; writing of the situation around Calais, Dr Albert Bourgeois reported that nine out of ten of the founders or principal donors of leprosaria were of seignorial rank. In contrast, in other parts of the Hexagon Benedictine abbeys predominated; in Aquitaine, abbots of great houses apparently saw the founding of a clutch of lazar houses with chapels dependent on the mother abbey as a way to increase the number of altars before which priestly nephews could serve. Somewhat similar was the situation in eastern cities colonized by German settlers from the Rhineland. In Pomerania (now in Poland) town councillors keen to provide posts for brothers, sons and nephews in holy orders frequently founded leprosaria, each equipped with its own chapel.

Obviously serving a multiplicity of purposes, once underway the leprosaria founding movement took on a momentum of its own. By 1200–50 any self-respecting lord, abbot or town corporation possessing a full range of jurisdictional rights was certain to have in hand a functioning leprosarium with its own chapel as well as a mill, a gaol and a gibbet.[57] The problem was to find enough "lepers" to justify keeping all these costly facilities going; to this issue I now turn.

At the Fourth Lateran Council in 1215 it was decreed that members of two deviant groups—lepers and Jews—should wear special clothes so that passers-by could see them in time to avoid contamination; the pairing is significant. Though anti-Semitic feelings went back a long time, the notion that Jews were aliens had been expressed with especial clarity by Peter the Venerable, the abbot of Cluny. Peter was esteemed by the zealous as a reformer second only in importance to Bernard of Clairvaux. Abbot Peter had questioned:

> whether a Jew is a human being, for he will neither accede to human reasoning nor his own tradition. I do not know, I say whether that person is human from whose flesh the heart of stone is not yet removed.[58]

During the years Peter was musing about the humanity of Jews—the 1130s and 1140s—the most pressing issue among job-hungry, Paris-trained, clerkly literati was career advancement. Earlier attracted to the university where the great Abelard had taught, after their course of studies was completed new-style clerks feared that Jews educated in synagogue schools would, through merit, win newly created posts in dynasts' and papal bureaucracies.[59] With its accusations of leprosy and removal from normal social intercourse, R. I. Moore's "persecuting society" would provide one way out of this difficulty.

Other than serving as learned clerks, another type of career for which Jews seemed particularly suited was identified by Roger Bacon, philosopher at the University of Paris. Writing before 1292, Bacon concluded that:

> the whole wisdom of philosophy was given by God . . . to the patriarchs and the prophets . . . complete in all its details *in the Hebrew language*; [those with access to the language of God would be able to utter incantations] in accordance with the intention of the rational [universal] soul, which receive in the mere act of pronouncing them the force of the heavens. . . . For by this power *our bodies are cured.*[60]

Following Baconian logic, *curing the sick* through invoking the power of the rational world soul in the Hebrew tongue would become a Jewish monopoly. Obviously, this would not go down well with literate Gentiles.

Among Gentiles likely to serve as accusers on leprosy juries, it was common knowledge that numerous medical practitioners were Jewish. Though Jews were of course not found in areas from which they had already been banished (such as England), elsewhere, as in Languedoc and Provence, Jewish practitioners might constitute nearly a third of the local learned medical community. Finding this intolerable, Gregorian and New Egypt clerks and bishops, gathered in provincial synods, repeatedly banned

Jewish doctors from treating Gentile patients.[61] The same end could be achieved by application of Construct leprosy and the removal of Jews to leprosaria.

The myth that Jews were particularly prone to leprosy seems to have been among the detritus of learning inherited (via Josephus) from Ptolemaic Egypt. Working from effect ("leprosy") to cause brings us to the ancient allegation that Jews were especially lascivious. This behavioral pattern was attributed to the Jewish prohibition on the eating of the meat of pigs, which in twisted logic, meant they shared the proclivity of pigs to breed often and have large litters.[62] During the Great Hunt, Jews' reputation as sexual giants readily translated into accusations that they were lepers. How often this accusation was made remains unknown; listings of inmates in Europe's several thousand lazar houses tended not to find their way into archival collections now extant.

Other than this absence of listings, another curious lacuna is the paucity of leprous skeletal remains dating from before 1350. Using the number of known leprosy asylums in 1300 as a rough guide, physician-historian A. Bourgeois calculated that in Pas-de-Calais there should have been two to three lepers per thousand. To date, this hypothesis is not supported by archaeology; disinterred Norman corpses indicated all sorts of illnesses but not Hansen's disease. Elsewhere, the principal find of leprous skeletons comes from a single leper hospital at Naestved in Denmark, located a long way from the heartland of the "leper" culture (the Hexagon). It is significant that most of the Naestved skeletons date from the tail end of the Great Hunt, at a time when its ideological motivation was in decay.[63] Other than this ambivalent Danish evidence, most of the few skeletal remains bearing marks of Hansen's disease found in leprosarium cemeteries elsewhere in Europe date from the late fourteenth through to the sixteenth centuries, after the Great Hunt had ended. In heavily governed England for the years of the Great Hunt itself, documentary evidence about the proliferation of lepers remains unsupported by disinterred leprous bones.[64] This is what one would expect if leprosy was a construct existing in the minds of accusers rather than a bacteriologically caused disease.

Another anomaly is that until the Great Hunt was over, stone carvers, sculptors, manuscript painters and other masters of the art of representation did not portray "lepers" with the collapsed noses, claw hands and other physical characteristics of the lepromatous type of Hansen's disease to which twentieth-century Europeans seem most prone. This artistic lacuna is nicely illustrated at Chartres. Lying a few kilometers outside the cathedral city was a large leprosarium, the Grand Beaulieu de Chartres, which presumably had as its clientele whoever local priests, magistrates and other accusers regarded as lepers. In the city center was the great gothic cathedral of Notre Dame, complete with north transept and its huge sculptured porch (erected after 1230) and south transept with porch (erected after 1224). These were donated by Louis IX, the royal foot-washer of lepers, and his mother. Sculpted on these porches were arrays of statues representing scenes from the Old and New Testaments and from everyday life carved by sculptors obviously capable of portraying human forms with great realism. Yet nowhere among these two great crowds of thirteenth-century humankind are there any recognizable sufferers from Hansen's disease, symbolizing the loving mercy of Christ (curing lepers), or suffering the curse caste upon them by a disgusted God. At the time these programs were being executed at the bequest of royal patrons, one would have expected scores of people bearing all the traces of Hansen's disease to have been living just up the road at the Grand Beaulieu de Chartres, bored out of their minds and more than willing to pose for a sculptor's sketch.[65] On the other hand, Construct lepers who were physically just like anybody else would not have been of particular interest to an artist.

In an economy increasingly based on hard cash and negotiable assets, an important issue in determining a medieval person's disease status was his or her personal worth. Though large leprosaria such as the Grand Beaulieu in Chartres had a few places for pauper-lepers supported by charitable trusts, most houses required inmates to buy their way in (operating in the way most sheltered housing for the elderly does in western countries today). Thus in 1508, King Johan of Denmark ordered the chaotically administered house at Naestved to accept only locally born male lepers who paid the entrance fee. It appears that in the recent past many entrants had been healthy priests or friars who regarded the lazar house as a free food trough. In a related example, rules written in 1344 for the leper hospital of St Julian near St Albans ordered that inmates leave two-thirds of their property to the hospital at their death; they could request that the remainder go to a family member. Here hospitalization was a privilege for the better off.[66]

On occasion "lepers" with disposable property were considered mere commodities. Françoise Bériac reports a case from around 1255 from Corbie in which the town fathers and the local abbot disputed which of them had the right to place a certain leper in the hospital. The first round was won by the town council: the victim was captured and thrown into the lazar house. The abbot then brought the case to a royal court which subsequently declared in his favor. Following the handing down of the judgment, a mannequin mock-up of the leper—who had died in the course of the proceedings—was ceremoniously carried from the leprosarium back to his former house.[67]

In considering the role of leprosy in the transfer of land, office, bags of gold or other forms of property, it should be borne in mind that during the Great Hunt each region was governed by its own unwritten, customary laws. On the Continent, the writing down, codification and imperfect standardization of regional law was undertaken only in the sixteenth century.[68] In some customs (such as those imported into England by its Norman duke-king), convicted lepers lost the right to inherit properties. Keeping one foot on the ground of local custom, we can fantasize about potential heirs improving their life-chances by having an inconvenient elder brother or cousin charged with leprosy, put on trial by a compliant literatus and removed from the scene. Rather late in the day, Guy de Chauliac in *La Grande Chirvrgie* (1363) reminded doctors on juries to make certain that authentic medical signs of leprosy were present, "because the injury is very great . . . [if] we thus submit to confinement those that ought not to be confined."[69]

Aware of the danger of atypical evidence, instances of politically motivated accusations of leprosy dating from the Great Hunt can be reported from southern England. One occurred in Winchester in the reign of King Edward II (murdered 1327). When gearing up finances for an assault on Scotland, the Crown ordered the expulsion of lepers from Winchester. Town bailiffs took this as a license to hunt down the former mayor, Peter de Nutle, who had presumably used his position to feather his nest and harass bailiffs. The bailiffs arrested Peter who, claiming the right to a fair trial, secured a writ from Chancery. The trial was duly held and after "inspection and examination before our council by the council and by physicians expert in the knowledge of this disease" Peter was found to be "whole and clean, and infected in no part of his body," free to live wherever he chose.[70]

Somewhat lower on the social scale, another action at law comes from the village of Brentwood in Essex and dates from 1468. Here neighbors accused Johanna Nightyngale of continually mixing with them though infected by "the foul contagion of *lepra*." Worried, Nightyngale secured a writ for a trial before the Court of Chancery. In due course physicians were brought to the place of hearing. Carefully following the list of "the forty or more distinctive signs of the species of *lepra*" set forth in their manual (Guy de Chauliac had listed only sixteen), the doctors pronounced Nightyngale "utterly free and untainted."[71] Though it is likely that all this cost Nightyngale a pretty penny in legal fees, things might have ended differently. Considering the date of the incident (the 1460s), her accusers were as likely to have charged her with witchcraft (the fantasy of the future) as with leprosy (the fantasy of the past).

Most historians have accepted that leprosy was brought under control by around 1550. According to the expert on knowledge, power and the body, Michel Foucault, this "strange disappearance" was "the spontaneous result of segregation."[72] However, studies written around the turn of the century by Charles Creighton and Jonathan Hutchinson, now supplemented by more recent works, make it possible to affirm that, contrary to Foucault, no permanent locking away of all of Europe's lepers (the Great Confinement) ever took place.[73] This can be demonstrated in several ways, beginning with the understanding that in the actual Middle Ages, lodgement in a leprosarium depended on good behavior. For example, according to the 1380 rules of St Lazare at Andelys, an incarcerated leprous man who had carnal knowledge of his wife would be expelled for a year and a day.[74]

Working towards the same end, rules of 1344 at St Julian near St Albans ordered that married lepers not be admitted unless their lawful wedded wife either became a nun (confined, sworn to chastity) or took vows to remain perpetually chaste. Also at St Julian, patients who grumbled about the way the hospital was run or engaged in any form of usury ("monstrous and hateful to God" according to "New Egypt") would be permanently expelled.[75]

In the French Hexagon, entry to a leprosarium might be a voluntary act. This was the case in the southern uplands in and around Montaillou where, by the third decade of the fourteenth century, the Inquisition had acculturated people to accept that leprosy was a special disease. Here it was commonly held that locals might disappear either because they were debtors, because they were Cathar heretics (living in fear of the Inquisition), or because they were lepers. If the last, they might first join sufferers from ringworm, scabies or St Anthony's fire (New Egypt again) at the sulphur baths at Ax-les-Thermes. If the disease worsened, they might find it convenient to enter one of the leper colonies at Saverdun or Pamiers.[76]

Even in regions well endowed with lazar houses, impoverished "lepers" could not always expect to find an institutional place. Lepers with nothing to offer but the (spiritually rewarding) sight of their ravished bodies might be forced to beg in front of churches, on bridges or at markets. Some towns regarded them as unseemly nuisances, yet in other jurisdictions old-fashioned values survived. As late as the sixteenth century, the great-hearted Habsburg prince, the Emperor Charles V, carefully distinguished between ordinary beggars, banned from public places, and mendicant friars and lepers (the favored and the poor of Christ) who were permitted to remind Christians of their charitable obligations towards people less fortunate than themselves.[77]

Standard antiquarian studies of leprosy in jurisdictions everywhere between Italy and Scotland have listed royal, ducal and municipal decrees threatening begging "lepers" with harsh punishment and have suggested that the frequent repetition of bans by the same authority demonstrated that decrees were poorly enforced. What has not often been noted was that leprosy decrees often stipulated that leprous beggars be allowed to enter the town during Holy Week and other major religious festivals. Similar attitudes allowed the movement of leprous pilgrims to healing shrines; after the late twelfth century the shrine of St Thomas à Becket in Canterbury Cathedral was a particularly favored destination for French "lepers." These permissive government decrees clearly showed that "leprosy" was regarded as a moral condition rather than as a threat to public health as that concept is now understood.[78]

Very little is known about living arrangements in twelfth- and thirteenth-century leprosaria. Some lazars were small and contained fewer than a half-dozen "lepers". Larger institutions numbered twenty or more inmates attended by mass priests and clerical assistants. Court cases from the leper asylum at West Somerton near Yarmouth in England give us some idea of the way an institution actually operated in the 1290s. Using proceedings dating from some decades after the house was founded, an historian found that though West Somerton was intended for thirteen lepers, only eight lived there, perhaps because of the terms of entry. Before they were admitted, "lepers" had to swear that they:

> [would] never go out of the hospital, not to look over the walls or climb trees to talk to their friends, or to complain in any way about their state, justly or unjustly, by which any plea or complaint could be begun against the prior or his successors.[79]

To frighten off the lepers' friends, the prior kept a guard dog before the gate. Presented in a court of law, besides this charge, the prior was accused of maintaining living accommodation for himself within the leprosarium, consisting of a hall, bed chamber, chapel and receiving room in which he frequently held large parties for:

> archdeacons, officials, deans and their beadles, the king's bailiffs and their assistants, with diverse other men and women coming every day and staying the night and dissipating and destroying the lepers goods.[80]

This lawsuit was followed by another. This time, the prior as plaintiff charged the priest at neighboring Mutford with allying himself with the inmates to help them recover their goods; obviously this lazar house was no longer a vibrant model of Christian charity. However, West Somerton's problems paled when compared to these faced in 1321 by lepers in the French Hexagon.

The horrendous events of 1321 can perhaps be understood as the end-product of a conjunction of abstractions: the leprosy Construct, the Construct of Jews as outsiders, the crusader ideal, and the looming Islamic threat. Interpreted by a centralizing head of state suffering from a wasting disease, these concerns were then translated into administrative action.[81]

Lying at the center of the web was King Philip V, the Long One (1316–22). As grandson of the failed-crusader king, Saint Louis IX, Philip was duty-bound to lead Christian hosts to recover lost holy places in Palestine. Using rumors that Muslims (now in occupation of the Levant mainland—Acre fell in 1291) planned to bring all Christendom under their sway, the king persuaded the tight-fisted Pope (John XXII) to grant the proceeds of a special tithe to a French campaign in the Middle East. Of more immediate royal concern however, was English-inspired unrest in Gascony to the south and in Flanders to the north. To act firmly in these areas, the Long One knew he needed to tighten royal control over fief and office holders within the core lands of his realm.

Since permanent financial arrangements with taxpayers in the localities did not exist (and would not until after the Revolution of 1789), Philip followed customary practice in calling a special assembly to meet him at Poitiers (300 kilometers south-west of Paris) in June 1321. People in the know expected the session to be stormy. The Long One had just promised to go off on a crusade and needed money. Obviously unwell, he had been predeceased by his only son and heir.

Topping off the general atmosphere of uncertainty was the hysteria which the idea of a crusade against enemies of Christ stirred up in northern heartlands. In the spring of 1320 unruly crowds of Norman youth invaded the Île de France before moving down the Garonne Valley. On their way they systematically slaughtered members of Christ's own ethnic group. Jews who survived were terrified of what this presaged; they had only recently been readmitted to the Hexagon after being expelled in 1306. Recalling the way the king's father had dealt with the rich crusader order (the Templars) in 1314 (trumped-up charges of sexual obscenities, show trials, executions and confiscation), Jewish leaders tried to win the Long One's protection; a financial arrangement was worked out in May 1321. Unfortunately, this did not save them once the killing of lepers was underway.

In the week before Good Friday, castellans and bishops in and around Pamiers (just north of the Pyrenees) sent reports to Philip V in Poitiers that a plot involving hundreds of lepers had just been discovered. This fantasy held that the leprous heads of lazar houses had met and decided to even scores with the people of France by causing them all to become lepers. This would be done by poisoning wells with a mixture of reptile parts and human excrement. Once everyone in France had become lepers, the plotters would become new rulers of the land.

To deal with this wild plot, leading ecclesiastics were called to meet the Long One. Consultants included Dominican inquisitors and the heretic-hunting expert, the Bishop of Pamiers, Jacques Fournier, of whom we will hear much more later on. Given the urgency of the situation, it was decided to torture leper suspects. Using infallible Inquisition techniques that only dead men can resist, the authorities learned that the Jewish community was paymaster to the lepers and that outside funding was coming from a mythic Muslim sultan of Babylon and the king of Granada.

Whatever his motives, Philip V acted as if he accepted the reality of the plot. Required as king and would-be crusader to take action, in a decree issued in Poitiers on 21 June 1321 he accused the lepers of *lèse-majesté* and ordered that they all be put on trial for their lives; those found guilty were to be burnt at the stake and their properties confiscated by the Crown. On 18 August the Long One followed this up with a decree ordering that the land be entirely cleaned of the "putridity" of the "fetid lepers."[82] Convinced that he meant what he said, hundreds of suspect lepers fled over the mountains to Aragon, only to find that the king there (Jaume II) also believed in the reality of the plot and had ordered the arrest of fugitives entering his realm.[83]

Everywhere in the Hexagon officials interpreted Philip V's decrees as license to kill. Though evidence is sparse, it is known that in many southern cities trials ended in massacres and that leprous women clutching babies to their breasts were burnt at the stake. In some places officials blamed an overwrought populace; at Rouen, it was alleged that lepers were slaughtered, "more by the people than by secular justice." Elsewhere the role of officials was more obvious; at the château of Esquerdes, a castellan imprisoned thirteen lepers and tortured them for sixteen weeks before handing five of them over to a mob. In the county of Artois, the count's officer took a leper from the Douriez leprosarium, put him on trial, then burnt him alive. In nearby Flemish towns, officials threw lepers into prisons while mobs railed outside. Violence against lepers also took place in Lausanne, to the east of the Hexagon. To the south, in the Crown of Aragon, local inquisitions were ordered to torture lepers and put confessed plotters to death; proceedings are known to have taken place in Huesca, Ejea, Tarazona, Montblanc and Barcelona.[84]

In the Hexagon proper, lepers were not the only victims of terror; Jews, the social non-conformists whom ecclesiastical authority had twinned with lepers in 1215, were also killed. In a particularly infamous incident 160 Jews were burnt in a large pit in the castle of Chinon in the bailliage of Tours. Twelve months later Pope John XXII ordered Hebrews banished from papal lands around Avignon. In the Hexagon as a whole, ethnic cleansing wound up in 1323 when the brother and successor of the deceased Long One, King Charles IV (the Handsome) expelled the Jews from the realm; he had already dealt with lepers.

Soon after his accession in 1322, Charles IV had instructed local office holders to lock all lepers permanently into leprosaria; indigent lepers were to be maintained at the expense of the parish. This financial demand, unprecedented in the history of France, proved the ruin of the project. No sooner had the decree been issued (31 July) than it became a dead letter, for fiscal reasons clearly unenforceable.

During the massacres which actually did take place, Construct leprosy impacted directly upon the consciousness of ordinary people in the towns and cities of France. An example comes from the burnt-over southern uplands. As recounted by Le Roy Ladurie, while being interrogated by a Cathar-hunting inquisitor, a worried middle-aged man, one Arnaud de Verniolles, confessed to sexual experiences while a student at Toulouse in 1321:

> At the time when they were burning the lepers one day I "did it" with a prostitute. And after I had perpetrated this sin my face began to swell. I was terrified and thought I had caught leprosy; I thereupon swore that in the future I would never sleep with a woman again; in order to keep this oath, I began to abuse little boys.[85]

Some years after the death of Charles IV, Jacques Fournier, Bishop of Pamiers, the cleric whose zealous efforts had led to the extermination of thousands of lepers in 1321, was elevated to the throne of St Peter as Pope Benedict XII. Concerned in 1338 about the fate of his soul, the now Pope admitted that the lepers who had been massacred in 1321 had been innocent and that the leper plot had been fabricated by scheming bureaucrats.

In an important related move, as part of his overall program of reform, Fournier as pontiff established (in the Bull *Benedictus Deus*) that God judged all souls individually as soon as they departed a cadaver, thus replacing the earlier biblical (Book of Revelation) idea that judgment would be put off until the end of the world.[86] Created in 1336, the new system of *instant* entry into heaven or into purgatory—the half-way house to heaven or hell—immeasurably sharpened survivors' interest in the fate of their recent dead. Long accustomed to saying prayers for long dead lineage members they had never met, lay people enthusiastically welcomed the new dispensation which held that "good works" would free a beloved wife, child or confraternity colleague from the miseries of purgatory and send them directly to heaven.

In its institutional aspects, Benedict XII's new dispensation encouraged wealthy donors to establish chantry chapels and altars before which priests could say masses for the repose of the recent dead.[87] Among jobs this created was a contract arrangement for a chantry priest to recite blocks of thirty masses (trentals) for a named person. Another was appointment as priest servicing a lay confraternity of the sort being organized in progressive French and Italian towns to ensure that members at death would have properly attended funerals and be assisted by prayers for their souls in purgatory. A further innovation was the creation of indulgences, which excused a soul from serving a stipulated amount of time in purgatory. Distributed by priests in exchange for a free-will offering to the Universal Church, indulgences offered priestly part-timers a way to top up their income. Taken together, chantry chapels, indulgences and the like significantly impacted upon Construct leprosy.

Since around 1260, the equivalent of Church marketing experts had begun to notice that donor interest in funding new leprosaria was dropping off. Given standard rates of attrition for leprosaria—closure after two to three generations—any slackening in the creation of new foundations meant a serious loss of potential places for priests. Fortunately for them, this falling away was made good by the increased demand for priests created by Fournier's papal bull *Benedictus Deus* (instant judgment).

Further impetus for rethinking "leprosy" was given by the Black Death; by killing numerous clerics in a few short months, the pestilence forced a hard-pressed Church to replace them with semi-literate acolytes. Emerging from this recruitment crisis was the gratifying assurance that wealthy donors still considered priests to be relevant to changing societal needs. This encouraged the Church to modernize the stereotype of the enemies of God against whom clerics preached. Serving as new stereotypes who made old fashioned construct lepers obsolete were witches, heretics and Jews. Following this change in targeting, in the decades after 1360 authorities made less and less effort to discourage medical doctors from serving as jurors at leprosy trials.[88] As we noted earlier, one-time papal physician Guy de Chauliac first published his list of the sure marks of true leprosy in 1363. Using these, humanitarian doctors could, and apparently did, prevent false accusations of leprosy from causing the removal of innocent people from civil society.

In writing his account of medieval leprosy in 1891, Charles Creighton assumed that the scare and the rash of lazar house foundings was merely the result of faulty knowledge. Medieval jurors had erroneously diagnosed as leprosy a whole collection of disease types including yaws, pellagra, "lumpus and cancer of the face, of scrofulous running sores, or of neglected skin-eruptions more repulsive to the eye than serious in their nature." From this it followed that:

> [i]n medieval England the village leper may have been about as common as the village fool, while in the larger towns or cities . . . true lepers can hardly have been so numerous as the friars themselves, who are supposed to have found a large part of their occupation in ministering to their wants.[89]

Living as we now do at the tail end of the twentieth century when ethnic cleansings are still being carried out in Europe in the name of religion and its semi-secular near relation, nationalism, we are perhaps wiser than was Creighton about the ways in which an emerging, still insecure elite built up a stereotype (the leper Construct), then identified deviants to fit it and had them taken care of by a Leprosarium Experience which, by chance, left few skeletal remains.[90]

Leprosy and Empire

The medieval link between dark hidden meanings and leprosy survived Enlightenment campaigns against the enemies of Reason,[91] and surfaced again in the mid-nineteenth century. In that age of rapid population growth in Europe, of mass migration to the Americas and of aggressive pursuit of opportunities for investment by capitalists from the City of London, Amsterdam, Paris and New York, the first renewal of interest in the taint of leprosy took place in Hawai'i.[92]

Located half-way between San Francisco and Australia, the Hawaiian islands had been settled by Polynesian peoples some 1,500 years before they were rediscovered by the English sea captain James Cook. From that moment, in 1777, white-introduced venereal diseases began to affect the reproductive capabilities of Hawaiian women. Adding momentum to Hawaiians' numerical decline were measles, whooping cough, influenza and smallpox. By 1853 a population variously estimated to have been anywhere between 242,000 and 800,000 in 1776, was down to 73,138.[93] Writing in *The Hawaiian Islands: Their Progress and Condition under Missionary Labours* (1864), the Reverend Rufus Anderson thought this decline a natural phenomenon, rather like "the amputation of diseased members of the body."[94]

After their first arrival in Hawai'i, American missionaries produced by the Great Awakening carefully recorded the transformation of a tiny white settlement into a booming colony. With the discovery of gold in California in 1848 and a massive surge in trade with China, Hawai'i suddenly became the provisioning station of the Pacific. To meet this demand, *haole* (mainlander) entrepreneurs bearing surnames such as Dole, Bishop and Judd introduced cattle ranching and crops like cane sugar and tropical fruits, but found there were not enough Hawaiians to supply plantation labor needs. Part of the problem was that the aboriginals were often sick, and, according to the report of Dr William Hillebrand of Queens Hospital, Honolulu, slow to accept the "sober unpretentious working of a scientific method in curing disease."[95] Their custom was to tell a plantation doctor they didn't feel well and ask for time off—a request it was standard procedure to refuse. Later in the day they would be found out in the fields, dead. To make up the Hawaiian labor shortfall, foreign field hands were brought in, including at first a few Norwegians who may have been sufferers from the disease Armauer Hansen would find amongst his fellow countrymen. After 1851 ambitious young immigrant men from Hong Kong and China were the main recruits for service in Hawai'i; when legislation blocked this source, laborers began to flood in from the Philippines.[96]

Some time after 1777, just when is unclear, leprosy was introduced into Hawai'i. Writing in 1897 (a few years before he became editor of the prestigious *Journal of Tropical Medicine*), leprologist James Cantlie quoted notes written up just after 1823 by a Reverend C. S. Stewart of the American Board of Missionaries. These reported "the frequent and hideous mark of a scourge, which more clearly than any other proclaims the curse of a God of purity . . . which . . . annually consigns hundreds of this people to the tomb." Stewart further said that most Hawaiians were:

> disfigured by eruptions and sores, and many are unsightly as lepers. Cases of ophthalmia, scrofula and elephantiasis are very common. [underlining by Cantlie][97]

Whether some of the "walking sepulchers" Stewart saw as unsightly "*as* lepers" were actually lepers or whether he was merely using figurative language is unknown. Quoting from a later missionary source, Cantlie recorded that a gentleman who had learned to recognize leprosy in Egypt reported that he had seen lepers in Hawai'i in 1840. Perhaps he had. However we are on safer ground in assuming that *haole* fruit growers recognized that it would be bad for the Hawaiian export trade to admit to the presence of leprosy. This is likely to be why no mention was made of it in publicity handouts issued when the Hawaiian Board of Health was founded in 1850 (the handouts however did admit to cholera).[98]

Then in 1863, finally braving the powers that be, Dr Hillebrand informed authority ("although it may not appear quite in place") that leprosy had become endemic among the native population.[99] Conveniently forgetting the presence of immigrants from Norway, the *haole* assumption was that leprosy had been brought in by Chinese workers—people for whom whites already had an aversion almost equal to that for Africans.

Following directions from *haole* eminences, the puppet Hawaiian king decreed rigid segregation of lepers in 1865 and within months a concentration camp for convicted disease bearers was in operation. It was located on a peninsula of the north coast of Molokai Island bounded on three sides by the sea and cut off from the rest of the island by a steep cliff which made it virtually escape-proof. In the dry-as-dust phraseology of a US Health Service official:

> To accomplish this [segregation] it is provided that individuals suspected of having leprosy shall be reported by anyone having such information to the Board of Health, which in turn must have the individual examined. The suspect is entitled under the law to have his examination conducted by three physicians. . . . one physician may be selected by him. Thus an impartial medical board is selected and the opinion of the majority of these is a final opinion.[100]

Once sentenced to Molokai, the expectation was that patients would never return; leprosy was thought to be incurable. In the absence of health provisions, fresh water, or more than the bare minimum of food, death soon after arrival from one disease or another was apparently common. Conditions improved marginally after the Belgian Catholic missionary priest, Damien, came to work among the lepers in 1873.

Missionary heroism being at the time good copy, when Father Damien himself became a leper, the world press lapped up his story. Of virtually no interest to non-locals were the many Hawaiians who discovered that they or their family were marked by leprosy. Though they had had no experience of the disease before 1777, now that it was among them they resolutely ignored Christian teaching about dark hidden meanings and continued to regard it as one illness among many. Left alone by authority, afflicted victims chose to live out their lives in normal fashion among their own people.

In the late 1880s, Judge J. Kauai, a leper, and some of his leprous friends slipped away from *haole* Health Board surveillance to live quietly in secluded Kalalau Valley on the island of Kauai.[101] They were joined around 1890 by a saddle-maker, cowboy and marksman named Koolau who was also suffering from the illness. A short time later the peace of the judge's little community came to an end. Settler rulers of what had recently been established as an independent Hawaiian Republic, aware of the notoriety that Father Damien's death had attracted, thought it good for their export trade to enforce leper segregation laws. Accordingly in 1893, sheriff Louis Stolz was sent over to Kauai Island to capture marksman Koolau and the other lepers; Koolau sent him to the next world with a bullet through the chest. In response Sanford Dole, now president of the Hawaiian Republic, declared martial law and dispatched a gunboat, howitzer and troops. Landing on Kauai Island, the army moved up Kalalau Valley to capture old Judge J. Kauai (by this time in his late sixties and bedridden) and fourteen other lepers. Then marksman Koolau—still not a dehumanized leper of the Christian stereotype—killed two soldiers; a third soldier accidentally shot himself dead. With three fatalities, the army of the republic felt it had had enough and, after firing nineteen howitzer rounds in Koolau's direction, withdrew. The leper hero survived the shelling and lived on in the valley until both he and his leprous son died in 1896. Koolau's famous rifles were buried with him in his grave.

After the annexation of Hawai'i by the USA in 1898 (part of the fallout of the Spanish-American War), Hawaiians continued to revere the memory of marksman Koolau and to defy *haole* rules about leprosy. In 1909 the US Public Health Service built a $300,000 leprosy research unit near the lepers' camp at Molokai. Working within the Christian paradigm that a person afflicted with leprosy loses all sense of her/his earlier social identity and becomes merely a leper, US Health Service personnel assumed that they could readily persuade Molokai's lepers to volunteer for live experiments. However the paradigm failed to take Hawaiians into account; only nine of the 900 lepers at Molokai felt sufficiently leprous (in the stereotypical way) to volunteer. Exasperated, the *haole* scientists packed up and went home, leaving their expensive laboratory equipment behind.[102]

This faint-heartedness—at the time hardly noticed in the world press—contrasted with the earlier rigorous, "benevolent and paternalistic" policies for which Hawai'i would remain famous.[103] Writing of *haole* success from the perspective of colonialized Hong Kong in 1897, James Cantlie had claimed that:

> No one can study the careful and accurate reports issued by the [Hawaiian] government and withhold a meed of pity and a word of admiration, for the oldest European state could not have shown greater zeal, wisdom, and self-sacrifice than this small nation, so recently risen from the savage state . . . so dreadful is the scourge [that] the Board of

> Health expenditure for the year ending March 21st 1894 was $337,300, the greater part being for the leper establishment [which in that year was coping with 1,152 lepers, 1,011 of whom were "native Hawaiians"].[104]

In short, according to Cantlie, what was being done by the government of Hawai'i was a dazzling example of a colonial regime bravely shouldering the white man's burden.

At the first World Leprosy Conference at Berlin in 1897, delegates, supported by leprologists Cantlie and Armauer Hansen, endorsed a policy of strict isolation for lepers everywhere in the non-western world.[105] During the next few years leper confinement controls were introduced in the American-ruled Philippines, in British-ruled Malaya and Singapore, in German south-west Africa (now Namibia) and in settler-dominated Cape Colony (after 1910, incorporated into the Union of South Africa). Neighboring Basutoland (now Lesotho) in turn attempted to enforce compulsory segregation and in 1914 made concealment of lepers a punishable offense. It was this enactment which sparked off Africans' first meaningful response.

Early in 1914 colonial police captured 657 Basuto lepers and imprisoned them at Botsalelo camp. Weeks later (in May) the victims recovered their sense of social identity and broke out in revolt; most escaped to their own villages to live out their lives hiding among their own people. In the next fifteen years lackluster white rulers (numbering only a few hundred men all told) fitfully tried to enforce the segregation order, but to little effect; at Botsalelo the numbers of inmates remained fewer than before the 1914 revolt.[106]

After the Berlin Leprosy Congress voted in 1897 for world-wide segregation, colonial rulers everywhere had to consider the financial implications. After doing their sums, some decided simply to ignore their leprous populations. In King Leopold's Congo—where international concessionaire companies were making huge fortunes from slave-labor-harvested rubber for American and British markets—no official interest was taken in lepers or, indeed, in keeping up any pretense that white men had a civilizing mission. With respect to lepers, until the 1920s, the same situation pertained in France's sub-Saharan colonies.[107]

In Egypt, a country conquered by the British in 1882 to guarantee foreign debt repayment (including a considerable chunk of the Prime Minister's personal investment portfolio), it was also clear that cost-conscious colonizers were determined to keep indigenous lepers out of sight and out of mind. In 1900, during the *de facto* rule of Evelyn Baring, Lord Cromer (member of one of Britain's leading banking families), only three cases of leprosy were treated at the government hospital in Cairo; this suggested that prevalence was of trivial dimensions. However, during the same year the hospital treated 570 cases of "syphilis." Since symptoms of syphilis commonly appeared only a few days after contact, and of leprosy not until several years after exposure, it was obvious which was perceived as the greater threat to the British-run Cairene sex scene. In 1927, a few years after an abortive nationalist revolution which had briefly focused world attention on Egypt, British official sources continued to deny that leprosy required serious government action and claimed that leprosy prevalence was less than 0.5 per thousand. But what the masters perceived as virtually a non-existent problem was recognized by Egyptians after the British finally left as a serious health menace. A post-imperial estimate found prevalence at around two per thousand.[108]

In Nyasaland (now Malawi), similar perceptual contrasts marked the era of British rule (when the colony was seen as a milch cow), and the era after independence. In 1908 an official estimate held that there were 769 lepers in the whole territory; by 1927 colonial masters admitted there might be 5–6,000. After independence, Malawian officials reported a prevalence rate of twenty-eight per thousand—one of the world's highest.[109]

From the perspective of bottom-line accountancy, somewhat similar was the situation in Sudan, the huge province the British forced Egypt to relinquish in the 1880s (when it was conquered by the Mahdi) then recaptured in 1898 at the battle of Omdurman. After escaping official notice for a quarter of a century, in the mid-1920s British investigators finally discovered that prevalence rates among animists living south of the 6th parallel exceeded forty per thousand. Months passed, then in 1928, spurred by an untypical burst of conscience, the regime decreed compulsory segregation. More than 5,000 lepers were rounded up and interred in three large camps where, on the Hawaiian model, they were detained under keepers' close supervision.[110]

Somewhat more complex was the situation in India where the British had been the dominant power since the late eighteenth century. Following the death of Hawaiian missionary Damien, purportedly from leprosy, and the establishment of the (British) National Leprosy Fund in 1890, public concern about leprosy as "Imperial Danger" required an on-site survey; a blue-ribbon commission was appointed in 1892. However, in choosing members, Government insured that financial considerations were not overlooked.

Accordingly, once out in India, after inspecting a couple of municipal hospitals which were run along the cost-effective lines suggested by Birmingham's Joseph Chamberlain, the commissioners decided that "the number of lepers has been greatly overstated, 110,000 [rather than an earlier estimated 250,000] being perhaps nearest the truth." This point established, they concluded that "Leprosy cannot, therefore, be regarded in the light of an 'Imperial Danger'."[111] Perhaps the commissioners were right or perhaps it was simply that they (and gentlemanly capitalists back home) did not want to know that a serious infectious disease problem existed. Except during a major crisis like the Indian Rebellion in 1857, the elementary rule of British imperial domination was that remittances be sent *from* the colony to the metropolitan power rather than the other way round.

Using the leprosy commissioners' count and the figure of 200 million as the population of India, the 1892 leprosy prevalence works out at around 0.5 per thousand; unpleasant for victims and families but not a threat to the Raj. However, this was obviously a underestimate. Spot checks of India's prison population in 1921 (after India had been battered for twenty years by bubonic plague and famine) revealed a leprosy prevalence of ten per thousand: a guesstimate based on this suggests an overall Indian rate of around four or five per thousand. Twenty-four years after independence a survey of lepers was made by Indian health personnel; this found a prevalence rate of 5.8 per thousand.[112] Same country, same disease, different perceptions.

In addition to the useful colonialists' phrase, "financial constraints," the neglect of lepers in imperialized territories could also be attributed to attitudes of western medical doctors. Writing from the Calcutta School of Tropical Medicine in 1931, Dr Ernest Muir, a medical missionary who had gone out to Palestine in 1905 and then to India, reported that most medical men looked at leprosy "as an incurable infirmity, rather than a disease . . . for fear of contracting the disease itself . . . [few of them] were willing to undertake its treatment." For professionals of this sort, it was best not to know what true prevalence figures were. Half a century later, the climate of opinion seemed not to have changed. Writing in 1983 from their laboratories in Oslo and New York, Bloom and Godal found that "it is virtually impossible to recruit physicians or health workers into the field of leprosy control and treatment."[113]

These comments seem to be borne out by the situation in the field. Around 1900, in a Cape Colony with a total population of 2.4 million (24 percent of them white), only one or two of the 720 registered doctors saw fit to work regularly with lepers. Characterized by E. B. van Heyningen as "overwhelmingly male, white, middle class, British-born and educated in Edinburgh," these medical "agents of empire" left it to the only woman doctor among them (Jane Waterston) to pay an occasional visit to convicted lepers on Robben Island.[114] On the other side of the world, in the British-run leprosarium in Singapore, medical doctors were also rare birds whose absence left patients to the attentions of lay staff. Asian warders used long sticks to prod lepers from place to place and gave them food in old tin cans slipped under the doors of their cages. In Singapore city, when rounding up lepers, attendants wore masks and gloves and liberally sprayed victims' houses and possessions with decontaminants. As A. Joshua-Raghavar (himself a leper) pointed out, these techniques seemed tailor-made to convert paramedics who might not before have feared lepers into paranoid leperphobes; the stereotype fed on itself.[115]

Westerners' fear of leprosy was a double-edged sword that cut both ways; when interviewed in 1931, village people in upland north-east India claimed that leprosy was actually caused by European medical doctors. Similarly in northern Nigeria in 1927, local people in the Tula Wango district which had only recently been taken over by the British told a white visitor that the disease had not been known before. Following the same logic—leprosy as white man's disease—it was claimed among the Natal Zulu that leprosy had been unknown until Afrikaners broke in upon them around 1840. Unfortunately for the Zulu, the colonizers were particularly keen upholders of paradigmatic Christian leprosy controls.[116]

During Boer expansion into the arable and pastoral lands of black Africans in the 1890s, leprosy among the latter was seen as irrefutable evidence of the Old Testament Leviticus account of the wages of sin. Bearing a double curse from God (skin color *and* stigmatizing disease) black lepers were obvious targets for compulsory removal by white police and tracker dogs. Victims were lugged to heavily guarded concentration camps ringed with barbed wire. One such camp was at Emjanyana in the Transkei; another was the Leper Asylum in Pretoria. Both admitted to annual death rates of 20 percent. Yet for whites concerned about escaping black lepers who might spread contamination, far better than Pretoria or Emjanyana was an installation on an inaccessible island such as the colony on Robben Island or that established by German colonial authority on Lunda Island in Lake Nyasa. Once dumped on either island it was expected that lepers would die from natural attrition, obviating the need for costly medical services or anything else.[117] Reporting on Lunda Island in 1909, it was found that:

> Some of the lepers had run away at first but the Government had punished the neighboring chiefs who had assisted them to escape so now their confinement seems assured. It was said that one poor woman in her fury had burnt down most of the houses . . . they complained of shortage of food.[118]

Yet in some corners of the tropical world, another form of assistance was at hand: white Christian missionaries.

In the last third of the nineteenth century, three phenomena—ancestral white ideas about leprosy, the expansion of white control over the tropical world, and the growth of a proselytizing impulse among a self-chosen few—made non-family work among lepers in the colonized world a near monopoly of missionaries and members of Christian voluntary organizations. Given the paucity of information about colonized people's attitudes, it is difficult to draw large conclusions about the ways they responded to these people. Obviously not all Africans were like those around the southern Nigeria Ossiomo Leper Settlement, who according to the medical doctor in charge, "In 1931 . . . were convinced that inside the settlement was a big hole into which lepers were pushed and buried alive [by the missionaries]."[119]

The missionaries themselves issued quantities of newsletters and articles about the meanings of leprosy. What is particularly significant is that these reports frequently referred to the notion that leprosy was the old biblical disease.[120] Typically, a learned French medical adviser to Emperor Ménélik II of Ethiopia, one Father Mérab, stated around 1920 that "to understand the rules governing this quintessentially biblical disease once common among the Jews, it is enough to read Chapter XIII of Leviticus."[121] The same point was made thirty years earlier by the Central Africa Anglo-Catholic missionary "H. W." who wrote: "looking at the nature and results of this disease, one does not wonder at the stringent laws against lepers among the Jews."[122]

With variations, this interpretation of leprosy as stigmatizing disease was taught to African medical trainees, who internalized it and passed it on to other Africans. Thus in Nyasaland in July 1927, an African medical assistant named Fred Nyirenda who had been taught by members of the Anglo-Catholic Universities Mission to Central Africa (UMCA), told a meeting of the North Nyasa Native Association that the English had banished leprosy from their land during the Middle Ages by the rigorous segregation of every leper. With a local prevalence rate of twenty or thirty per thousand, before Christian missionaries had come on scene the common Nyasaland response was to allow lepers to "to dine in the same dish and drink from the same cup with others . . . [and to] carry other people's children in their arms."[123]

Looking at the disease in world historical perspective in 1970, Gussow and Tracy contended that:

> The relationship of missionary activity to world leprosy has become a remarkable chapter in the . . . bringing to life of a modern parable. . . . In discovering [lepers] missionaries discovered . . . a name that linked the present with some of the most poignant teaching and practices of Christ. This association of idea and disease made "lepers" of persons with the disease leprosy. . . . Thus leprosy began, more and more, to be thought of . . . as a moral condition . . . as a disease with a moral diagnosis. . . . [T]he status of leprosy came to be colored by the status of the care-takers, *the religious, not the physician.*[124]

Depending on accidents of time and place, the success with which missionaries brought these universal (to them) truths to bear on actual lepers varied. In East and Central Africa, where the phenomenon of colonialism appeared nearly eighty years after India had come under British rule, before local people had time to appreciate that missionaries were the forerunners of tax collectors and of settlers who would confiscate their land, they were sometimes willing to listen to Western teachings. One early success in converting an ordinary disease into a moral category dates from 1891 when the UMCA head office opposite Westminster Abbey was informed that missionary Clement Scott had successfully convinced local "savage tribes . . . to have a more pronounced horror of leprosy" than they had had before.[125] However, within a couple of decades Central and East Africans caught up with Indians and came to realize that mission medicine was a "key element in white power," best used only for those few diseases (such as yaws) that whites had proved they could actually cure. At that time the colonizers had no effective cure for leprosy.[126]

Within India, a principal agency of western concern was the London-based Mission to Lepers, founded in 1874. Much to the disappointment of its workers, it made little progress among Indians of the better sort. In 1920, the Revd E. Cannon bluntly stated that the lepers who came to their asylums "are most low caste Hindus, very ignorant, very superstitious, thinking only of the disease with which they are affected . . . they are generally paupers."[127] Another volunteer who was troubled by continuing Hindu concern with caste was W. C. Irvine. Addressing a meeting of asylum superintendents in 1920 Irvine complained that:

> In . . . India, with its all-powerful caste system the true Christian will find little or no difficulty (whatever his caste has been) in treating his brethren in Christ (whatever *their* caste may have been) in the true spirit of Christian brotherhood IF (and oh how much depends upon that "if") he sees those already professing Christ saved from the thraldom of caste and living as brethren. We had to fight the matter out in our Asylum and a sharp fight it was for the first three to be baptized were Mahars (a very low caste).[128]

Founded as a voluntary organization by independently wealthy Anglo-Irish, the Mission to Lepers doubtless did ease the last painful years of deformed leprous cripples. It also gave satisfaction to Protestant longings to do Good Works. Possibly aware of the fourteenth-century Catholic use of lepers as supplicants for the souls of the founders of leprosaria, in 1920 Irvine argued that:

> Perhaps someday we shall wake up to the fact that within our asylums is a marvelous latent force ready for use, longing for employment . . . a band of praying lepers who will . . . give themselves continually to definite prayer and thus become a mighty force in the ranks of Christ's army.[129]

This suggests that the missionaries needed their lepers more than the lepers needed them. The same would be true in Africa.[130]

In British West Africa early in the era of colonial rule, personnel and revenues were in short supply, with the result that work among lepers was somewhat haphazard. In southern Nigeria (an area seized on behalf of London-based gentlemanly capitalists in the late 1890s), a non-missionized leper village at Asaba in Iboland was described in 1905 by a government medical officer, E. Moore. Moore calculated that in this collection of rude reed huts there were, on average, thirteen women and sixteen male lepers supervised by a "native" overseer who, as Moore took pains to point out,

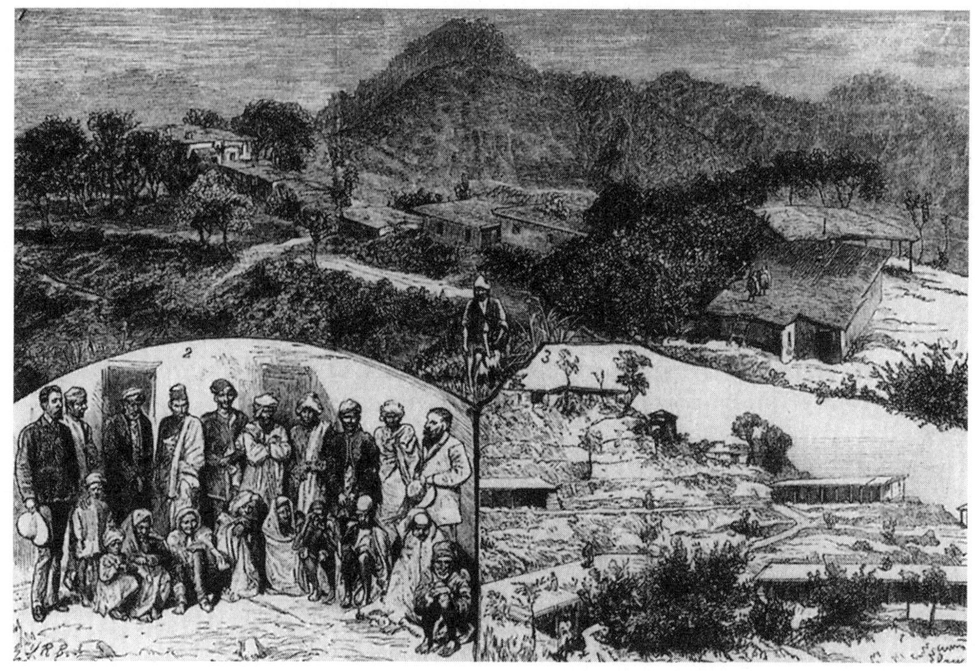

6. Three vignettes: missionaries and lepers in India. A wood engraving, *c.* 1900, by R. B.

was "extremely gentle to the patients." In the absence of police, guard dogs or barbed-wire fences, the patients "wandered through the markets when they feel inclined." Moore was troubled by this lack of discipline and looked forward to the establishment of an enclosed compound for at least 1,000 lepers at Onitsha—pending availability of funds.[131] Elsewhere in Iboland, the new colonial government had already begun to impose order on lepers. At Igboka in 1904:

> The king called a meeting of the town to give them the new laws from the Government and tonight a boy has been going all round the town calling out loudly that those who were lepers were to be taken away.... But there are very few even among the Christians who confess there are lepers here.[132]

With the "opening" of Africa by Livingstone, Lugard and others after 1875, an old service distinction remained in place. Administrators, military officers, medical doctors, missionaries and other professional sorts whom home authority considered first rate went out to India; the rest went "somewhere else," which is to say to Africa.[133] Writing in the late 1880s, big-game hunter Sir John Willoughby reported that the Church Missionary Society (CMS) missionaries he encountered in East Africa were:

> manufactured out of traders, clerks and mechanics. The process is not a difficult one: a man, thinking he can improve his position by missionary work, has only to go to a school for a year or two and learn a certain amount of medicine and carpentry, flavoured with a little theology, and he is turned out a full-blown missionary.[134]

If CMS recruits were as intent on upward social mobility as Sir John suggested, they knew when leaving England that because of the perils of tropical disease their chances of making the return trip were at best 30 percent. Yet there seemed no shortage of recruits. Between 1896 and 1906, the number of CMS mission stations in West Africa increased from 51 to 72; reputed converts increased from 21,000 to 32,000. In addition to the CMS there were other missionary societies—the Sudan Interior Mission, Primitive Methodists and Catholics of various sorts, all vying with each other for converts.[135]

In an Africa in which the full impact of white expansionism only hit in the 1880s and 1890s, the timing of culture contact was crucial. To learned ideas about leprosy as moral condition were added the insights of Social Darwinism. This claimed that modern science had proved that created humankind was divided into higher (white) and lower (black and colored) racial types. Typical of the discourse in this alliance between Christ and Herbert Spencer was an article in 1902 in the journal of the Universities Mission to Central Africa, *Central Africa*. Entitled "The Black Man as Patient" it pointed out that:

> Taking a broad biological view of the different races of man, and regarding their relationship with the animal world, it is impossible not to remark that, starting from the more highly organized races and going down the scale, the acuteness of pain experienced seems to grow less and less . . . the blunted feeling of pain . . . give us some clue to the vitality as a race exhibited by the negro. . . . But the sick negro has many amusing ways. . . . Dying he creeps out into the sun, or hides away in the long grass, like some animal.[136]

Other Social Darwinist tendencies that missionaries were likely to take with them to African dark corners were suggested in an address leprologist James Cantlie gave before the graduating missionary class of Livingstone College in May 1906. Cantlie held that:

> When we send out our missionary he is looked upon as one who knows something of medicine, in the first place, *from the very fact that he is a white man*; and in the second place, seeing also that he is a learned man and religious, he is believed to possess the attributes all natives are accustomed to associate with religious teachers, namely the power of healing.[137]

Writing for a missionary readership, Ronald Ross (of 1897 malaria fame) only slightly changed the emphasis and in the process constructed a usable history of medicine. According to Ross:

> During the beginning of civilization in Egypt, Greece, and Rome, the priests were also the physicians. . . . In my opinion, the missionary of today may still hold a similar position among the barbarous peoples he is called upon to educate. . . . Often called upon to live in the remotest districts, far from hospitals, municipalities, health departments and officials, he is now exactly in the position of the priest of old, and to him still belongs the double duty of curing both mind and body.[138]

For missionaries who had chosen to heal the wounds of Africa (brought about by the slave trade) by curing the disease of tainted souls, Ross's words must have cut home. In 1909, the missionary journal *Central Africa* reported the work being done in the small UMCA leper colony near Zanzibar. It asked:

> Can any life be so miserable than that of the black man afflicted with this dire malady, or any vocation so dull as that of a white "religious" dressing foul sores. . . . Yet the picture of the Crucified above the bed . . . speaks eloquently of Hope and Joy and Peace.[139]

"Manufactured out of traders, clerks and mechanics," few of the missionaries who went out to Africa had more than a smattering of training in medicine. In 1898, the *Journal of Tropical Medicine* attempted to recruit young graduates by appealing to their altruistic instincts:

> We have seen the doctors in Egypt and in South Africa showing forth the spirit of loving helpfulness to the leper and to the starving suffering native. . . . What is needed . . . is a desire to make professional skill an instrument for the amelioration of the sufferings of the heathen world. . . . Reward does not come in the shape of wealth, but the income of these missionaries is adequate to their needs and the sense of freedom from financial care is far greater than among many of their professional brethren at home.[140]

Notwithstanding similar recruiting attempts, medically trained missionaries remained a rarity in black Africa. Typically, of the 525 missionaries (getting on for a fifth of the total white population) in the Nigerian regions in 1927, only eighteen were professional doctors. Commenting a few years later on leprosy-control work in Central Africa, a visiting expert commended medically untrained missionaries for their "noble relief work" but concluded that they contributed little to the ultimate control of the disease.[141]

In the Nigerian regions during the first twenty years of British rule, some leper camps were under government control while others were run by missionaries assisted by small grants in aid. Then in 1926 (when only 3 percent of the missionaries had medical qualifications) government gave the missionaries control of the leper stations in the south, followed ten years later by control of the northern stations at Zaria, Sokoto and Katsina. The director of medical services admitted that this was done with "some hesitation in the first instance" knowing that local people in the largely Muslim North might not take kindly to having proselytizing Christians in charge of their lepers. However, coached by gentlemanly capitalists in London, the medical services director and the governor recognized that mission-run leper stations were good value for money. Though Nigerians numbered more than a third of Britain's sub-Saharan African subject population, they generated less than an eighth of its total British-managed revenues.[142]

In the fifty years between 1890 and 1939, many missionaries were—in Ronald Ross's words—"called upon" to serve in districts far from the corrupting influence of white settlers and of white-run towns, bars and brothels. Most Protestant missionaries who chose Africa seem to have done so after experiencing a revelation centering on an overpowering sense of personal sin and of alienation from the European or Euro-American society from which they had sprung. As evangelical Christians, they were revolted by the flood of scholarly, death-of-God books (Strauss, Renan, Nietzsche) that called immutable religious truths into question. If they happened to be high church ritualists of an authoritarian bent, they were also disturbed by their home countries' recent democratic enfranchisement of ordinary people.[143]

In "being called upon to live in the remotest districts" missionaries put themselves in positions where they could establish "authentic" communities modelled on the (mythic) ordered hierarchy of village life in the Middle Ages touched up with a whiff of the "New Egypt" of Robert of Arbrissel. As in these imagined pasts, the missionary knight and priest could command the unquestioning loyalty of leprous patients, black helpers and ordinands.[144] Because many inmates were dependent on their white benefactors for basic subsistence needs, leper villages had great potential for giving missionaries the sense of a task well done.

As exemplified by leper settlements at Uzuakoli, among Ibo people in the Calabar region, and at Itu (re-established in 1928 under the directorship of the Primitive Methodist A. B. McDonald, and used as a model for leper-control camps in the Belgian Congo), leper villages were laid out with a view to visual and psychological order. Neat rows of leper huts segregated by sex, disease phase or by tribal grouping, faced onto straight streets with cross-roads at 90-degree angles. At Itu, the morals of the whole village were kept tidy by twelve policemen and a police court. Itu and Uzuakoli were both intended to be self-sufficient in foodstuffs not only as a means of cutting down costs (Itu charged patients an entrance fee), but also to give lepers an opportunity to share in the Protestant work ethic which the German sociologist, Max Weber, claimed gave people a feeling of social worth. In both Nigerian leprosaria, exposing patients to frequent sermons and other forms of moral uplift was seen as a another way to restore self-respect to people whose social identity had been swallowed up by their disease.[145]

In the mid-1930s, leprosy officials in search of funding from benefactors in the West claimed that in those parts of Africa which lacked the progressive, civilizing influence of large numbers of settlers of the sort found in South Africa and the Kenyan highlands, well-run leprosy plantations served as centers of "enlightenment" for whole regions. With its 1,100 patients, Uzuakoli in Nigeria was arguably:

> a center of training and a demonstration model of village conditions as they should be . . . an agent for reconstructing villages, making new roads, giving practical demonstration of improved methods in agriculture, improving the diet of the people and in every way spreading enlightenment and hope.[146]

Yet in perverse fashion, inmates of African leprosaria sometimes failed to respond to western goodness in the way which their improvers thought they should. At well-ordered Itu in 1940 two decades after founding, it was reported that the more than 2,000 inmates still lacked the entrepreneurial zeal that institutionalization under whites was supposed to provide. To rationalize this failure it was explained that most of the patients were from minor tribes, "apparently of a servile race, having formerly been slaves and sufferers from the slave trade." Obviously, such people could not be expected to be converted into progressive urban tycoons overnight.[147]

Also rather disappointing was the record of the leprosarium at Uzuakoli in Iboland, Nigeria. As visiting missionary Armstrong noted in 1935, a work-study-prayer schedule had been devised to keep lepers so busy "that they have no desire to return to their native village." The ideal being invoked here was that the mission community should be the only society to which inmates felt they really belonged. However, Armstrong let slip that links between patients and their villages had not in fact been broken. Supplemental funds given to lepers to buy food at the plantation store were often spent "on the maintenance of other relatives in outlying villages."[148] Here was a confession that Africans enjoyed a pluralism of identities which, to the missionary mind, smacked of apostasy.

Tension between competing ideals was also found in a community modelled on Uzuakoli. Writing of the leper community at Ngomahuri in Southern Rhodesia, a leprosy inspector noted that: "The natives of this part of Africa possess a close family bond, and are very fond of their children."[149] Here the missionary act of "bringing to life of a modern parable" by separating lepers from their families was regarded by local people as a denial of their cultural identity. After the mother house at Uzuakoli was wrecked in the Civil War, Nigerians made clear that the place was a painful reminder of a colonized past which they, by choice, would leave an unreconstructed ruin.[150] It is against this understanding that the role of leprosy as a re-enactment of the Judeo-Christian parable must be seen.

As we saw, James Cantlie, editor of the *Journal of Tropical Medicine*, assured missionary students in 1906 that primitive people everywhere would recognize that a missionary knew something of medicine, by "the very fact that he is a white man." Yet when confronted with leprosy—the quintessential medieval European biblical disease—Europeans had no practical cure. Admittedly, this was not for want of trying to find one. In the late nineteenth century western doctors experimented with chaulmoogra, a derivative of the oil of the hydnocarpus tree, used by curers in India for several hundred years. Yet as was noted in 1895, "in cases in which a cure results, the cure is not due to the treatment [with chaulmoogra], but is the natural development of the disease."[151]

A breakthrough of sorts occurred in the early 1920s when a way was found to inject chaulmoogra oil into patients. To boost this technique Leonard Rogers (later knighted) founded the high-profile British Empire Leprosy Relief Association (BELRA) in 1923. Yet results were disappointing; self-cures continued to be more common than cures medically induced. As Rogers reluctantly admitted in 1927, "there is still no specific cure for leprosy in general."[152]

Yet for missionizing purposes the new chaulmoogra technique was a godsend. To receive a continuing series of injections—as at Itu paid for by five hours' work in the fields—patients were required to live in the leprosy village where their semi-voluntary labor contributed to the success of the plantation's palm oil, cotton and other export-crop production. But more important, their payment in labor service was intended to strengthen their faith that the white man's medicine would cure their leprosy. It was in this sense that John Iliffe considered the chaulmoogra treatment was a *permissible* "confidence trick." Not all would agree.[153]

It remained for the non-missionary leprologist Robert Cochrane to prick the chaulmoogra balloon. Writing of the situation in India in 1927, Cochrane announced that in most asylums, two out of three of the leper inmates were burnt-out cases who were no longer infective. Though he regarded the provision of homes for these now harmless destitute lepers as "a great humanitarian work," it did "little or nothing to reduce the incidence of leprosy." Cochrane enlarged upon this insight in his 1931 Cameron Lecture at Edinburgh University which attracted wide press coverage. Ironically, as early as 1910 the asylum fallacy had been exposed, but the journal article in which this was done had fallen stillborn from the press, presumably because the author (Dr Khan Babadur N. H. Choksy) did not have the skin pigmentation required of those who were experts in modern medicine.[154]

By the inter-war years, disinterested medical observers in the West recognized that compulsory segregation in camps was not having much effect on leprosy prevalence. Well and good in itself, this finding did not take into account the career interests of camp professionals out in the colonies. Typical of expats who needed a solid twenty or twenty-five years in service before they could receive pensioned retirement back home were high-grade leprosy workers in the American Philippines. In 1928 their representatives at the Cairo Conference on Tropical Medicine boasted that their regime was spending a third of its health budget on punitive leprosy controls. In 1935, after the financial crash of '29, Philippine authorities were even more forthright: "[leprosy] control *must* be based" on "the *accepted* fact [emphases theirs] that the disease is infectious and that it is transmitted by contact . . . evidence is accumulating that [this contact might be brief]." This claim (unsupported by objective science) was made in the face of a report showing that the impounding and maintenance of 13,000 victims in the Culion Leper Colony between 1906 and 1921 had had no appreciable impact upon leprosy prevalence rates.[155]

Leprosy impoundment in the approved Hawaiian way could also be seen as one way to authenticate a colonial regime which needed to prove that it was in the mainstream of civilization. Typifying this attitude was Portuguese Goa (India). Seeking to demonstrate its role as an outpost of western values, the Goa regime submitted plans to the Cairo Conference in 1928 for a get-tough scheme for the confinement of all its lepers.[156]

Also feeling on the defensive in a hostile world were South Africa's million and a half whites who lived among a black population twenty times as large. Certified as "guarantors of a Christian Civilization upon the Continent of Africa," the South African government felt obliged to spend heavily on leprosy. In the mid-1920s they let it be known that they had introduced Sir Leonard Rogers's new disease treatment in their five leprosy centers. Then in 1940, they claimed that they had spent £2–3 million on leprosy, at a per annum cost per patient of £40 to £50, and in the last twenty years had discharged 4,502 "cured" lepers. Obviously, for this white minority regime, the old "Imperial Danger" announced by the Archdeacon of Grantham in 1885 was still a useful prop. In reality however, the major killer among rural and urban black South Africans was tuberculosis; for this disease the government made available only token funds.[157]

On the other side of the world, in Singapore, another colonial regime also found Archdeacon Wright's "Imperial Danger" thesis useful. While in Singapore in the 1920s, a Brazilian leprologist learned that non-infective burnt-out lepers were not being released from the local internment camp because the leprosy-control decrees written in the last century had made no provision for discharge—except through death. Some years later, in 1931, this continuing situation was adversely commented upon by an editorial writer on the *Straits Times*. Aware of Europeans' curious obsession with medieval leprosy, he reminded readers that tuberculosis was "five times" more infective than leprosy. As in South Africa, the regime was spending hardly anything at all on TB.[158]

Within the western spectrum of things "civilized" as opposed to "barbarous," there was considerable ambivalence about the bounding capacities of leprosy. Writing as medical superintendent of Robben Island asylum in 1890, a Dr Ross (not he of malarial fame) held that:

> the pure native races, like the Zulus and Kaffirs, are seldom effected [*sic*] with leprosy; but among the Korennes and cross-breeds between native women and the nomadic Boers . . . are to be found a large number of cases.[159]

This was another way of saying that leprosy was caused by miscegenation.

Some years later, Edward Muir, sage and medical doctor at the Calcutta School of Tropical Medicine, claimed that incidence of leprosy was a barometer of the state of civilization. Among hill tribe primitives who had yet to be corrupted by modern ways, leprosy was little known. According to Muir, it was also little known among urbane educated middle-class Indians. But, as he went on to say:

> where we get contact between the primitive and the more advanced, there, at the point of contact we find leprosy . . . unfortunately the more easily adopted features of civilization are often the less credible and are apt to be physically and morally dangerous when not countered and controlled by its [civilization's] less easily acquirable safeguards.[160]

Dr Muir's mix of Christian parable and medical truth was perhaps harmless *except* when it affected research priorities and set the next generation of leprosy workers off on the wrong track. In his capacity as Christian, the sage made clear his loathing of Belgian Congo African males who were polygamous; yet in his capacity as medical doctor he claimed that venereal disease was not a predisposing cause of leprosy. Such however was the nature of discipleship that Muir's Indian student doctors took it for granted that venereal diseases were a predisposing cause of leprosy. This erroneous understanding—which mimicked the twelfth-century teachings of the Cluniac abbot, Peter the Venerable—was an unattractive part of the legacy of colonialism.[161]

Central to the thinking of western workers in leprosy before 1980 was the idea that civilized people everywhere shunned lepers; any cultural group which didn't behave in this way was barbarous or at best semi-civilized. Using this criterion, seen as backward were the Kigezi in Uganda. A. C. Stanley Smith worked among these people in 1931 and in his patronizing way was impressed by their knowledge. At his request they brought in victims in the early stages of the disease which "I [Smith] would have hesitated to accept as such until a positive scraping from the nose revealed the bacillus lepra and proved these primitive diagnosticians correct." What however rendered these people barbarous was their habit of mixing freely with lepers. To his disgust, Smith discovered "it is common to find lepers marrying *untainted* wives."[162]

Other ethnic groups who neglected to fear lepers and so were uncivilized in western eyes were found in the strange country that was Ethiopia—until 1935–36 the only African land unconquered by Europeans. As recounted by Richard Pankhurst, before the Italian invasion, leprous beggars were everywhere, thronging markets and the court of the Emperor, and on occasion breaking into private palaces demanding alms. In the 1880s the German representative of the Church Mission to the Jews, Henry Aaron Stern, admonished the Emperor that he should lock away the leprous beggars lying around everywhere in promiscuous confusion. To this the Emperor famously replied "Do I not already bear enough infamies on my conscience?"[163]

Perhaps most troubling for missionaries ministering to what they *knew* were the needs of lepers—following the Christian parable—was that learned Muslims did not place its sufferers in a special moral category. Wherever they went, missionaries encountered Islam—in India and Dutch Indonesia, in Sudan and West Africa, in East and Central Africa. They also found that for every convert they made, Muslims made ten. In 1906 Friedrick Shelford attributed Muslim success to the biological fact that "Mohammedan" missionaries were natives, whereas Christian missionaries were Europeans with no immunity to tropical disease and, accordingly, were often "not on seat." Typically at Malindi, Nyasaland, after the abrupt departure of the sick UMCA missionary priest in 1906, Christian converts and ordinands had gone over to Islam *en masse*.[164]

Following the dismemberment of the old Ottoman Empire by Allied treaty arrangement (1919) and the triumphant defense of the Turkish homeland against West European invaders, a flood of popular books on Islam appeared in Europe, among them *The Moslem World in Revolution* and *Young Islam on Trek*. Their central message was that the Muslims most closely in touch with Western civilization were disillusioned with the orthodoxies of their own faith but were not yet open to the truths of Christianity. In the missionary perception, "Mohammedans" thus remained a volatile and worrying force.[165]

For leprosy workers what was particularly distressing about this Muslim Other was that Islam challenged the Christian parable. For believing Muslims, the disease held no terror. A *hadith* of the Prophet witnessed that, "He took the hand of a leprosy patient and put this hand in a dish from which he was eating and said 'eat with me, and I believe in Allah and the disease will not catch me unless Allah wants it'." Another *hadith* held that: "The disease will not pass from one to another."[166] More distressing yet, among the common people sayings translated into actual practice. Thus while visiting Nigeria in 1930, Dr T. F. Mayer found that, "Among the Mohammedans of the north there is no fear of the disease. It is even difficult to keep friends and strangers from sleeping in the leper camps at night."[167] Differing attitudes towards leprosy, for Christians a disease of the soul, for Muslims a disease only of the body, added weight to missionary fears that in African and Asian regions where the illness was common, the future might not belong to them.

The credibility of western science as a benign, secular force was strengthened by post-World War II breakthroughs in the treatment of leprosy, the sulfide drugs in the 1950s giving way to multiple drug therapy in the 1980s. Now the West at last had an effective cure, what was medically required was that sufferers be recognized in the very early stage of the disease and encouraged to come voluntarily to leprosy out-patient clinics to learn how to take drugs regularly on their own. It was presumed that if this medical approach won through, channels for new infection would be cut off and leprosy could be wiped out, region by region, until it followed smallpox into extinction.[168]

Yet as Gussow and Tracy foresaw in 1970, now that effective scientific treatment was possible, to regard leprosy as a "no-fault disease" without stigma or blame threatened to destroy what Christians regarded as a potent spiritual resource. Writing in 1988 an Indian anthropologist at the University of Ranci found that:

> Unfortunately, the fear and stigma against leprosy still persists, more so among the more educated urban class, including even the medical profession. It is nothing short of [a] disgrace for humanity at large.[169]

3 Smallpox in the New World and in the Old: From Holocaust to Eradication, 1518 to 1977

Introduction

Most epidemiologists and historians admit that in the absence of smallpox pathogen in the New World, pre-Columbian people had no opportunity to develop immunity to the disease. However, any statement which goes beyond this is likely to be contested.[1] Here I adopt a moderate position. Accepting that 80–90 percent of any virgin soil (non-immune) *local* population might have died when smallpox first appeared, I then ask why populations of survivors failed to recover their numbers.[2]

This inquiry is in two parts. Beginning with a foray into cultural history during the era of the Renaissance, I examine the role of the Ancients (for our purposes, Aristotle and Christ) in the making of the humanist idea that New World peoples didn't have the mental potential to develop into rational, European-type adults. Formulated in the upper strata of society, this learned concept meshed nicely with the popular notion that white settlers should have full mastery over American lands regardless of whoever happened to be there already. I then examine the attitudes and behaviors of New World peoples themselves as they tried to cope with the physical presence of Europeans, the diseases the Europeans introduced, and the Construct which held that indigenous native "Americans" were sub-human barriers to the acquisition of wealth.

In this chapter, I openly accept the thesis of "American Exceptionalism." On no other continents in historic times has a combined disease and Construct phenomenon led to the collapse of an entire indigenous population. Varying in its timing with the pace of white penetration (late in the Pacific North-West, early in Hispaniola and Meso-America), before smallpox dealt its initial blows Native Americans constituted perhaps a fifth or a sixth of the population of planet Earth. Then soon after smallpox hit Meso-America in 1518, the Iberian conquerors began to use slave labor in newly discovered gold and silver mines. Their first ploy was to force Native American miners to work in environmental conditions which led to mass deaths from smallpox and other lethal things.[3] To make good the resulting labor shortfall, the Iberians imported Africans. As it happened, many of these Africans had previously acquired immunity to smallpox through a childhood brush with a mild pathogen. This meant that they remained virtually untouched in the midst of the smallpox epidemics that decimated indigenous local people. Smallpox & Co. were thus inexorably linked to the creation of the New World institution of black African slavery.[4]

All this contrasted markedly with what would happen in colonialized India (with approaching a fifth of the world's population), and in western-bullied China (with its quarter of humankind). In both Oriental societies, notwithstanding the best efforts of whites in the eighteenth and nineteenth centuries, indigenous people always outnumbered invading Europeans by a hugh margin and in the long term controlled the ways in which their societies re-created and renewed themselves. This, despite the presence in India and China of smallpox, influenza, measles, typhus, malaria, leprosy, cholera, bubonic plague and other pestilential diseases which even conservative modern-day scholars reluctantly admit had been absent from the pre-Columbian New World.[5]

Turning to Europe after Columbus crossed and recrossed the Atlantic in the 1490s, we are confronted with the imponderable dynamics of a non-human force. Some time in the mid- to late seventeenth century smallpox transformed itself from a mild childhood disease most Europeans underwent—hence the initial immunity of Europeans in America—into a virulent disease threat. One authority claimed that by the early eighteenth century smallpox "represented a more regularly occurring check on the growth of population than plague had been."[6]

Fortunately (for Europe), this was only a temporary phase. At some point in the eighteenth century a European-wide demographic revolution occurred in which mortality permanently fell well below birth replacement rates. Linked to this revolutionary change—in ways on which a scholarly consensus has yet to emerge—were campaigns to induce immunity to smallpox, through inoculation, variolation and vaccination. In the nineteenth century, associated with these campaigns, and with the actions of the disease itself, was a huge increase in surplus Europeans who found *Lebensraum* in the vast spaces of the Americas which were all but empty of descendants of the original inhabitants. At the end of the chapter, we conclude on an upbeat note by recounting how in recent times western-trained health personnel dealt the smallpox virus the same fate met by the Taino of Hispaniola after 1518–19: eradication from the face of the earth.

The Disease and its First Impact on New World Peoples

In 1720, a virulent form of smallpox appeared among the 200 inhabitants of tiny Foula Island, north of Scotland. Genetically these descendants of ancient Picts and Norsemen were no different from other north European peoples. But living as they did by fishing and subsistence farming, the islanders had been cut off for years from anyone suffering from any form of smallpox. In consequence—atypical of Europeans generally—they had no immunity. When smallpox struck, 90 percent of the Foula folk died; this was similar to mortality rates common during epidemics among Native Americans.[7]

The high mortality in Foula suggests that the virus involved was either fulminating smallpox with standard 100 percent mortality or malignant confluent smallpox with 75 percent mortality. In its fulminating form "life was terminated either by massive vomiting of blood, intestinal or uterine hemorrhage, or more peacefully, by blood poisoning." Malignant confluent smallpox, sometimes known as the black smallpox, was characterized by

> relentless deterioration. . . . Many patients lived until the fourteenth or fifteenth day when the stripping of the cell tissue of the outer surface of the body became so widespread that life was ended by blood-poisoning or a hemorrhagic catastrophe.[8]

Smallpox could be caught by inhaling infected air breathed out by suffering victims. After contact was made, the virus remained dormant for eight to twelve days; then the sufferer was laid low by headache, nausea, eruptions on the skin, and other horrors. Another way of catching the disease was through contact with its characteristic pustules and scabs; scabs remained infective for a fortnight or more.[9] They survived longer in a warm dry climate (such as that on the Pacific coastal plateau of the Andes) than in a cool damp place. Infective scabs might be found on the body and clothes of the smallpox dead. Conflating the actual dead with the spiritually dead, the much-pestered Amazon Yanomamö alleged earlier this century that "when the whites undress, they leave the illness in their clothes."[10]

As of 1996 there were some 450 strains of smallpox virus in cold storage in the Centers for Disease Control in Atlanta, Georgia, USA. Eight or ten of these were varieties of *Variola major* and the rest were variants of *Variola minor* or *Variola intermedius*. Most forms in this wide spectrum were genetically equipped to transmute into something else, depending on the availability of appropriate environmental niches.

Though a mild form of smallpox was described by the Islamic scholar Al Razi around 910 CE (he thought the disease was part of the natural process of the thickening up of children's blood), smallpox was unknown to Greco-Roman physicians. The profession being what it was in the early modern period (dependent on past authority for legitimization), in standard western texts the illness remained virtually unnoticed. This meant that early European adventurers in the New World had little information on which to draw when they witnessed epidemic smallpox among Native Americans. Sometimes, as in Mexico during the catastrophe of 1521 and in the Inca Empire in 1527, what they described was clearly smallpox. At other times they listed symptoms which might have been caused either by some form of smallpox or alternatively by measles, typhus or some other illness. Confronted with simultaneous epidemics such as those that hit the remnant population of the Inca Empire in 1585–91, even medically informed Europeans were at a loss to know what was going on.[11]

In the decades before the Spanish arrived in Meso-America with their horses and pigs, swine flu, typhus, measles and smallpox, people in many of the polities there and in South America were beneficiaries of sophisticated forms of socio-economic organization. Writing of the situation in the Andes, Suzanne Alchon reported that 27 percent of the pre-Columbian remains excavated were of men and women who had lived past the age of forty. After the Spanish came on the scene (following the conquest of the Inca Empire by Francisco Pizarro in the early 1520s), fewer than 12 percent of the indigenous population lived that long.[12]

Further north, in Meso-America in pre-Columbian times, four mainland societies had developed systems of writing: the Maya, the Mixtec, the Zapotec and the Aztec. The Aztecs were the first of the literate societies to undergo the trauma of epidemic smallpox, and the first highly militarized state to fall to the Spaniards.

In 1519, the Aztec state was centered on the capital city at Tenochtitlán, built on land reclaimed from swamps in the 1320s, some twenty years before the bubonic plague first ravaged Europe and the Mamluk Middle East. The Aztec capital had a population of 200,000 to 250,000, about half the size of pre-plague Cairo, but four times the size of the Seville or the Genoa known to Christopher Columbus. Tenochtitlán was supported by a complex food provisioning system based on irrigated agriculture and on local and long-distance trade. Its many two-story stone houses, stone towers and temples, its great public squares and markets, its myriad crowds, its canals and bridges, its high aqueduct bringing in fresh water for drinking and for baths, all combined to create an urban place which in Europe might only have been challenged by the city of Rome 1,500 years earlier after it had been newly rebuilt by Augustus. Of course by 1519 old imperial Rome lay in ruins and was inhabited largely by pigs and sheep, swine-herders and shepherds.[13]

Reporting on his first visit to Tenochtitlán while he was a guest of the Emperor Mutezuma, Hernán Cortés told his own king that:

> in order to give an account to Your Royal Excellency of the magnificence, the strange and marvelous things of this great city and of the dominion and wealth of this Mutezuma, its ruler, and of the rites and customs of the people, and of the order there is in the government of the capital as well as in the other cities of Mutezuma's dominions, I would need . . . many expert narrators.[14]

Back at the main Spanish base on the island of Hispaniola, a highly contagious disease which a celibate in holy orders recognized as akin to the smallpox known in the fatherland, but much more virulent, first broke upon

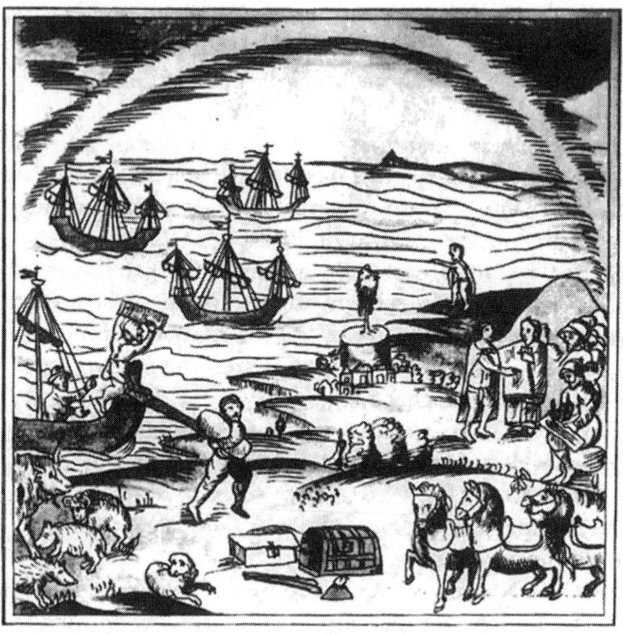

7. The landing of disease-laden Spaniards and their farm animals. After a reconstruction, 1894, by Paso y Troncoso.

the indigenous Taino people late in 1518. By 10 January 1519, when the friar wrote to the Catholic Kings telling them what was going on, smallpox had already carried off nearly a third of an already greatly reduced population.[15]

It is now known that in 1492 when Columbus came among them as the herald of the end of their world, the Taino had numbered at least a million and perhaps even 5–6 million people, equivalent to the combined populations of the British Isles and Scandinavia. A short time after they landed, the Spanish began to search for gold among their hosts and to exact labor and tribute requirements. They followed this by sharpening their swords in the bellies of pregnant Taino women and urging dogs to eat living Taino men. While these sadistic sports were underway, the Taino were attacked by an epidemic of swine flu brought in from south-west Spain. In precipitous decline already because of the swine flu and Spanish massacres, for the Taino the arrival of smallpox in December 1518 proved to be their penultimate crisis. Indeed by 1550, after a final turning point marked by their unwillingness or inability to reproduce, the Taino people had become extinct.[16]

In the same letter in which the anonymous friar announced the recent arrival of virulent smallpox among the Taino, he also mentioned that the disease had already leaped from Hispaniola to Puerto Rico and killed a third of the population there. This feat was soon repeated in Cuba. Later in the spring of 1519, Hernán Cortés (since 1504 secretary to the Spanish governor) led a troop of conquistadors from Cuba to mainland Meso-America and the land of the Aztecs. Though given a friendly welcome in Tenochtitlán by Emperor Mutezuma, the Spanish soon proved treacherous guests. After they began murdering unarmed dancers, the Aztecs forcibly turned them out. In the battle that followed, the Aztecs killed 900 or so of the 1,200 Spanish and sent the survivors scurrying back to the coast. Man for man, Aztec warriors were as good as any *human* thing sixteenth-century Europe could hurl at them.[17]

In the interval between Cortés's first visit and his triumphal return when he took Tenochtitlán by storm (13 August 1521), smallpox devastated the Aztecs. According to tradition, the disease was brought to the Yucatan mainland by Pánfilo de Narváez's counter-expedition which had been sent to recall Cortés to base. When this smallpox passed northward through the central zone of the Valley of Mexico in 1520 it left more than half the population dead. These gruesome happenings were recorded in words transcribed from the Nahuatl language by an early sixteenth-century Spanish historian, Fray Bernardino de Sahagún. Fray Bernardino's informants claimed:

> And before the Spaniards had risen against us, a pestilence first came to be prevalent: the smallpox. It was [the month of] Tepeilhuitl when it began, and it spread over the people as great destruction. Some it quite covered [with pustules] on all parts—their faces, their heads, their breasts, etc. There was great havoc. Very many died of it. They could not walk; they only lay in their resting places and beds. They could not move; they could not stir; they could not change position, nor lie on one side, nor face down, nor on their backs. And if they stirred, much did they cry out. Great was its destruction.[18]

This then was the sort of crisis in Tenochtitlán when Cortés and his Tlaxcallan allies arrived before the city. Yet even in their straitened condition, Aztec warriors made certain that Cortés did not win the battle unopposed. Angered that pagans *in extremis* should resist, Cortés applied the tactics of terror. In his own words: "We did them so much harm through all the streets in the city that we could reach, that the dead and prisoners numbered more than eight hundred."[19] During the next twenty-four hours the Spanish slaughtered 40,000 men, women and children. Cortés later boasted that "in those streets where they were we came across such piles of the dead that we were forced to walk upon them."[20] Token resistance continued, then on 13 August 1521 ceased entirely. On that day, sacrifice to Huitzilpochtli (the Aztec God of Life) was banished from the land.[21]

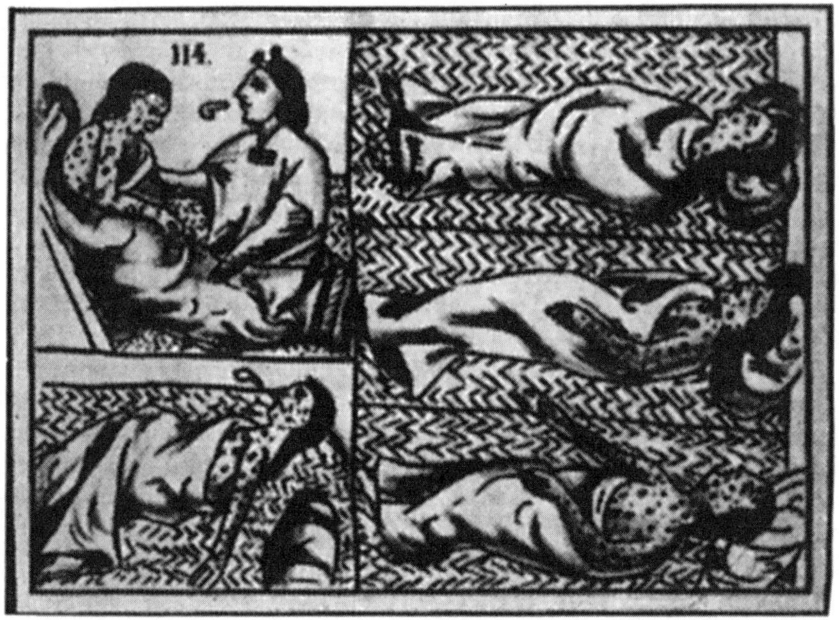

8. The smallpox and the Aztecs. After a reconstruction, 1894, by Paso y Troncoso.

Smallpox again attacked the much-shrunken Mexico Valley populations in 1531–32 and periodically thereafter. By 1605 a people that specialists in Nahuatl studies claim had numbered 25.2 million in 1518 had been reduced to a mere 1.1 million.[22]

After the Aztec state collapsed in 1521, smallpox followed trading networks to penetrate Native American lands hundreds of miles from Tenochtitlán. Perhaps moving southward down the coast, it arrived at the Rio Platte in the Argentine where the city of Buenos Aires (good air) now stands, and then followed Native American stone-built roads northward into the high Andes, the heart of the Inca lands; at the time the Inca Empire was the most extensive in the world.

Arriving in 1524–25, smallpox killed the Inca leader, Huayna Capac, together with his potential heirs and thousands of warriors, commoners, women and children. Disease holocaust and dynastic crisis was followed by civil wars which, in a re-run of the Mexican disaster of 1519–21, opened the way for the conquistador, Francisco Pizarro. Blitzed by smallpox, Inca forces who in normal times would have been more than a match for Spanish terrorists were unable to put up a fight.[23]

Ironically, in 1518 when smallpox entered the New World and moved on to ravish the Aztecs, the virus found in Europe had yet to become a serious threat. Instead it manifested itself in a little unpleasantness children suffered as a matter of course; survival rates were 90 or 95 percent. However, this partially changed: in 1544, smallpox in a lethal new form was reported in Spanish Naples. A few years later (in 1570–71) smallpox carried off 10,000 people in Venice and in nearby Mediterranean cities. Yet one should not exaggerate the extent of the crisis. Co-existing in Europe with localized attacks by virulent forms which might kill off 30 percent of its victims were more widely distributed *endemic* milder forms which exacted far lower tolls. Children who survived a mild form acquired lifelong immunity. Those who later went to the New World—with its virulent smallpox—took their immunity with them. Thus throughout the seventeenth and eighteenth centuries, Europeans commonly exposed to immune-rendering endemic smallpox as children appeared to receive preferential treatment when compared to Native Americans.[24]

From our own perspective, it might be assumed that whites out in the New World would want to learn from American indigenous curers about the strange new disease environment in which they found themselves. Local intestinal parasites, for example, were not necessarily the same as those in Europe. In the event however, it seems that those few university-trained medical doctors who actually did venture across the Atlantic during the first century or so made little effort to consult with local health provisioners. One reason lay in the negative attitudes about Native Americans created by Spanish humanists back home and by Spanish terrorists in the field. Another was learned physicians' fear of *empirics*. Any doctor in the New World who dared experiment with new drugs or practices under the guidance of a Nahuatl speaker ran the risk of being regarded by colleagues at home as an empiric who had forfeited respectable social status.[25] In any case, in that New World, there were far easier ways to acquire respectable status than by following a painstaking career in medicine.

While on the American mainland, the conquistadors soon came into possession of silver mines. In 1545 they discovered what was then the richest find in the world, a sugar-loaf-shaped mountain of silver in the uplands of Bolivia, at Potosí. In short order, these mines were being worked by slaves. In such matters the Spanish followed simple rules of cost-efficiency. They found that since replacement costs were virtually nil it was unnecessary to attend to the slaves' creature needs. This policy led a contemporary to report that: "If twenty healthy Indians enter [a mine] on Monday, half may emerge crippled on Saturday" leaving the dead half behind.[26]

Within the shafts themselves, life expectancy was usually too short to allow smallpox to catch and kill new victims. However, the viruses raging about above ground were readily transported hundreds of miles away through the activities of slave-labor recruiters. Unending Spanish labor requirements, long-distance recruiting squads, and the epidemics they spread led to the demographic collapse of the Andean population. By 1630 it was only 7 percent of what it had been before 1524.[27]

Elsewhere, with minor variations, the tale was the same. Before smallpox hit in 1524–25, the 2,000-mile-long Pacific coastal shelf of Peru was inhabited by perhaps 6.5 million people who used their fertile land and genius to grow foodstuffs for Cuzco and other major Andean cities which were far larger than Seville or Genoa. Unfortunately this range of rich arable outcrops alternating with desert provided an ideal bio-setting for the spread of smallpox. Whipped over by epidemics several times, by 1590 the Pacific shelf lay deserted. Only now are archaelogists beginning to uncover the mute testimony of an extinct people who before 1518 made this place a paradise of fertile fields and gardens on the order of the Tuscan landscapes painted by Renaissance artists.[28]

In the 1520s, smallpox also moved far to the north, but just how far is in dispute. Ann Ramenofsky and others have suggested that Native American runners passing along well-used trade and communication routes may have brought the disease all the way to west Texas. Bearing in mind that the smallpox virus lay dormant in a victim's respiratory tract for eight to twelve days, each runner had time to move the smallpox front forward by 300–400 kilometers or more. With mortality rates sometimes exceeding 85 percent (as at Foula Island in 1720), it has been conjectured that smallpox may have reduced many North American tribal groupings to shattered remnants long before they were actually visited by whites.[29]

Yet several examples of depopulation likely to have been directly caused by record-keeping whites are known. Thus in 1539, Hernando De Soto travelled through the lower Mississippi Valley searching for gold and came upon large settlements of people belonging to what is now called the Mississippi Culture. None of the flourishing cities, towns and temple complexes De Soto claimed to have seen still existed when white settlers arrived in the early 1700s. Further north, Jacques Cartier found heavily populated townscapes complete with wood-built long-houses at Stadacona and elsewhere along the banks of the St Lawrence River. In the winter of 1534 he recorded that shortly after his arrival at their settlements Native Americans began to die of some strange disease to which his own men were immune; later historians suggest this was smallpox. Despite his inability to identify the illness, Cartier was not a medical incompetent. He reported that his French companions were laid out by a sickness he identified as scurvy. He also reported that the Native Americans knew how to treat this effectively: their practice was to drink a mess of boiled pine-tree bark and pitch. Seventy years later Samuel de Champlain travelled along the same canoe route but found Stadacona denuded of all living humankind. From what has been said, it is pretty obvious that the absent tribesmen had not died of scurvy.[30]

And in the Dutch colony of New Amsterdam (the future New York City), in 1650, Native Americans claimed that they had been ten times more numerous "before the arrival of the Christians, and before the small pox broke out amongst them."[31] In coastal Massachusetts, an epidemic disease which some scholars recognize as smallpox wiped out the Patuxet people just before the Pilgrims arrived at Plymouth in 1620. It was all so convenient. Instead of squads of hostile warriors standing by to drive them back into the sea, Miles Standish, John Alden, Priscilla Mullens and other whites found arable fields all neatly cleared and waiting the planting of crops.

As interpreted by one of the Pilgrims: "The good hand of God favoured our beginnings . . . in sweeping away the great multitudes of the Natives by the Small Pox."[32] Other first-generation settlers also marvelled at the way smallpox carried off pagan Native Americans like flies while leaving people like themselves untouched. At Plymouth Plantation, William Bradford reported in 1634 that:

> This spring, also, those Indeans that lived aboute their trading house there fell sick of the small poxe, and dyed most miserably. . . . [Yet] not one of the English was so much as sicke, or in the least measure tainted with this disease.[33]

From this Governor John Winthrop concluded that: "For the natives, they are neere all dead of small Poxe, so as the Lord hathe cleared our title to what we possess."[34]

Catholic writers viewed the phenomenon in much the same way. In the Portuguese colony in Brazil, during the months in 1562–63 when 30,000 Native Americans were dying from smallpox in and around mission stations and slave labor camps on the captaincies given out to private Portuguese owners along the coast, the Portuguese themselves remained untouched, witnesses to what N. D. Cook called "the secret judgment of God."[35] Similarly among French Catholic commentators: "Touching these savages, there is a thing that I cannot omit to remark to you, it is that it appears visibly that God wishes that they yield their place to new peoples." So wrote an observer of the once mighty Natchez whose numbers had been cut back by a third in the 1530s–40s.[36]

Yet as we now know, differing rates of mortality from smallpox between the two main ethnic groups did *not* in themselves cause the *generality* of Europeans to regard the inhabitants of the New World as *homunculi*, creatures who had only vestiges of humanity about them.[37] Instead, the *homunculi* image should be seen as a flower emerging from the rich humus of religious and philosophical teachings present in learned discourse in Europe even before 1492.

Earlier we saw how difficult it was for Renaissance scholars to accept that first-person empirical observation might capture the essence of the real world better than did the writing of the Ancients. So it was that because none of the Authorities writing before 1492 had mentioned the existence of (still undiscovered) Native Americans, the easy supposition well after that date was that these two-legged creatures were inferior beings. It followed that New World peoples, whether as converts to Christ or continuing as worshippers of idols, should be kept subordinate to the lowest order of Europeans. Typical of this attitude, after nearly a century of Spanish rule, the moral historian of the Indies, José de Acosta, held that: "All those who are scarcely men, or only half men, must be taught how to become men, and be instructed as if they were children". Even Bartholomé de Las Casas, Dominican defender of the Indians against Spanish genocide, regarded them as having the permanent mental age of children of ten or twelve.[38]

In such matters, the experience of the Spanish was of critical importance. Not only were they the first Europeans to come into permanent contact with New World peoples; in their time they were also the world's only superpower. Like the dominant Europeans and Euro-Americans of the recent past who dogmatically adhered to the truths of the Enlightenment, late fifteenth- sixteenth- and seventeenth-century Spanish Humanists believed that they alone possessed the attributes of fully "civilized beings." Included in this concept were virtues of the sort discussed by the Stoic emperor Marcus Aurelius (*fl.* 173 CE), a pagan Roman philosopher many Humanists held in high esteem. In his *Meditations* the emperor had praised attributes such as "thrift, compassion, sincerity, carefulness, orderliness, energy, watchfulness, hard work, obedience, humility, grace, discretion, good memory, modesty, courage and resolution." Ironically, these particular virtues were those a high-born Aztec survivor of the Spanish massacres and smallpox of 1519–21 claimed had been most esteemed by *his* own people.[39] Yet as the Spanish priest who recorded this list was well aware, neither the Aztecs nor Marcus Aurelius had known the Christian God. For the Spanish, possession of that knowledge alone set fully civilized man apart from all others.

Uniquely blessed by their transcendent God, during the months when Columbus was preparing to sail west across the Atlantic, Spanish Christians conquered the rump of the old Muslim kingdom of Granada (it surrendered on 2 January 1492). In the same year, in a second vindication of their faith, Spain expelled its Jews. Preparatory work for these ethnic cleansings had been completed a few years earlier when the centralizing Catholic monarchs, Queen Isabella of Castile (reigned 1474–1504) and her husband King Ferdinand of Aragon (r. 1479–1516), finally ended centuries of squabbling between weak monarchs and factious nobles. After 1480, the strength of the Catholic Kings was greatly enhanced when the Spanish Inquisition began to function as their committee for ideological purity. Its most public manifestation was an *auto da fé* at which heretics were burned at the stake.[40]

Significantly, a high proportion of first-generation Spaniards going out to the New World were impecunious adventurers from Extremadura and Andalusia. Born in frontier regions facing what at the time of their birth was still *Muslim* Granada, from an early age they were trained in religious truths and the mindset of guerrilla terrorists. Their cult heroes were accustomed to ambushing at night, destroying whole libraries of books, burning the enemy's storehouses and crops, cutting down able-bodied prisoners in cold blood, and slaughtering old, blind, deaf and crippled civilians and infants.

Writing of what was presumably the mirror image of these terrorists, it was noted that the local police leagues, the *hermandades*, called into being to maintain a semblance of order on behalf of the Catholic Kings, used tactics scarcely different from those of the bandits. According to the queen's personal physician, standard *hermandades* procedures were:

> so severe that it appeared to be cruelty, but it was necessary because all the kingdoms had not been pacified. . . . There was much butchery, with the cutting off of feet, hands and heads.[41]

With the military conquest and surrender of Granada on 2 January 1492 (at the cost of a third of the Muslim population dead), and the spread of ferocious police leagues intent on maintaining the Kings' peace everywhere between Castile and Gibraltar, Christian men at arms in search of quick wealth through plunder suddenly found themselves without much to do.

Considerations such as these were taken into account by impoverished young hidalgos (sons of second-rank nobles) when considering career opportunities. Especially attracted to the loot offered by the New World were the youth of two Extremadura towns: Cáceres and Trujillo. Trujillo was the hometown of Pizarro, disadvantaged son of an unwed mother and later conqueror of the Incas. As Ida Altman has shown, in the sixteenth century 921 members of fifty-six families from Trujillo emigrated to the New World, 27 percent of the total emigration from Extremadura. An additional 14 percent came from nearby Cáceres, the *pueblo* (hometown) of the second governor of Hispaniola.[42]

Some Extremadura and Andalusia hidalgos casting about for careers, and driven by what Las Casas identified as avarice and ambition, had reason to be aware that the Catholic Church was becoming increasingly intolerant of the Jewish minority. Jews had been banished from Andalusia and southern cities in 1482–83, a decade before the general expulsion. Accordingly, a man of Hebrew birth concerned about his future in Spain might decide to profess his conversion to Christianity. Yet even if a New Christian married into an Old Christian noble family, all might not be plain sailing. The judicial arm of the Catholic Church—the Inquisition—remained extremely suspicious of New Christians and in the years before 1490 caused 2,000 of them to be burnt at the stake. Aware of the importance of setting, the Inquisition had 700 victims burnt in Seville, the gateway to the Americas.[43]

Some New Christians, like Saint Teresa of Avila, won universal acclaim through their obvious devotion to the mysteries of the Christian faith. Others, like St Teresa's seven New Christian brothers, realized that they could never meet the criteria of purity of blood needed to acquire high status in Spain and, accordingly, went out to the New World. At least one of the brothers returned to Spain a wealthy man, bought a large estate near Avila and, as befitted a noble, styled himself *don*. Other New Christians whose movements were recorded by the Inquisition were in the party that reputedly brought smallpox from Cuba to Yucatan in 1519. These included Bernardio de Santa Clara, son or nephew of an earlier royal treasurer in Hispaniola, and the quartermaster, Pedro de Maluenda, a merchant from a well-known Burgos New Christian family.[44]

Whether Old Christian or New, the overriding aim of adventurers accompanying Columbus to Hispaniola in 1493 was to discover gold and then to high-tail it back to Spain to live the life of a respectable gentleman. For them, it was immaterial how they achieved this goal. This in part explains the behavior of the Spanish who, shortly after they landed, turned on the Taino of Hispaniola whom they suspected of hiding great quantities of gold. In a famous account Bartolomé de Las Casas tells us what happened next: systematic genocide under the direction of Admiral Columbus himself.

> Once the Indians were in the woods, the next step was to form squadrons and pursue them, and whenever the Spaniards found them, they pitilessly slaughtered everyone like sheep in a corral. It was a general rule among Spaniards to be cruel; not just cruel, but extraordinarily cruel so that harsh and bitter treatment would *prevent Indians from daring to think of themselves as human beings* or having a minute to think at all. So they would cut an Indian's hands and leave them dangling by a shred of skin and they would send him on saying "Go now, spread the news to your chiefs."[45]

The same policies were followed by Cortés after the fall of smallpox-blitzed Tenochtitlán, except that there genocide was followed by the systematic destruction of the Aztec libraries, the temples, and artifacts sacred to the Aztec and to Nahuatl speakers generally. Following the departure of the conquistadors, cultural annihilation was continued by the long-robed missionary priests and *encomenderos* (concessionaires) who succeeded them as rulers of the land.[46]

Since all Spaniards in the New World professed to be followers of the Christo-Pauline religion which accepted the old Jewish commandment "Thou shall not kill," they sometimes tried to explain why they took such obvious pleasure in killing, torturing and raping Native Americans and putting them in environments where they were certain to die of disease. Aside from heathen Roman martial precedents of which Latin scholars everywhere were aware, one rationale was that the end of the world was at hand and that it was the duty of all Christians to kill pagans preparatory to the Last Day.

This was the position taken by the Franciscan order of missionaries and by the well-connected literate adventurer Fernández de Oviedo. Writing in the second decade of the sixteenth century, Oviedo hailed the death of most of the Hispaniola Taino as a significant event which had purged the island of the influence of Satan. As he further explained in his *Historia General y Natural de las Indias*:

> The devil, being so ancient an astronomer, knoweth the times of things and . . . maketh them [the Indians] believe that they come so to pass by his ordinance, as though he were the lord and mover of all that is and shall be. . . . By reason whereof, the Indians . . . honour him in many places with sacrifices of the blood and lives of men.[47]

Oviedo's *Natural History* quickly established itself as a key source in the shaping of Europeans' perceptions of the New World. It was deliberately rushed into print in summary form in Toledo in 1526, and appeared in an Italian version in 1534, in French in 1545, and in an edited English version in 1555. An entrepreneur who did not hide his light under a bushel, Oviedo was acutely conscious that his was an important pioneering work: "I know that my writings will not vanish, for they have passed through the doorway of truth, which is so difficult and heavy that it will sustain and prolong my vigils."[48] Rival accounts, hand-written and stowed away in libraries, remained forgotten until the nineteenth century. We will meet Oviedo again in Chapter 4 as a syphilis profiteer under the Crown.

Other Spaniards, who regarded Native Americans as something more than elements in the local bio-system (as they were in Oviedo's jaundiced view), thought in terms of a mirror image, an Other. According to an early sixteenth-century Dominican friar:

> On the mainland they eat human flesh. They are more given to sodomy than any other nation. There is no justice among them. They go naked. . . . There is no obedience among them, or deference on the part of the young for the old. . . . They exercise none of the human arts or industries. When taught the mysteries of our religion, they say that these things may suit Castilians, but not them and they do not wish to change their customs.[49]

In addition to their strange religious ideas, another Native American cultural attribute which the Spanish and later the English held to be bestial was the absence of western-style private property. In most indigenous societies, the community allotted use-rights to arable land proportional in quantity to the requirements of each family at various stages of its life-cycle. But according to humanists such as Juan Ginés de Sepúlveda (*fl.* 1547), Francisco de Vitoria (b. 1486), and later social philosophers such as Thomas Hobbes (b. 1588) and John Locke (b. 1632), the Philosopher (Aristotle) held that private property was a defining characteristic of civilization. The other seminal Ancient, Christ, had been somewhat ambivalent about the meanings of property; this enabled synthesizers to give Aristotle full marks. Summing up the Truth which emerged from this exercise, and using the Aztecs as his example, Sepúlveda contended that:

> they have established their commonwealth in such a manner that no one individually owns anything, neither a house nor a field that one may dispose of or leave to his heirs in his will because everything is controlled by their . . . kings. They live more at the mercy of their king's will than their own. They are slaves of his will and caprice and they are not masters of their fate. . . . For numerous and grave reasons these barbarians are obligated to accept the rule of the Spaniards by natural law.[50]

From this "natural law" it followed that any land management system not based on private property was a barbarous, slavish anomaly and a standing invitation to outsiders to come in and put things right.[51]

Among the general populace of Spain and its sister crusading state, Portugal, similar arguments held. On any city street, along any pier, in any warehouse, were Iberians who held that private property was synonymous with "human freedom." To achieve this freedom for themselves, tens of thousands went out as emigrant missionary priests, friars, *encomenderos*, ranchers, mining entrepreneurs, sugar-cane slave-plantation owners, land surveyors, farmers, merchants, and other types bent on gaining personal wealth.[52]

Aside from aborigines' unacceptable ideas about property, further proof that they were depraved was the custom—found particularly among the Caribbean islanders and Eastern Woodland tribes—of permitting chieftains several wives. By an unfortunate coincidence, Native American polygamy was similar to the multiple marriage forms earlier used among the Muslims of Granada. Worse, rather than being merely a historical curiosity which had been made extinct by the conquest of 1492, multiple marriage was *still* being practiced in the aggressive young Muslim empire contesting Christian control of the Balkans and eastern Mediterranean: that of the Ottoman Turks. The parallelism was impossible to resist. Driven by binary Manichaean impulses they inherited from St Augustine, neo-scholastics had no difficulty in concluding that New World peoples were Satanic agents who could best serve humanity by becoming extinct.[53] With this in mind, a friar out in New Spain held that:

> concerning the plagues that we see among [the Indians] I cannot help but feel that God is telling us: "You are hastening to exterminate this race. I shall help you to wipe them out more quickly."[54]

Among the God-fearing of New England, the notion that Native Americans were tools of Satan, best exterminated, was exemplified in their culture-clash with the pagan Pequot of the Connecticut Valley. In 1634 the Pequot were savagely mauled by an epidemic of smallpox in which no English person died. Convinced that their extermination was foreordained, in 1637 colonial and English troops made a surprise raid on the Pequot and slaughtered most of the men, women and children who had survived the epidemic. As one of the colonials later recalled:

> It was a fearful sight to see them thus frying in the fire and the streams of blood quenching the same, and horrible was the stink and scent thereof; but the victory seemed a sweet sacrifice [to Almighty God].[55]

To erase the memory of these people, the Connecticut colonists renamed the Pequot town New London and forbade the handful of survivors to call themselves by their old tribal name.

Yet with the passage of time, and the weakening of the fires of the religious and cultural enthusiasm that early seventeenth-century English settlers had brought from the Old World, alternative attitudes towards the denizens of the woods sometimes began to creep through. In the late seventeenth and early eighteenth centuries, in New England, in upper New York colony, and in Pennsylvania, the concept of Native Americans as Other was, at least in a few minds, no longer pejorative.

These few select included the several hundred whites who had been captured by Native Americans and violently forced to live among them. Accepting the validity of *empirical* observation (not one of these people was a learned scholar whose perceptions were established by ancient Authority), they decided that, on balance, they much preferred Native American modes of life. Given the chance during periods of truce to come back to white settlements, hundreds of these former captives voted with their feet and, after briefly visiting home, returned to live permanently among the Indians.

As in the case of the captive Eunice Williams (seen by her parson father as a traitor), this rejection of white ways reflected a dim awareness that the forms, structures and ideologies of the no longer new English colonies were coming to replicate the disorder and gratuitous brutality found in the island kingdom the settlers' ancestors had deliberately left behind.[56] However, among the generality of American-born whites this dim awareness often led to defensive attitudes which in time would ripen into aggressive patriotism. Certainly in the 1780s, Tom Paine, America's first intellectual, would not make himself popular with white triumphalists when he wrote:

> Among the Indians of North America, there is not . . . any of those spectacles of human misery which poverty and want present to our eyes in all the towns and streets of Europe. [Poverty is a creation of what] is called civilized life.[57]

In the absence of written testimony by whites who had themselves returned to live among the Native Americans (practical literacy was one of the things they chose to do without), some features of their life were publicized by travellers such as Jonathan Carver. After sojourning among the Ojibway of the Lake Superior region in 1766–68 (when he was in his fifties, no longer a naive, impressionable youth) Carver reported that:

> we . . . see them sociable and humane to those they consider as their friends and even to their adopted enemies, and ready to partake with them of the last morsel, or to risk their lives in their defence. . . . [In all things] they are possessed of virtues which do honour to human nature.[58]

This possibility of living in the alternative world of aboriginal North America all but ended with the collapse of Chief Pontiac's resistance movement in 1763—when General Sir Jeffery Amherst, commander of the British army in North America, directed that smallpox-laden blankets be sent among the Native Americans to speed their extinction.[59] Among its intended victims, white behavior of this sort was not unexpected. As an Ottawa chieftain reported, just before the epidemic of 1757 decimated his people:

> the small-pox which they brought from Montreal during the French war with Great Britain . . . was sold to them shut up in a tin box . . . after they reached home they opened the box; but behold there was another tin box inside . . . when they opened the last one they found nothing but mouldy particles . . . a great many closely inspected to find out what it meant . . . pretty soon [there] burst out a terrible sickness among them.[60]

In the years after the conquest of Quebec city and the rest of New France by Britain (1763), followed by Euro-American rejection of hereditary British kings (1776), and their achievement of political independence (1783), the new rulers of the land recognized that they no longer needed Native American allies to swing the military balance against a (now non-existent) white foe. Accordingly, the aboriginals who occupied territories in the Ohio Valley and in the Deep South which the new rulers intended for Development were sent packing to marginal lands in the west. In such matters, the Euro-American hero was President Andrew Jackson, with his Indian Removal Act of 1830. This was followed by the Removals of 1837–38, the Trail of Tears, and other disasters, including frequent attacks of smallpox.[61]

North of the Great Lakes where the Ojibway lived, the tale was the same: smallpox devastated the Ojibway in 1781–82. However, the ending here was somewhat different. Until 1781, European and Euro-American traders in animal pelts (for the beaver hats fashionable London and Continental gentlemen wore) had been dependent on the Ojibway for their foodstuffs, birch-bark canoes, traps, tools and technology as well as the pelts needed for trade in Montreal, Albany and New York. The Ojibway did not let white dependency go to their heads and continued to maintain a diversified economy. They mixed settled agriculture, hunting, the gathering of wild products such as maple syrup, birch syrup and berries, and trading locally and far afield. Communities numbering scores of extended families wintered in heavy log-built cabins.

All this was imperilled by the smallpox epidemic of 1781 which worked its way east and north from the Missouri River country, through what are now the Dakotas, Minnesota, Wisconsin, Ontario, Manitoba and Saskatchewan all the way to Lake Athabasca near the Arctic Circle. A decade later, travelling through northern Minnesota, David Thompson reported that:

> This great extent of country was formerly very populous, but [now] the aggregate of its inhabitants does not exceed three hundred warriors; and among the few whom I saw it appeared to me that the widows were more numerous than the men.[62]

After smallpox slashed Ojibway numbers and population recovery faltered, tribal organization fell apart. Now for the first time, dependent on the white man's bounty (rather than the other way around), the Ojibway were eager customers for alcohol, iron wares and trinkets. Craft skills were forgotten and they came to resemble the despondent, lazy Indians the white man's stereotype held them to be. Yet notwithstanding their broken numbers and psyches, the Ojibway were able to hold fast to their ancestral lands near the trading post of Grand Portage on the shores of Lake Superior near what is now the Canadian–US border. As of this writing, they are still there.

Tribal groupings further west were less fortunate. Their common fate after being attacked by smallpox was to be uprooted by white military and sent to marginal land where their numbers rapidly declined. Setting this in train was the 1837–40 smallpox epidemic which swept the Great Plains from Kansas north to Prince Rupert's Land on the Pacific coast, killing 40,000 Blackfoot and all but exterminating the Mandan. Twenty years later, smallpox introduced into Victoria (Vancouver Island) by a passenger shipping in from San Francisco led to similar results. After the virus caught hold among Indian traders encamped around the town, the authorities evicted them, thus perhaps inadvertently ensuring that the disease followed each trader back to his family lodge. Once set in motion, smallpox swept the Pacific coast northward to Alaska, killing 60 percent (20,000) of the Native American population. It has been suggested that had white authority held the infective traders in quarantine, the epidemic would have been contained. This of course would not have freed up the land for white Development.[63]

Caged up in reservations, and prey to smallpox and typhus, between 1890 and 1910 Native Americans reached their demographic nadir. Their guardians in the Bureau of Indian Affairs in Washington, DC sat on their hands collecting their salaries like gentlemen, but doing little else. In an era of rampant Social Darwinism, ordinary Euro-Americans confidently assumed that Native Americans would soon become extinct.

Mindsets and Practices

As we saw, during the smallpox epidemic which swept over Foula in 1720, nineteen out of every twenty islanders died. This high mortality among Caucasians is an historical fact which invalidates arguments that the ethnic (genetic) peculiarities of Native Americans account for smallpox mortalities of 50 percent or more. Yet it must be admitted that certain *cultural* traits may have contributed to the toll.

During their first century of contact with smallpox, New World peoples had less experience in coping with the sickness than did, for example, the inhabitants of some parts of India, where smallpox was possibly endemic. In one such region, Bengal in the early eighteenth century, competent adults recognized that a child suffering from mild smallpox—perhaps induced by the process of variolation (see below, p. 112)—must be kept in isolation and cared for by someone who had already had the disease, lest it leap forth and ignite a full-scale epidemic.[64] But in New World contexts where smallpox and other crowd diseases were unknown before the coming of the alien whites, the idea of quarantining the sick was culturally repugnant. When smallpox first broke out in an Algonquin encampment in the 1630s, adults felt duty-bound to visit the sick. While offering moral support, they crowded into victims' lodges, inhaling the air. Similar support systems were still in place among the New Mexico Pueblo in 1898. Buffeted on all sides by encroaching whites, the Pueblo were determined to hold the custom of visiting the sick inviolate.[65]

During the ten to twelve days while victims of virulent smallpox were semi-delirious, unable to move about without knocking off bits of their disease-blackened flesh, they still had to take in water and food; in the absence of help they would starve to death. After 1518, white observers sometimes noted that in a Native American settlement engulfed by an epidemic, family and community nursing care seized up. Considering that the virus was entirely new to the Americas and that no old experienced curers could have acquired long-term immunity through surviving mild cases of the sickness while they were children, neglect of this sort could be expected. Then too, however deeply entrenched the culture of curing might be, whenever disease incidence went beyond a critical point, curers would flee for their lives, leaving the sick to the attention of carrion birds and dogs.

Terrifying situations of this sort occurred in the Andean city of Arequipa in 1589. According to one report, during the Arequipa disaster while pain-crazed victims ran shouting through the streets health provisioners fled: the visitation left more than a million dead.[66] In Tenochtitlán in 1521, an informant observed that very many Aztecs "starved, [for] there was death from hunger [for] none could take care of [the sick]; nothing could be done for them."[67] A more detailed description of what could happen comes from Plymouth Colony in 1634. Here the Algonquin:

> fell down so generally of this disease as they were in the end not able to help one another, no not to make a fire nor fetch a little water to drink, nor any to bury the dead. But [they] would strive as long as they could, and when they could procure no other means to make fire, they would burn the wooden trays and dishes they ate their meat from, and their very bows and arrows. And some would crawl out on all fours to get a little water, and sometimes died by the way and not be able to get in again.[68]

In contrast, nineteenth-century Euro-Americans struck down with smallpox while living in settled communities might expect to lie "in heated or ventilated homes . . . attended by physicians, nurses, or family members" who provided nourishment, medicines, changes of bed linen and "encouragement against the torment, fever, delirium, despair, purulence, stench, fear of disfigurement" which accompanied serious cases.[69] Typical of the white system at its best was the response by authority in Richmond, Virginia in December 1790 when a black slave owned by Isaac Lane but working for another white took sick with smallpox. Immediately it was notified, the Richmond Common Council gave order that the victim be placed in an isolated house, provided with bedside attendants and "every thing necessary for his recovery" plus a guard to prevent him running mad through the streets spreading contagion. All this was paid for by municipal funds.[70]

Beginning with Las Casas, Spaniards immune to smallpox through childhood exposure were convinced that the grotesque hygiene habits of Native Americans contributed to their smallpox deaths. From their historical experience as neighbors of Islamic Granada, the Spanish identified all bathing as a ritual proceeding a Muslim's act of worship. Accordingly, people observed bathing were reported to the Inquisition. In addition to the prohibitions on all-over bathing which were specific to the Iberian peninsula, Europeans generally held that dousing the body in water opened the pores to evil forces which might come in and upset the balance of the four humors, causing illness or death.[71]

During New World smallpox epidemics which left white communities intact but killed off native peoples wholesale, whites everywhere held that aboriginals who washed their rotting bodies in hot or cold water were appealing to the healing power of a pagan god. Justly punished by the Christian deity, these bathers could expect to die in large numbers. Among other examples of the evil practice, it was found that aboriginals in the Valley of Mexico at Ocopetlayuca customarily bathed at midnight. Similarly seen as a ritual element in the worship of the Devil was the twice-daily bathing practiced at Tepoztlán. Fully convinced of the evilness of bathing, the Spanish were ruthless in their efforts to stamp it out. For their part, confronted with this welter of enforced prejudice, Native Americans became seriously depressed. Accustomed to being physically clean, they felt sick when their bodies began to stink. In such a state, husbands and wives may well have chosen not to engage in the intimacies of sexual reproduction.[72]

Other psychological factors also contributed to the inability of Native Americans to recover population numbers lost to smallpox. One of these concerned the scarring suffered by survivors who—unbeknown to themselves—had become immune to further assaults from the virus. Among egalitarian North American Eastern Woodland males whose pride was in their personal appearance, it was customary to spend hours plucking out unseemly facial and body hair. Thus pockmarked survivors of smallpox were unable to grow beards to cover their scars. Writing of what he had observed during the epidemic of 1738, James Adair reported that scores of Cherokee survivors took a hurried look at their pox-marked faces in trade-good mirrors and "being naturally proud" committed suicide. Perhaps more commonly, men who were disfigured or rendered blind by smallpox were rejected by women as suitable marriage partners.[73]

At the physiological level, smallpox attacked tender parts of the flesh; some surviving males were left impotent, without viable sperm. This may have something to do with a claim made by one of the giants of the Enlightenment, George, Comte de Buffon. Writing his definitive study of New World flora and fauna, Buffon asserted that every natural thing was bigger and better in Europe than in America. As a sub-category of this, he held that the genitals of Native American males were too small to enable them to reproduce. Less biased commentators noted that a surprising number of Indian couples remained childless. A recent calculation found that among seventeenth-century populations in the Andes, a quarter to a half of all couples remained childless; during the same period among the gentry of Northumberland in England, fewer than 6 percent of all married couples had no children. Then too, smallpox in its virulent American forms was often sex- and age-specific. Among adults, pregnant women were severely hit—experiencing a 50 percent mortality rate rather than the 30 percent common among menfolk over the age of twenty-five. This suggests that not all childless Native American couples were childless by choice.[74]

In New Spain, regional governments offset the cost of ruling conquered peoples by levying tributes. Among the imponderables they ignored was that a population slashed by smallpox, famine and typhus might not be able to pay up. Dramatic examples of Spanish incomprehension on this point were found in the Yucatan. Here between 1648 and 1656 epidemics of yellow fever overlapped with smallpox. When informed that thousands of Mayans had died, the authorities refused to cut back their demands. More extreme was the situation during the rule of Rodrigo Flores de Aldana as governor in 1664–65 and 1667–69. An exquisite exemplar of Spanish greed, Flores de Aldana made clear he was in the Yucatan to exploit the natives and retire to Spain a wealthy man. In response, hundreds of tribute-worthy Mayan youths and maids fled to the outlands beyond his reach. This led to a situation in which population losses due to flight, disruption, smallpox and yellow fever threatened the very survival of the people.[75]

Aware that absentees assessed for tribute could not readily be made to pay up, the Spanish eased the task of collection by forcing populations into centralized villages or "congregations" modelled on Spanish pueblos back home. In regions such as the Valley of Mexico where pre-conquest peoples had been urbanized already, this involved only a bit of tampering here and there. Elsewhere, where "congregations" were entirely new, they were tailor made for explosive epidemics. People who had earlier lived in semi-isolated places would have had little exposure to any endemic, mild form of smallpox. In silver-mining regions in Peru, Bolivia and Mexico, most "congregations" were in fact slave labor camps; here deaths from smallpox might equal the number of fatalities in the mines. To keep these "congregations" in being, they were topped up with recruits brought in from distant places by crews who spread smallpox wherever they went.[76]

Some of the communities the Spanish established in Ecuador appeared to be purpose made death camps. For example, in 1559 a village group from near Anaquito was forcibly relocated to a windy mountainside without access to safe drinking water. This was done at the end of a smallpox epidemic when many survivors were still weak. During and immediately after the move, many of them died. This and similar Spanish acts helped to ensure that the Ecuadorean population surviving into the late 1560s was only a third of what it had been at first contact.[77]

Five thousand kilometers to the north, in the old province of California, beginning in the 1590s Spanish friars established mission compounds and compelled would-be converts to come in for the good of their souls. Unaware that smallpox and other diseases were spread by anything other than the will of God, missionaries failed to connect their congregating practices with the collapse of aboriginal populations. Writing in 1678, a Jesuit reported that though 500,000 converts had been won since proselytizing began, only one in nine remained alive.[78] Here, in cruel contrast to the situation in the Islamic Middle East where believers dying of bubonic plague were assured of instant entry into Paradise, Native Americans dying of smallpox knew that they had been struck down because they had deserted their ancient gods.

Among the cultural attributes that set the Catholic Kings and their successors apart from the Tartar, Genghis Khan (killer of millions), was their fascination with categorization and definition. Thus in the middle years of his reign, aware that conditions in New Spain were not what they might be, King Philip II (great-grandson of Isabella) ordered that priests interview elderly Nahuatl-speaking survivors. Question 5 in this Grand Inquest of 1577–86 asked

> whether the district is inhabited by many or few Indians and whether in former times it had a greater or lesser population; the causes for the increase or diminution and whether the inhabitants live permanently together in regular towns or not. State also what is the character and condition of their intelligence, inclinations and modes of life.

Question 15 asked "whether they used to be more or less healthy anciently than they are now, and what reasons may be learned for this."[79] Serge Gruzinski recently analyzed survey replies and made some unexpected discoveries.[80]

Nahuatl-speaking elders claimed that in the days before the Spanish, people had lived longer and been less troubled with diseases than they were now. This response was not, as might at first appear, one made by misty-eyed oldsters harking back to a mythic golden age, but was a matter-of-fact account by informers whose lived experience showed that the old Aztec regime had been psychologically and physically *more demanding* than the new order imposed by Spain. In former times, gradations of power had shifted rapidly. Nobles had not inherited rank but instead had to earn status through prowess in battle: if they failed their tests they would be cast down among the commoners. Similarly, among the middle ranks, status had to be won by displays of competence. Thus for proper Aztecs accustomed to striving for rank, disciplined personal activity had been required: all was "austerity, frugality and incessant work." This had had important demographic consequences. Because proving skills and competencies had required long years of striving, men and women had married late—men around thirty, women in their mid-twenties.

Under the present rule of the Spanish, the situation was quite different. Former social divisions had been erased and everyone had been ground down to the dark, equal rank of serf. Under this alien "easy and convenient life," there seemed no purpose in anything. Bored out of their minds, young people now married early and according to the informants were simply too lazy to keep babies alive. The elders saw this as an important cause of population decline.

Survey informants exposed to missionary endeavors for half a century and interviewed by priests, dared not openly say that population decline also had been caused by the neglect of old gods who had punished defectors to Christ by sending down smallpox. Strengthening this contention were the adaptive responses of remnant cultural groupings like the Zapotec. These denizens of the once densely populated region of Ocelotepec (400 kilometers south-east of Mexico City) had retained their independence from the Aztecs, but then fallen under Spanish control. During the survey years they were struck by smallpox: 1,200 of them died. Jolted by this crisis, the Zapotec took remedial action. Abandoning the worship of Christ and his mother, they re-erected the altars of the old gods and honored them with customary sacrificial rituals. Their morale much boosted by this flagrant defiance of Spanish prohibitions, the Zapotec freed themselves from the melancholy and fear which, according to some medical teachings, heighten disease morbidity and mortality.[81]

As it happened, the Grand Inquest took place during the most serious epidemic to break over Meso-America since 1519–21. Though medical opinions vary, the chief killer was probably smallpox topped up by typhus and famine. Particularly hard hit was the archdiocese of Mexico where half the population died. Back in Spain, Philip II interpreted this epidemic and its twin disaster, the loss of the Spanish Armada, as evidence that God was angry with his Spanish. To cool the Almighty's wrath, the Inquisition decreed that no further writing in the Nahuatl language be allowed.[82] With this compulsory winding up of literacy in a Meso-American language, a great spike was driven into the coffin of aboriginal culture. Others were being driven in as well.

Left temporarily vacant when Native American populations fled in the face of smallpox, communally held lands were seen by incoming white ranchers as free for the taking. With this theft, Native Americans lost the arable land they needed to grow basic foodstuffs. After they were dispossessed and left destitute, they often fell under the legal protection of a missionary or farmer to became the progenitors of the lazy, shiftless types reported by Henry Dana along the Mexican and Californian coasts in the 1840s.[83]

Though it did not happen in core territories in Meso-America, extinction of whole groupings within a century of contact was common in North America, the Caribbean Islands, and in Brazil. In South Carolina, smallpox swept away an entire nation of coastal Indians in 1699 causing the half-dozen survivors to run away, leaving their unburied dead to the mercies of jet-black ravens and carrion crows. In Virginia, twenty-eight of the sixty tribes listed by Captain John Smith in 1607 had ceased to exist by 1680. In the coastal regions of Portuguese Brazil, by 1798 only 250,000 Indians, most of them dispirited human wrecks, were officially known to exist; by that time they were outnumbered six to one by black African slaves. Writing of the huge Amazon River basin, Claude Lévi-Strauss holds that before First Contact it was occupied by complex civilizations encompassing some 7 or 8 million people. By the early years of this century, when serious anthropological work got underway, these civilizations had been reduced to shattered remnants, each numbering only a few hundred people. Principal killers included the Portuguese *bandeirantes* and the smallpox.[84]

Fortunately for cultural preservationists, in the centuries after Spanish rule gradually became regularized, the population of the Valley of Mexico was never in immediate danger of extinction. However, there were several nasty scares. In 1797–98, smallpox returned in epidemic form. It had last been present eighteen years earlier, which meant that everyone under the age of eighteen—rather more than half the population—was without immunity. In the central city, smallpox swept away 7,000, mostly young, victims. For their part, local Spanish authorities recognized that during a disease crisis 80 percent of the populace were too impoverished to look after themselves. Choosing not to interpret this as an indictment of 270 years of civilizing rule, they took refuge in the notion that aboriginals were by nature lazy, hence poor.[85]

Out in the hinterland during the 1797–98 crisis, the populace were convinced that the Spanish and their God had caused the smallpox. Strengthened by this belief, they resisted Spanish disease-control techniques—compulsory inoculation and the isolation of infected children. The uncomprehending Spaniards had little sympathy. As a priest put it: "These people are the most stubborn in the world. . . . Some say that God sent the disease to the town but they will not permit the Spaniards to give it to any more of their children."[86] On the eve of the main epidemic, in the town of Teutitlan del Valle, the authorities captured sixteen young victims and put them in an isolation hospital, only to have them rescued by an angry crowd who feared that their incarcerated kin would be left to starve to death. Similar rescue attempts happened elsewhere.

Ten thousand kilometers to the south, epidemic smallpox appeared in 1791 among the 200,000 people living beyond the Bio-Bio River in Chile. Until then they had resisted conquest, even though on wall maps in Madrid their territory was marked out as belonging to the Spanish Crown. Thinking to profit from the distress of these "ignorant and superstitious barbarians" who were "moved by whim not by reason," when smallpox hit the Spanish offered to send in missionaries and medical assistance. Denying ulterior motives, the Spaniards "let it be known that . . . the fathers in brown habits [Franciscans] have no desire for your lands, your estates or your women." The Bio-Bio people knew better and replied that they would "continue to refuse to admit the fathers, saying that they would kill them in boiling water, as has happened to other Spaniards."[87]

Left to their own devices, the Bio-Bio people closed off access across the river between themselves and the Spanish, the Spanish God, and the men in brown habits. To explain why smallpox had broken out, they claimed that a smallpox-dead young man named Cayullanca had robbed the Bishop of Concepción's travelling party four years earlier (in 1787) and that the bishop had retaliated by declaring a state of feud and sent in the smallpox which now threatened the entire people. In the event, because the south Bio-Bioians scattered themselves about the countryside, the smallpox touched them only lightly. Two years on, however, the clever Spanish governor, Ambrosio O'Higgins, was able to play on the divisions that had developed during the smallpox crisis. In a treaty concluded in 1793, the Spanish were granted permission to build mission stations, forts and connecting roads wherever they chose in Bio-Bio country, on the tacit understanding that they would not again send in smallpox through witchcraft.[88] But in the New World Order, capitulations of this sort were inevitably followed by white men's broken promises.[89]

The African Connection

Europeans in the New World after 1492 coming upon mineral deposits, cleared fields, grasslands and forests realized that hordes of laborers would be needed to convert all this raw potential wealth into high-value goods marketable at home. Following the Philosopher (Aristotle) in holding that manual labor was appropriate only to slaves, whites assumed that Providence intended that the millions of *homunculi* in the new lands be enslaved to produce goods for Europeans. Then, finding that Native Americans were dying from smallpox and other diseases at an alarming rate and that even when alive they didn't function well, it became obvious that an alternative supply of slaves was needed. This too Providence provided.[90]

In the mid-sixteenth century, Portuguese traders began drawing on their privileged access to an apparently inexhaustible source of sturdy servile labor in what is now Angola. Conveniently enough, this source was located only a few weeks by sea from Spanish America and the Portuguese colony founded after Alvarez Cabral made landfall in Brazil in 1501. In fact, the West African slave-collection stations were only a part of a much larger Portuguese trading empire. Starting in a small way some years earlier, Portuguese sailors had rounded the Cape of Good Hope and crossed the Arabian Sea to establish a fortified trading base at Goa, on the west coast of India. From Goa they had crossed the Bay of Bengal and established a network of connections in Malacca (in Malaya), Macao (in China), Nagasaki (in Japan) and in Manila (in the Philippines). As a result of their frenzied activity, by 1550 the Portuguese were unique among the polities of Europe in having control of a commercial complex that straddled the globe. Through the accidents of European dynastic and papal politics, for many years they were the principal suppliers of slaves to Spanish America.[91]

Even as it was coming into existence, the Portuguese trading empire won the support of those African rulers of kingdoms on the western coasts who were prepared to sell slaves captured in inland parts to seaborne white traders. Building on their West African networks, by the 1490s the Portuguese were sending 1,200–2,500 slaves a year to Lisbon, Seville and the Italian cities. Then with the transfer of the technology of sugar-cane cultivation from the Old World to the New, beginning in Brazil, most slaves caught in Africa were sent to America rather than to Europe.[92] Between the 1670s and the late nineteenth century, some 30 million captives were "sent down the Path" to collection points on the African west coast. About half of them survived this ordeal and shipment across the Atlantic ("the Middle

Passage"). Nineteen out of twenty survivors were consigned to buyers in Brazil, or to the West Indies (now with virtually no inhabitants of pre-contact descent).[93]

As early as 1519 Spanish friars commenting on the conquest of Meso-America and its devastation by smallpox claimed that the human agent who first brought smallpox to the mainland was an African slave. Though the Spanish had very confused ideas about contagion, they seem curiously unanimous in concluding that the person who brought smallpox from Cuba to the Yucatan was an African slave owned by De Narváez who had been lodged with a family in Cempoala where he had taken sick. From that household the disease had spread throughout Cempoala village, then to other villages, then throughout the region, and up the Valley of Mexico to Tenochtitlán where it had arrived late in October 1520.[94] But at this point, a word of caution is in order. As late as 1894 when assessing the worth of similar accounts of how a particular disease outbreak had come on the scene through a named agent, the Army Sanitation Commission in India made it clear that the evidence presented was circumstantial, based on hearsay, and lacking in elementary empirical worth.[95] In considering the tale of the African slave owed by De Narváez, it would perhaps be wise to follow the ASC lead.

Rather than linking the spread of smallpox from Africa to the New World with enslaved persons of color, it is far more probable that the agents were the whites who worked the slave ships. As Herbert Klein and others have pointed out, among the crew members of the white-owned vessels that plied the Middle Passage, mortality rates from smallpox and other crowd diseases were often higher than those of their slave cargoes.[96]

In part, this mortality differential reflected the sort of treatment the smallpox sick were likely to receive; whites generally would be given preferential care. Rather than being trussed up while still alive, dragged to the side of the ship and tossed overboard—the common fate of sick black cargo—sick whites tended to be given crumbs of food and tumblers of water by their mates. Depending on the carers' immune status, this close contact might spread the virus widely among them.

Differential behavior ashore also suggests that black slaves (in trade terms "pieces") were not particularly efficient carriers when compared to white crew. Most whites on landing in a New World port after four to six weeks on a putrid slaver were starved for sex with a woman. Finding their way into a brothel, they were often serviced by Native American girls in town to earn money for their families in the hinterland. During the intimacies that followed, a smallpox virus might be transmitted that, when the girl returned home, would infect the local population.

For their part, newly unloaded, shackled, exhausted black African slaves were unlikely to have shore leave in a brothel or to enjoy the geographic mobility of a sailor with money in his pocket. In addition, many slaves from inland Africa captured by raiders from coastal tribes had already become immune to smallpox, either through variolation or through undergoing a bout of the disease as children. These slaves would not be carriers.[97]

Epidemiological studies suggest that the form of smallpox found in principal catchment areas for slaves later sold in the New World was *Variola intermedius*. With standard mortality rates at between 2.8 to 10.9 percent, it was less lethal than *Variola major* (with mortality rates from 30 percent upwards) though somewhat more lethal than *Variola minor*. *Variola intermedius* was able to maintain itself within a small population of pastoral peoples or nomads for years, with a case here and a case there, leaving most people free to go about their everyday affairs. *Variola intermedius* was usually transferred over longish distances through close contact between overnight guests and their hosts, but was seldom picked up simply by being downwind of a victim.

However, during periods of social disruption caused for instance by the arrival of a slave-raiding party from the coast and the flight of local people to escape capture, *Variola intermedius* might suddenly transform itself into an epidemic. Epidemic *Variola intermedius* seemed to choose more of its victims from among young people of fifteen to twenty-five years of age (ideal catches for slave traders) than among the middle-aged or among five to fourteen-year-olds. And depending on where the new virus had originated, epidemic *Variola intermedius* might be joined by the far more deadly *Variola major*.[98]

By around 1650 (when slaving was still at low-level intensity) the only part of the continent where human numbers were *already* far fewer than local forms of agriculture might have supported was West Africa.[99] This low density was possibly related to the cyclic appearance of smallpox epidemics. Before slave raiding really took off in the 1690s, a likely source of epidemics would have been the movement of large numbers of people southward across the inland sea which was the Sahara Desert. Among the groups of people periodically linking Arabia, and its endemic smallpox, with the southern shores of this desert were Hausa Muslims returning from their once-in-a-lifetime pilgrimage to Mecca.[100] Mass population movement was also caused by climatic irregularities. Touched off by an exceptionally short or an exceptionally long wet season, migrations of whole peoples north or south would be made in response to shifts in the frontiers between desert and savannah. In the course of these migrations, smallpox might spread.

More certain is our knowledge that in the late seventeenth century—when the mass capture of slaves far inland from the coast was just getting underway—the only part of Africa in which a special smallpox god was already known was Yorubaland. This suggests that smallpox had for some time been well established there. Writing about the history of the rituals performed to placate this god in what is now south-western Nigeria, Dahomey and Togo, Donald Hopkins confirmed information given me a few years ago by my local Shopona priestess at a shrine near Oshogbo. The god

Shopona, otherwise known as Overlord of the Earth, was the elder brother of the God of iron and meteorites (Shango) and could either bestow fertility on lands given over to the cultivation of grains or demonstrate his anger by making people's skins come out in grain-like pustules followed by death. Offerings encouraged Shopona to withhold smallpox.[101]

Elsewhere in Africa where there were no deities specific to smallpox (suggestive of a situation in which smallpox had been largely absent), new rituals had to be devised to cope with it when it finally arrived. Some of these were first reported in the nineteenth century and may have originated only a few decades earlier. For example in Kikuyuland (now in Kenya), women living on one ridge would shout and yell to drive the smallpox spirit to the next ridge where another group of loud-voiced women would drive it further on until it was forced beyond the lands used by inter-communing villages.[102]

Rather different was the practice recorded by Arab traders along the East African coast; here the custom was to "buy off" smallpox. James Bruce described this in the 1770s:

> The women . . . from time immemorial . . . are the conductors of the operation in the fairest and driest season of the year. . . . Upon the first hearing of the smallpox anywhere, these people go to the infected place, and wrapping a fillet of cotton cloth about the arm of the person infected, they let it remain there till they bargain with the mother how she is to sell them. . . . One piece of silver or more be paid for the mother . . . this being concluded, they go home and tie the fillet about their own child's arm; certain, as they say, from long experience, that the child infected is to do well, and not have one more than the number of pustules that were agreed and paid for.[103]

Epidemiologically this "buying smallpox" might work; virus in smallpox scabs caught in clothes and bedding remained alive for a fortnight or more. A related practice was to introduce a bit of pus from a smallpox sore into a cut in another person's skin to ensure that the latter would have a mild case of smallpox. This practice was known as variolation or inoculation. A Hausa woman described how she had been inoculated as a child around 1892:

> they used to scratch your arm until the blood came, then they got the fluid from someone who had the smallpox and rubbed it in. It all swelled up and you covered it until it healed. Some children used to die.[104]

As we now know, African and Middle Eastern forms of inoculation were problematic ways to control the spread of smallpox. Success depended on not cutting the flesh too deeply and not causing a secondary infection. More important, it depended on keeping the inoculated person in isolation during the period when she or he was undergoing the induced case of smallpox; let loose too soon the patient might spread the contagion. Confronted with an epidemic caused by an accident of this sort, in pre-colonial Africa the most common response was to break into small groups and take to the bush until the danger passed. Then, some months later, local health provisioners might again inoculate some of the children. It seems very likely that measures such as these were being undertaken by inland people in what is now Burkina Faso in the 1670s and 1680s.[105]

Half a generation later, on the other side of the Atlantic in the colony of Massachusetts, Old World illnesses such as smallpox were belatedly beginning to take hold among American-born whites. We now know that this rise in disease prevalence reflected the normalization of what had been an atypical demographic regime. The earlier situation, credited by the Pilgrim Fathers and Puritans to the working of a special Providence, had been marked by the near absence of virulent crowd diseases. This lacuna had had significant results. Though the colonists who had come to New England and other northern colonies between 1620 and 1642 constituted less than 6 percent of all the English people arriving in mainland and Caribbean island North America, left unpestered, they had successfully raised large numbers of children who survived to produce another large generation. Replicated nowhere else in the New World, this reproductive feat meant that by 1700 the descendants of the well-favored first settlers made up more than *half* of the white population of English North America.[106]

The emergence of a New England disease pattern very like that in colonies further south gave rise to much speculation about why God had deserted his chosen people. One of the men with leisure to come up with suitable explanations was the Reverend Cotton Mather of Boston's Old North Church, the well-known author of a tract attacking witches. Beside scapegoating witches, Mather also targeted Native Americans. Recalling the blissful state known in the time of his grandfather when whites were immune to crowd diseases, Mather waxed eloquent about the great epidemics that had killed ninety-five of every hundred Algonquin Indians "so that the Woods were almost cleared of those pernicious Creatures, making room for a better growth." A representative of this "better growth" himself, Mather was well respected by his parishioners.[107] As a mark of their esteem, in 1706 they gave him a black African slave. With this gift the scene was set for an important intellectual breakthrough.

Mather named the slave Onesimus. Then, worried lest the African bring smallpox into his household, he asked if he had ever had the disease. Onesimus replied yes and no; like all of his age grade he had been inoculated as a child in what is now Burkina Faso and had come down with a mild case of the disease which gave him lifetime immunity. This information set Mather thinking. Inquiring among other slave masters in Boston he found that many blacks from West Africa had also been inoculated as children.[108] With this knowledge, a behavioral practice which had long been common among non-western peoples entered the perceptions and discourse of colonial elites.

Towards Eradication

Encouraged by Mather, Euro-Americans of consequence came to accept that smallpox control through inoculation was feasible. However, imperial attitudes being what they were, in England the better sort disdained to be taught anything by colonials. Accordingly, in Britain full recognition that non-westerners were using some form of inoculation had to wait until 1714 and the publication of Emanuel Timoni's treatise on the practice in Istanbul.[109]

In Europe, what finally tipped the balance in favor of human intervention against smallpox was the shocked realization that in its newish virulent forms the disease was not properly respecting distinctions of hierarchy and rank: it was just as likely to kill the aristocratic holders of great estates as the sons and heirs of street sweepers. In England smallpox slew the Stuart queen Mary II (of the royal pair, William and Mary) and in 1700 carried off the last of her sons. These events led to the parliamentary legislation which transferred the right of succession to the Protestant ruler of Hanover and in time (1707) led to the parliamentary union of England and Scotland. Incidentally, with this last event, medical graduates from Edinburgh University found it a bit easier to acquire practices in England.[110]

Shortly after the Union, the great smallpox scare of 1721 provided an opportunity for an aggressive social climber to claim that she had introduced the idea of inoculation to Europe. Recently returned from Istanbul where her husband represented British interests at the Sublime Porte, Lady Mary Wortley Montagu let it be known that she had had her daughter inoculated using the Turkish method. Influenced by Lady Mary, Queen Caroline had her own children inoculated. Royal patronage made the process respectable. Thereafter in France, Sweden, Spain, Prussia and the Italian lands, rulers made a great show of having their families inoculated and encouraged deferential subjects to follow their lead. The *philosophe* Voltaire made much of what he termed this "medical breakthrough," and true to the effervescent spirit of the Enlightenment, suggested that *medical experts* would soon be able to conquer all diseases.[111] In this, muddled as usual, Voltaire was unaware of mainstream professional medical thinking.

During much of the eighteenth century, university-trained doctors steadfastly opposed inoculation. Insecure in their social status, ranking just above high-class tradesmen, they continued to legitimize their calling by claiming reliance on the theories of the Ancients. In 1765, a survey of Scottish medical doctors (seen then as the world's best and most innovative), found that only a third had taken to inoculating clients. On the Continent, even thirty years later, most physicians were still clinging to Greco-Hellenistic humoral theories which, on the face of it, seemed to rule out innovations in preventive medicine. Yet in this pre-modern medical world, ultimately it was the fee-paying clients who had the last say.

What happened was that perverse persons of quality, without whose continuing patronage the medical profession would have withered, privately insisted that their own children be inoculated. Accordingly, by the tail end of the century medical doctors found that, with a bit of juggling and fudging, the processes of inoculation could, after all, be made compatible with old theories. As practiced by medical doctors after around 1790, inoculation became a two- or three-week in-house vacation in which the patient was first prepared by a special diet and regimen (the word itself a legacy from the Middle Ages), and then allowed to recuperate in similarly favorable circumstances.[112]

Among ordinary people who obviously could not afford an inoculation regimen of this sort, the situation was quite different. If carried out at all, the inoculation of children was performed by amateurs or empirics. Contrary to what at first might be assumed, opening this field to empirics did not elicit much protest from medical professionals. Long accustomed to accept that mothers, midwives, village wise-women and other unorthodox curers already provided health care for ordinary children, doctors were not especially concerned that this particular clientele didn't come their way.

In south-east England, famous non-medically trained inoculators included Thomas Dimsdale and the Suttons, Robert and his son Daniel. In the Shetland Islands, admitting to have successfully performed several thousand inoculations was the jack of all trades John Williamson. Williamson claimed that his technique was to dry smallpox scab materials over a peat fire and bury them for seven or eight years (!) before using them to inoculate patients. In this island grouping, which included Foula where in 1720 smallpox had wiped out all but ten of the inhabitants, local people provided an enthusiastic clientele. However, in many other parts of Europe, ordinary people were less keen. Long experience with quacks from outside the village had taught them that avoidance was the high road to survival. Only when an epidemic was just over the horizon would they rush out to have their families inoculated by visiting empirics, deciding that the lesser risk (death by inoculation) subsumed the greater (death by virulent smallpox). In the nature of things, inoculation campaigns by unlicenced empirics very often escaped official notice. They thus failed to provide later historical demographers with the secure statistics they would need to reconstruct with any confidence the changing nature of past reality.[113]

Between 1750 and 1800 Europe's population increased from around 140 million to 180 million, and by 1900 it stood at 390 million. Seeking to explain this unprecedented growth, Eric Mercer draws on the work of the Cambridge Group for Population Studies who in turn attempted to tease out the relationship between declining mortality rates, and changing marriage and fertility patterns.[114] Well aware of the danger of rash generalization,

Mercer did, however, feel able to point out that in some regions human intervention against smallpox seemed to have had a significant impact on the well-being of a particular age cohort. For instance, in authoritarian late eighteenth century Sweden where smallpox sometimes counted for nearly a fifth of all deaths, between 1779 and 1782 94 percent of all these smallpox victims were children under nine. In response to this clear threat to the perpetuation of Swedes as an ethnic group, agents of the regime encouraged rural parents to have their children inoculated, and indeed made the process compulsory. Gritting their teeth, heads of households by and large conformed to state dicta. This led to a situation where the number of non-immunized population was significantly reduced; for some years the prevalence of lethal smallpox was also much reduced.[115]

Once underway—assisted by unsystematic inoculation campaigns—the momentum of population growth was helped along by another innovation in smallpox prevention techniques. In 1796 Edward Jenner, a medical practitioner in Gloucester, became aware of a process used a few years earlier by a Dorset yeoman farmer named Benjamin Jesty. Jesty admitted to using infectious matter taken from the udder of a cow suffering from cowpox to inoculate his wife and family. Finding all the relevant young Jestys still alive, Dr Jenner co-opted the process and called it "vaccination." Through well-publicized applications of the new technique, Jenner, already a man of recognized status, made himself wealthy. As well as the small marks of esteem which came his way, in 1803 the East India Company sent him a purse of £7,000. At the time, the annual earnings of a fully employed craftsman might approach £100.[116]

Medical historians who follow Peter Razzell now accept that the lymph Jenner used contained a curious mixture of things. One of its disadvantages was that because the infective agent had been watered down to make it safer, vaccination during childhood had to be followed up by re-vaccination during young-adulthood.[117] Yet historians who view society from the top down consider Jenner's breakthrough a turning point in western medicine. For instance, Yves-Marie Bercé of France regarded Jenner's work as an inspiring example of Enlightenment giants' "audacity." Announced to the world a few months after the Marquis of Condorcet wrote the brilliant manifesto, *On the Progress of the Human Mind* (1794), Jenner's work led *tout le monde* to assume that Europe could rid itself of its most dangerous scourge.[118]

Jenner's breakthrough took place at a time when much of Europe was under French military occupation. Borne aloft by Enlightenment optimism now represented by Europe's first modern dictator—Napoleon Bonaparte—clerics, magistrates, prefects and others with power over other peoples' lives persuaded subject populations to have their children vaccinated free of charge. An unspoken assumption was that the youths thus kept alive would provide the cannon fodder needed for the next war. In Prussia, after royal armies were smashed by Napoleon at the battle of Jena in 1806, vaccination

Curse on these Vaccinators we shall all be starved, why Brother I have matter enough here to Kill 50,
And those would communicate it to 500 more
Aye Aye. I always order them to be constantly out in the air, in order to spread the contagion
Oh Brothers Brothers, suffer the love of Gain to be Overcome by compassion for your fellow creatures, & do not delight to plunge whole Families in the deepest distress, by the untimely loss of their nearest and Dearest Relatives
The curse of human kind
VACCINATION against SMALL POX or Mercenary & Merciless spreaders of Death & Devastation driven out of Society

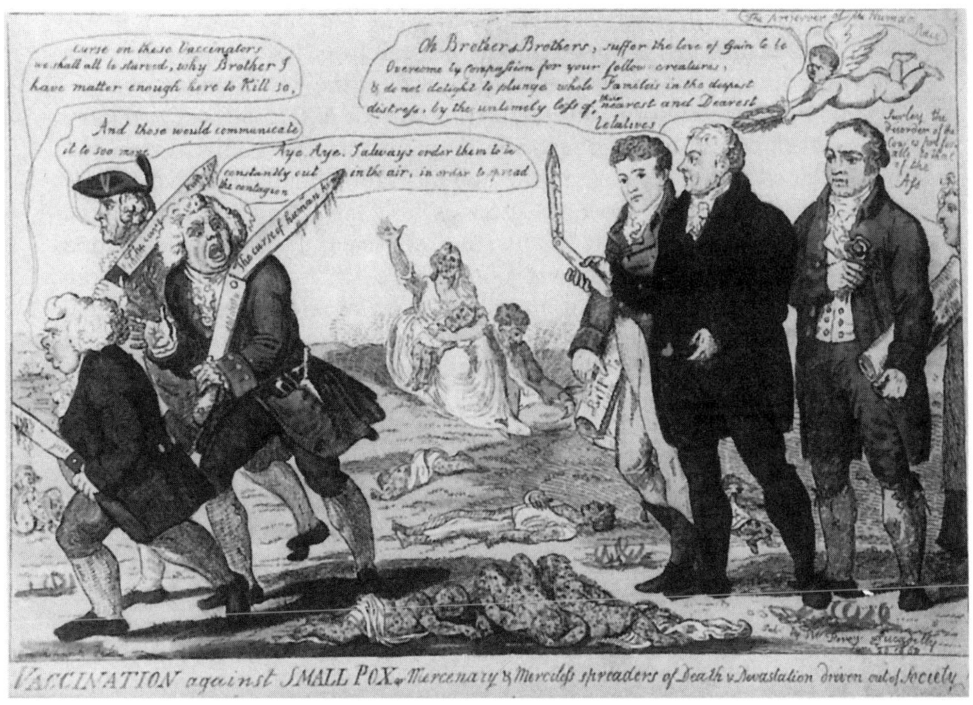

9. The heroic Jenner crushing his opponents. Colored etching by I. Cruikshank.

clinics were established in most sizeable settlements. In metropolitan France, agents of the Catholic Church on the payroll of the State encouraged families gathered at baptismal ceremonies to have their other children vaccinated after the service.[119] In Naples, typical scenes were described by a degree-holding British vaccinator who would soon return to Gloucester to work with Jenner. Here:

> It is not unusual to see, in the mornings of public inoculation at the hospital, a procession of men, women and children conducted through the streets by a priest carrying a cross come to be inoculated . . . the common people expressed themselves certain that it was a blessing sent from heaven, though discovered by one heretic and practiced by another.[120]

It has been argued that in this more sophisticated form, human intervention against smallpox contributed to the momentum of mortality decline. In any case, as a direct result of dropping mortality, particularly among children, there were huge population increases in Great Britain, the Germanies, the Habsburg lands, Italy and Scandinavia. Emerging from these lands after

1840 were restless young people who could not find places at home. Between then and 1913 more than 35 million Europeans went out to North America; another 3 or 4 million settled south of the Rio Grande.

Once in the New World, this population surplus to Europe occupied more and more of the lands earlier set aside "in perpetuity" for Native Americans. In the United States, the government administration humiliated by the Sioux who defeated Lt.-Col. George Custer at his "last stand" in the Dakota Territory in 1876 retaliated with the Allotment Act. This legislation removed 17 million acres of land from Native American control. Between 1887 and 1934, an additional 69 million acres were confiscated. Principal beneficiaries of this pillage were the immigrants from Europe, many of whom had been vaccinated against smallpox before they left.

By the 1890s the United States began to recognize its destiny as a great world power. One of its acts of self-assertion was to gobble up what was left of Spain's New World and Asian Empire. In 1898, at the end of the Spanish-American War, the US found itself in possession of Puerto Rico, the second of the Caribbean islands (after Hispaniola) whose Native American population had been decimated by Spanish smallpox in 1518–19. Bubbling over with the twin forces of nationalism and Social Darwinism, the Americans interpreted Puerto Rico's continuing difficulties with smallpox as a clarion call for action. In the words of the US commanding officer, Major General Guy V. Henry:

> Hardly had the last representatives of Spanish misrule turned their back upon the island before the American military administration . . . set on foot, as an act of beneficence to the newly subordinated people, the vaccination of the entire population.[121]

In fact, as early as 1803 the Spanish king had organized the transport of Jenner's vaccine to his subjects in the Caribbean. Twenty-two orphan boys had been packed aboard a small brig and two of them vaccinated seriatim every six or eight days using the arm-to-arm method to keep the vaccine fresh during the long voyage across the Atlantic. Following the first vaccinations in Puerto Rico, in the 1880s an Institute of Vaccination had been established and a compulsory vaccination program put in place. However, because ordinary Puerto Ricans saw medical doctors as representatives of centralizing authority, they were loath to come to town-based clinics for vaccinations. To encourage compliance, Spanish government administrators had fined the recalcitrant. This then was the program of state medicine which the New Men from mainland North America held up to scorn.[122]

In their determination to shoulder that "share of the white man's burden that has fallen to [them]" and to cleanse the pest-hole on their threshold, the US military closed the Puerto Rican Institute of Vaccination and began a draconian program intended to demonstrate their conviction that "comprehensive *compulsory* vaccination, properly conducted, will *alone, certainly* eradicate smallpox from *any* region or people."[123] In the event, after three years, Yankee enthusiasm faltered and the eradication campaign petered out. On the mainland, white jokesters took to calling cases of smallpox among sailors in US ports, "Puerto Rico scratches" or "Puerto Rican chicken-pox." Smallpox had become the disease of the colonized, the dispossessed, the Other.[124]

During the months when US military health authorities were showing what could be done in the fight against smallpox in liberated Puerto Rico, the last of the great smallpox epidemics in a modern developed country struck thirteen of the nineteen Pueblo settlements in New Mexico. Six hundred Native Americans died, with overall population loss in the worst-affected settlements running at 13 percent. Since the Bureau of Indian Affairs in Washington, DC regarded Native Americans as expendable, bureaucratic blockages effectively prevented the dispatch of qualified health professionals. Such assistance as there was was provided by local white volunteers. One of these reported that:

> I find the Inds very pleasant in their greeting but they look and act as if they had cried themselves dry. I asked one man who came to chop wood . . . how many children were sick in his house. "None" he replied; "I have buried them all. Three we had but they are all gone."[125]

After the epidemic passed, surviving Pueblo leaders (who knew that the disease had been caused by witchcraft) pleaded with well-meaning volunteers to go home and leave them in peace.[126]

In the late 1950s officials of the World Health Organization estimated the annual global incidence of smallpox at 13 million. By that time the disease had all but disappeared in Europe and North America, but remained endemic in Brazil, Colombia, Ecuador, Bolivia, and in most of Asia and Africa. Then one year after it launched the world's first artificial earth satellite (1957), the USSR sponsored a WHO resolution calling for global smallpox eradication. Following the priorities of the Cold War, eight years later the United States took up the challenge. Together the two superpowers pledged to free humankind from the smallpox scourge.

By this time, public health in the developed world was firmly in the hands of a highly professionalized medical elite for whom it was axiomatic that non-western approaches to disease control were based on ignorance and superstition. Working within this paradigm, in 1967 the WHO smallpox leadership decreed that eradication would be achieved through a saturation vaccination campaign. Though not openly stated, this campaign would be similar to that set up by General Guy V. Henry in Puerto Rico in 1898. Put into effect, it would mean that a vaccination scar on the upper arm, the "Mark of the West," be inflicted on 80 percent of the denizens of the underdeveloped world.[127]

Curiously enough, the scientific credibility of the freeze-dried serum used in WHO vaccination was less than secure. As the soon to be president of the American Association for the History of Medicine pointed out in 1978:

> We do not even know the origin of the vaccinia virus currently used in vaccination which is produced in laboratories by scarification of the skin of calves and sheep. Some believe it was derived from variola virus attenuated through continuous passage in human skin, others that it is a hybrid derived from simultaneous human infection with variola and cowpox, and others believe it is a laboratory virus derived from natural cowpox by continuous artificial propagation.[128]

If the genesis of the materials used was a mystery, the fact remains that the WHO campaign did vindicate at least one strand of western scientific thought: Sir Francis Bacon's empirical method. The early seventeenth-century Lord Chancellor had advised that any initial assumption which did not hold up in the face of practical experience should be junked. And so it was. While at work in eastern Nigeria, Dr W. H. Foege found himself running short of vaccine. He then made the crucial decision to limit vaccination *only* to those people with whom a known smallpox victim had come into contact, and to put the patient him/herself in strict isolation. Foege then sent out surveillance teams to discover which settlements were smallpox free and required no vaccinations. Thereafter surveillance, isolation of patients, and vaccination limited to immediate contacts became the guiding strategy of the WHO campaign.

Though the level of discipline and thoroughness of application differed and though the scale was much larger—a region, a nation state, a continent, the globe—essentially this was the way in which West African, Bengali and Arabic-speaking village and urban peoples had been coping with smallpox for hundreds of years. In another unspoken admission of the value of non-western precedents, reformed WHO strategy came to accept traditional healers as assistants in the eradication campaign; in the US campaign in Puerto Rico, these people had been seen as part of the problem rather than as part of the solution.

By combining notification, the isolation of known cases, and vaccination only of those in contact with known victims, smallpox was finally made extinct in Meso-America, and in South and North America. These were the regions in which smallpox, assisted by genocide, measles, typhus and famine, had killed off a sixth of humankind in the sixteenth and seventeenth centuries. In 1976 the world's last remaining infective smallpox out in the field was found among nomads in Somalia. In October 1977, Ali Mallin, a hospital cook in Merka, became the last earthling to develop a naturally acquired case of the disease.[129]

Vaccine stored in vaults in the Centers for Disease Control in Atlanta and in the Russian Research Institute for Viral Preparations in Koltsovo in

Novosibirsk in the Urals (for security reasons moved out from Moscow) remained, as of 24 January 1996, the only smallpox virus *known* to exist. Though anti-terrorist arrangements at the summer 1996 Olympic Games at Atlanta obviously left something to be desired, officials insist that the Centers for Disease Control in the same city can effectively insure that the virus in their custody will not be liberated by anyone bent on mass murder. At the January 1996 meeting of the WHO executive, it was decided to destroy the remaining Atlanta and Koltsovo stocks three and a half years later, on 30 June 1999.[130]

4 The Secret Plague: Syphilis in West Europe and East Asia, 1492 to 1965

Introduction

While compiling the *London Bills of Mortality* in 1662, the pioneer demographer John Graunt put his finger on a central issue in the study of syphilis during much of its 500-plus years' reign in Europe: its *near invisibility*. As he explained:

> Forasmuch as by the ordinary discourse of the world it seems a great part of men have, at one time or another, had some species of this disease, I wondering why so few died of it, especially because I could not take that to be so harmless, whereof so many complained very fiercely; upon inquiry I found that those who died of it out of the Hospitals . . . were returned of Ulcers and Sores . . . from whence I concluded that only *hated* persons, and such whose very Noses were eaten off, were reported by the Searchers to have died of this too frequent malady.[1]

In a world like Graunt's in which syphilis had become the most shameful of all diseases—replacing stigmatizing leprosy—it seems to have been common for surviving friends and family to bribe or bully searchers so that the officially recorded cause of death would not harm their own "good repute."

Other useful insights into the near invisibility of syphilis can be found in the swampy frontier lying between objective medical "truth" and subjective, culturally derived, perceptions. One of these hinges on the fact that in its "medical" first stage, syphilis showed itself in open sores on its host's penis or vagina. Then in its second stage (when the sores had healed) it lay latent, causing general debilitation. While in this stage, syphilis was often "medically" confused with gout, with tuberculosis, or some other socially acceptable affliction. In many cases perhaps, this confusion was caused by genuine medical misunderstanding.

Still in the frontier between real-world "objective" perceptions and those which were clearly subjective, it is known that unlike "the small pox" which killed in a matter of days, "the great pox" remained latent for anywhere between three and thirty years. Given that in Europe until the nineteenth century, life expectancy at birth was between thirty-five and forty years, syphilis acquired *after* sexual maturity (at thirteen or fourteen) which decided to remain latent for a long time stood a good chance of being short-changed as the listed cause of death by a more quick-footed killer. Entered into the record, this typology (which in the strict sense may have been perfectly correct) masked the fact that the person involved was a syphilitic.[2]

The impact of syphilis on past societies has also been masked by the nature of surviving source materials and the purposes they were meant to serve. Parish registers, for example, generally only listed live births (recorded as baptisms performed) and deaths (burials) of recognized human beings. Omitted from parish register listings were fetuses aborted early in pregnancy. Also omitted were the disease processes which led to the sterilization of women so that they could no longer bear children.[3]

To clarify how these omissions tied in with syphilis, let us run through a chain of events. Some months after a woman was impregnated with a man's sperm (it need not necessarily be her husband's), the *Treponema pallidum* disease agent she had acquired through the small syphilitic sores on the man's penis penetrated the wall of her womb and either killed or maimed the fetus she was carrying. About half of the women so afflicted aborted, while many of the others gave birth to a child with congenital syphilis. Most mothers who underwent either trauma then found themselves sterile for life.

Accepted in Europe as a central pillar of marriage until very recent times was the authority of the husband to *insist* that his wife join him in a sexual act—even if he happened to have sores on his penis. Buttressing this was the "dual standard" which held that a proper man entering his first marriage should already have had sexual experience with women. Another element of the dual standard held that a married man stuck with a wife unable to give him sexual satisfaction could use the services of a prostitute or take any woman who took his fancy providing, of course, he didn't cause a public disturbance. On the other hand, dual standard conventions held that no honor-conscious man would deign to marry a woman who had a prior sexual history. Following on from this was the rule that once married, a wife was always to be loyal to her husband.[4]

Until very recently in the West, it was customary to think in Cartesian binary terms. Standard pairs included: fact versus value; objective vs. subjective; medieval darkness vs. Enlightenment truth; ethical considerations vs. pure science. However, in dealing with venereal syphilis, the plague which society chose not to discuss, we enter an area where old binary distinctions are no longer particularly useful.

In his works on sexuality, the historian/philosopher Michel Foucault frequently employed the phrase "power/knowledge" which he derived from Sir Francis Bacon.[5] In Foucault's words:

> No power is exercised without the extraction, appropriation, distribution or retention of knowledge. At this level, we do not have knowledge on the one hand and society on the other, or science and state; we have the basic forms of "power-knowledge".[6]

Here, when dealing with the five centuries after syphilis first put in an appearance (in 1493), I accept the notion that knowledge is power, and see *control over the sexuality of other people* as a determining force in the making of Europe. But in my hands, unlike those of Foucault, the word "knowledge" is usually synonymous with *false knowledge* of "the earth is flat" variety. Sometimes, when drawn from the fount of ancient wisdom (Plato, Aristotle, Galen), this false, flat-earth knowledge was well-intentioned ignorance.[7] On other occasions it was an act of duplicity deliberately practiced to reinforce authority.

In this chapter, going beyond conventional interpretations of gender relationships, I will tease out linkages between syphilis and the repression of masturbation. It is my contention that in those milieux where it was pounded into the consciousness of young males that it was far better to use the services of a prostitute than to engage in solitary self-release, opportunities for the species survival of *Treponema pallidum* were much enhanced. I will also explore ways in which anti-masturbation campaigns sharpened the disciplinary skills of parents and tutors in households, of masters in schools, of sergeants and officers in the armed services, and of the medical pioneers who ventured into what they regarded as the "sinister" world of sexuality.

In the real world of objective fact, the sexual authoritarianism that began to flower in the mid-eighteenth century (greatly assisted by the anti-masturbation scare) led in the next century to the near demise of literature about actual human reproductive processes. Even if tinged by flat-earth-type platitudes drawn from ancient writers, this literature might have enabled *ordinary* people to avoid falling prey to syphilis. Unfortunately, under the influence of the Enlightenment with its cult of "human progress," the dark shadows grew darker yet.[8] With the development of "mass society" in the nineteenth century and its deliberate manipulation by authorities who both despised and feared it, the wet blanket of repression nearly stifled the European mind.

Flourishing between 1493 and *c.* 1935 in the fertile bed of repression, secrecy, shame and flat-earth pseudo-science were hosts of entrepreneurs who made a living from other people's misery. Seen from the perspective of our own post-modern era and its questioning of the authority of many of yesteryear's renowned councillors (Sigmund Freud, Carl Jung), it will come as no surprise that many of the entrepreneurial healers who called themselves medical doctors were frauds.

Towards the end of the chapter I examine how, beginning in the mid-nineteenth century, universalizing European doctors and missionaries introduced western moral entrepreneurship into China. Filled with a righteousness born of Sinophobia and power/false knowledge, they found venereal syphilis on a scale unknown anywhere else. What in fact they confronted was Construct syphilis. This consisted of two elements: (a) Sinophobic delusion; and (b) genuine medical confusion between authentic, sexually transmitted, venereal syphilis on the one hand and on the other, yaws and endemic syphilis (both non-sexually transmitted). As we will see, after some initial hesitation, Chinese elites, who already regarded people from the West as barbarians, managed to find an appropriate response to what they understood was the western sickness: entrepreneurship born of syphilis.

Initial Perceptions

Beginning in the 1490s, a highly contagious venereal disease (ancestral to syphilis if not syphilis itself) raced through port cities and towns in Spain, southern France and Italy and then spread out on a broad front which moved eastward beyond Vienna and north beyond Leipzig, Bergen and Aberdeen. Writing in 1497, the medical doctor to Pope Alexander VI, Alexander Benedetto of Venice, reported that he had seen victims who had lost eyes, noses, hands and feet. According to Benedetto, "the entire body is so repulsive to look at and the suffering is so great, especially at night, that this sickness is even more horrifying than incurable leprosy or elephantiasis, and it can be fatal."[9] Some decades later (in 1539), Ruy Díaz de Isla, a Spanish surgeon at Lisbon's All Saints Hospital, claimed that the new disease "has caused so much damage, that there is not a village in Europe with one hundred neighbors without ten of them dead of that ailment."[10] Though this particular claim was doubtless much exaggerated, at least it reflected a medical man's concern with a disease phenomenon which—though he dared not openly admit it—was entirely beyond his ken.

In their initial attempts to cope with the epidemic, learned doctors turned to their books to find out what ancient authorities had written; they drew a blank. This led the arch-Hellenist Niccolò Leoniceno, the leading medical professor at Ferrara, to aver that:

> when I consider that humanity has the same nature, is born under the same sky, grows up under the same stars, I must conclude that we have always been subjected to the same illnesses, and I absolutely cannot believe that this illness is born suddenly only now and has infected only our epoch and none of the preceding.[11]

Unwittingly, Leoniceno had laid bare a central, shocking truth; venereal syphilis was indeed a new disease. This leads us to the contentious territory of disease types and origins.

The discovery in Madras late in 1992 of an entirely new strain of cholera which resists all known vaccines (*Vibrio cholerae 0139*) is a reminder of the frightening rapidity with which disease viruses can transform themselves, following principles publicized by Charles Darwin in 1859.[12] An analogous mutation apparently brought into being the disease complex that contemporaries reluctantly concluded was new to West Europe in 1493–94. Only in our own century have scientists finally unravelled its complexities.

In 1905, Fritz Schaudinn and his colleagues in Berlin discovered that the causal agent of modern syphilis is *Treponema pallidum* (Treponema S). This breakthrough was followed by Aldo Castellani's identification of the treponema which caused yaws (Treponema Y) and later by F. Leon Blanco's discovery of the treponema agent of pinta (Treponema C). Experts also found that *non-sexually* transmitted syphilis (bejel or endemic syphilis) is caused by Treponema M. So in all, *circa* 1910, four different diseases were recognized as being caused by a treponema. Only one of these, venereal syphilis, was sexually transmitted. The three others, yaws, endemic syphilis and pinta, were transmitted by non-sexual means. However, as of this writing (1996) experts are still uncertain of how many disease agents there might be; under high-powered microscopes all the treponemae appear to be the same. The agents reveal their differences only when they cause a specific disease in a particular human host.[13] Also confusing experts is the ability of the "same" agent to cause different diseases in tropical as opposed to temperate settings.[14]

Almost from the beginning of its 500-plus-year stint in Europe, syphilis was perceived as a disease harbored by a culpable "Other" and then inflicted on innocent people. Closely parallel to this, beginning in 1526, was the assertion that the disease had been found among the indigenous people of Hispaniola, whence it was first brought to Europe by the ship crews serving under Christopher Columbus. By the eighteenth century, the American origins of veneral syphilis had become part of the European identikit. Thus in *The Spirit of Laws* (1748), the Enlightenment giant Montesquieu took it for granted that syphilis had come from the New World and that it had wiped out most of the great families of southern Europe. Similarly, in 1777 when the ink on America's Declaration of Independence from the king of Great Britain was barely dry, the highly respected Scottish historian and British patriot, William Robertson, asserted that by contaminating Europe with syphilis, America had forfeited all benefits which might have resulted from its "discovery" by Europeans.[15]

Though prejudiced readings of the meanings of syphilis persist in our own day, at least some of yesterday's chestnuts have been relegated to the shelves of the museum.[16] One is the old notion that the indigenous inhabitants of Hispaniola in 1492—the Taino—infected innocent intruders from Europe with full-blown syphilis. Instead, what seems to have been the case was that non-sexually transmitted yaws had spread earlier among Taino girls and boys while they were playing together. Years later, some of the little girls who had matured into women still carried their yaws. Then they were raped by Spanish males. While each rape was in progress, the long-unwashed and probably tender skin on Spanish groins, bellies, chests and penises was breached by *Treponema pertenue*, the yaws causal agent. Once the *Treponema pertenue* found itself in a new kind of human host and in a new climatic regime—the temperate Europe to which the alien Spaniards returned in 1493—it seems to have mutated into its new form, *Treponema pallidum*, to become venereal syphilis.[17]

That venereal syphilis was both an entirely new disease and a disease new to Europe is supported by its initial behavior—its spectacular skin manifestations were massively contagious and quickly lethal. Some medically informed writers hold that this first epidemic was a multiple-disease syndrome combining yaws, venereal syphilis and gonorrhea (an altogether different disease which in the male causes sperm to discharge from a flaccid penis). Then with time, what has been defined as "the typical thickening of the skin, bleeding fissures, spontaneous fractures of the bones, gangosa and other pathognomonic symptoms [of yaws]" dropped away, leaving venereal syphilis in complete control of the ecological niche provided by Europeans in their homelands.[18]

As we saw in earlier chapters, pre-medically modern Europeans (before Robert Koch went into high gear in 1882) sometimes explained the causes of a disease in terms we now find difficult to understand. In fifteenth-century Italian universities where astrology was a serious academic subject, one supposition was that syphilis was the result of the conjuncture of the planets Jupiter and Saturn in November 1484. Among the learned, another supposition was that it was some form of the "leprosy" common amongst the ancient Hebrews. Then too, many commentators saw a clear relationship between syphilis and "lewd or impure sexual gratification." Burdened with this prejudice, it would be a long while before it was fully realized that husbands engaged in copulation in marriage (a sinless activity) could also infect their wives. At the popular level, it was sometimes thought that syphilis was caused by eating pork (with its leprous and Jewish connotations), or by drinking a woman's menstrual blood.[19]

The first of the many "Others" that fear of syphilis would produce dates from the 1490s. A generation or so earlier rural Europe had begun to recover from the hemorrhages of bubonic plague, with the result that in many villages there were young people surplus to local labor needs. Confronted with a situation unprecedented in the recent past—overpopulation—community elders took a dim view of illegitimate baby boys. If these unwanted males survived to adolescence they were very often encouraged to join a troop of mercenary soldiers in the hope that they would disappear forever. In mountainous Switzerland (which after 1690 played a disproportionately large role in creating hysteria about sexual activity outside marriage), this technique enabled whole cantons to keep the size of their populations within manageable bounds.

According to commentators who despised mercenary soldiers, the new venereal disease had first taken off among the 30,000 hirelings who in 1494 accompanied the French Valois king Charles VIII on his momentous invasion of Italy. For *Treponema pallidum*, the progress of the Valois force was a precious boon. Moving south from Milan, the ill-disciplined army had dallied for some weeks in papal Rome, where it was said that prostitutes outnumbered clerics, and then moved on to Naples, one of Europe's largest cities. After Naples capitulated without a fight there was much fraternizing between the conquerors and available sexual fare. The Valois forces then moved north to Fornovo (not far from Milan) where they fought an inconclusive battle with Habsburg and Venetian armies. After that, the Valois hirelings disbanded. Some found new jobs as mercenaries; other returned to civilian life in towns on the northern side of the Alps.

The ever-widening circles where the *morbus gallicus* (French disease) struck in the 1490s are marked by government decrees and scholarly pronouncements in Paris, Edinburgh and Leipzig. Most of the rest of the world was also at risk. Travelling with sailors, merchants, missionaries and other agents of Europe's age of exploration, the disease established bases on the Mediterranean coast of Africa, then moved on to India, Ceylon and the Malay peninsula. By 1504 it was found at the great emporium at Canton where it came to be known as the "plum-tree ulcer."[20]

Once the initial disease completed its mutation to become *Treponema pallidum*, the venereal disease situation in Europe *may have* settled down. Conventional histories of medicine remind us that in a book published in Mainz in 1519 Ulrich von Hutten, a sufferer from syphilis, claimed that "when it first appeared it caused a far more loathsome stench than it does now, as if the sickness involved were of a different type altogether."[21] However, this modification of the symptoms apparent to an experienced nose does not mean that the at-risk population declined in size. On the contrary, it increased precipitously.

During the sixteenth century, rural population increase and general restlessness encouraged young country people who were not immediately in line to inherit parental lands to go to a town to find work, even if this meant risking a brush with syphilis. Writing in 1585 of his ten years as a medical doctor in London's St Bartholomew's Hospital, William Clowes claimed that one entering patient out of every two was syphilitic and that in five years he had treated more than a thousand patients. What we know of ordinary urban people's attitudes to hospitals and learned medical doctors—utter revulsion—suggests that Clowes's figurative thousand patients were only a small proportion of the actual number of Londoners racked with syphilis.[22]

Yet so long as settled *country* people (80 percent or more of the overall population) stayed clear of cities, it was unlikely that they would be much troubled with the disease. Unlike urban folk or mercenary soldiers, rural

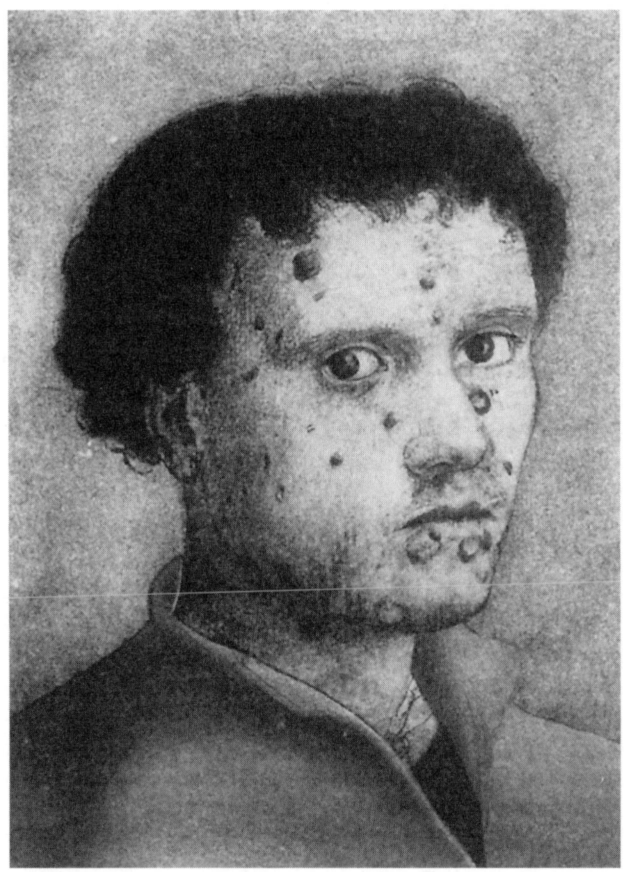

10. A young man afflicted with syphilis. Colored drawing 1523, by Hans Holbein the Younger.

people who spent their lives within a day or two's walking distance of their place of birth generally followed behavioral patterns which excluded casual sex, and with it the risk of syphilis.

Counselled by village elders who were reluctant to clutter up their village with surplus mouths to feed, rural youths and girls generally waited until they had found the partner they intended to marry before they had carnal knowledge of another person; according to demographers, partners would have been in their mid- to late twenties. Rural bastardy rates, generally under 4 percent and sometimes under 1.5 percent, support the thesis that for country people sexuality was a great iceberg.[23] Suggestive of this is the fact that around 1550, 10–15 percent of the population aged forty and above were still unmarried and, as far as the world knew, chaste.

The Commercialization of Syphilis

In his throwaway remarks about syphilitic America and its gift to Europe, Montesquieu noted that "It was thirst for gold which perpetuated this disease; people were continually going to America, each time bringing back new seeds."[24] This can be interpreted as meaning that in this age of nascent capitalism in Europe, some men and woman were minting money from syphilis. Among the earliest of these entrepreneurs was the genocidal terrorist, Gonzalo Fernández de Oviedo (1478–1577), and his business associates, the Fuggers of Augsburg, leading financiers to Charles V, the Habsburg Emperor.[25] This brings us to the making of a great fabrication.

It is important to remind ourselves here that reports made by Columbus and the medical doctors who accompanied him on his travels in 1492–93 made no mention of anything particularly lethal in the disease environment of Hispaniola. Similarly absent was any mention of shipfuls of men suffering from some sort of fast-acting syphilis on the return voyage home. Yet in his publication of 1526, the famous *Summary* of the *Natural History of the Indies*, Oviedo boldly asserted that "Your Majesty may rest assured that this disease came from the Indies."[26] This was the first time that the American origins of syphilis were set forth in print. Thereafter this allegation became the commonplace of learned discourse.

Oviedo belonged to a powerful aristocratic Spanish family and after 1513–14 was in the Americas as the Emperor's superintendent of silver and gold mines. While in Hispaniola he served as governor of the castle of Santo Domingo and presumably held properties in what became the town of Oviedo 190 kilometers to the west. Some time after 1516 Oviedo learned of a reputed cure for syphilis—wood of guaiac—grown on Hispaniola. Aware of the old doctrine of correspondences, he knew that the public believed that for every poison, God had placed a cure nearby. A well-experienced entrepreneur, Oviedo accordingly claimed that Hispaniola peoples had long been affected with full-blown syphilis, and that they cured the disease with the guaiac wood so conveniently near at hand.

The centerpiece of Oviedo's publicity campaign was the chapter in his treatise entitled "Of the Palo Santa called by the Indians Guayacan" (guaiac wood). Lest rich syphilitics miss the point, the guaiac was termed "Holy Wood," suggestive of God's willingness to remit punishment for the sin of sex. While writing up was in progress, Oviedo arranged for his Fugger partners to receive monopoly rights from Charles V to import and market the wonder cure throughout the Empire. From this, Oviedo and his friends netted handsome profits. But in the long term, of far greater consequence was the smear that this vicious literate Spaniard inflicted on the reputation of Hispaniola.[27]

Other entrepreneurs for whom venereal syphilis proved profitable were Europe's booksellers and printers. As sixteenth century media watchers knew, once a statement was laid out on a printed page it acquired a higher

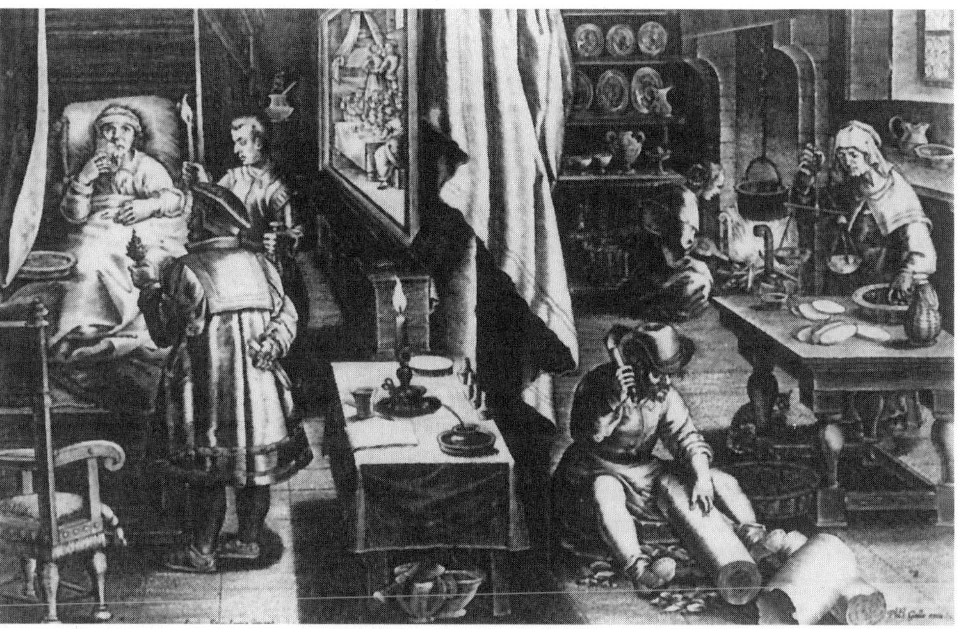

11. Guaiac wood, prepared and administered. Engraving, *c.* 1600, by Philip Galle after J. van der Straet.

level of authenticity than was possessed by a statement communicated merely by word of mouth (witness the impact of Oviedo's made-in-America claims). Yet as a means of making a living, the European form of printing—not invented until the 1450s—was still somewhat uncertain. Though the number of staff required were small compared to the gangs of copyists needed to produce handwritten books in quantity, capital costs were much higher. Hindering investment return was the inevitable long delay between printing a standard text—a Bible or commentary—and its sale to a customer.

In the early 1490s, bursting in on this stifling atmosphere, was the first epidemic of syphilis. Immediately, the demand for newly printed books boomed. Sales were fuelled by the reluctant recognition that the new illness was not mentioned in Ancient or Arabic medical texts previously printed and gathering dust on merchants' shelves. Responding to demands for information on how to cure the illness (or about quiet places where one could find a partner for casual sex), innovative printers devised a new method of production. Without going through intermediaries, authors now handed over their script directly to the printer/compositor.[28]

One of the earliest commercially successful syphilis texts was written by Joseph Grunpeck. An ambitious, well-connected young scholar from the university at Augsburg, Grunpeck had travelled to sinful Rome where he became personal secretary to the German Emperor, Maximilian. Somewhere along the line Grunpeck lost his footing in a whorehouse and found himself a victim of the dread pox. In his printed confessions of 1503 he describes the plight of soldiers:

> Some are covered from the head to the knee with a rough scabies dotted with black and hideous lumps. . . . Some . . . moaned and wept and uttered heart rendering cries because of the ulceration of their male organ.[29]

Whether sensationalism or accurate reportage, such books were welcomed by the literate public. Small though this public was, within a few years of its first publication, the *Libellus Josephi Grunpeckii de Mentalagra, Alias Morbo Gallico* went through five Latin editions and then was translated into German where it ran to a further two editions. But perhaps more to the liking of German commercial travellers was Johannes Haslbergk's poem "Von den Welschen Purppeln" (On the Southern Pox), published in Mainz in 1533. Under the guise of moralizing about the dangers of loose women and syphilis, the poem gave a detailed listing of haunts of prostitutes in the German lands. With this guide in hand, any male traveller was guaranteed his night of fun.[30]

Even more rewarding for its author was *Syphilis Sive Morbus Gallicus*, published in 1530 by Girolamo Fracastoro of Verona (1478–1553). A student of philosophy and medicine (in university curricula medicine was counted part of Natural Philosophy), Fracastoro spent much of his time pandering to those in high places. He was a regular correspondent of Fernández de Oviedo, the self-advertised Pliny of savage America. But it was to gentlemen with even greater clout that Fracastoro dedicated his *Syphilis*. The men so honored were the Roman pontiff, Pope Leo X (Giovanni Medici), and Cardinal Pietro Bembo. Bembo, a distinguished Venetian Humanist and a rising power in the Roman Curia, gave Fracastoro editorial guidance and suggested corrections that may have reflected his personal anxieties; the cardinal was a well-known womanizer on intimate terms with Lucrezia Borgia, the daughter of Pope Alexander VI.[31] Doubtless aware of Bembo's sensibilities and possibly also knowing of Martin Luther's devastating accusations of moral corruption in the Roman Church, in his *Syphilis* Fracastoro managed to avoid mentioning that the illness originated in genital contact. His then was an exercise in literary escapism rather than a medical conundrum resolved or a study of sinful lust and moral decay. For this and other services to Catholic humanity, after 1545 Fracastoro was appointed official medical doctor in residence to the fathers of the Church at the Council of Trent. His *Syphilis* continued in print during the remainder of the sixteenth century. Meanwhile his essay on contagion (*De Contagione et Contagiosis Morbis et Curatione*) of 1546 quickly fell into oblivion. There it remained until the late nineteenth century when Whiggish writers suddenly saw it as a precursor of their modern ideas about germs as causal agents of disease.[32]

Aside from booksellers, inspired authors and guaiac wood monopolists, venereal syphilis was also a money-spinner for some categories of low-status health provisioners. Proper medical doctors, possibly aware that their cures were ineffective and sometimes lethal, tended to send inquiring sufferers off to barber-surgeons. In London the Company of Barber-surgeons was incorporated in 1540.

Within the English metropolis and in most sizeable continental towns, barber-surgeons' shops were centers of male sociability. As everyone of any importance knew, a scabby-faced cripple was a rotter to be avoided, while a well-formed, well-dressed man with clear skin and freshly trimmed beard was obviously to be trusted. So finding himself in an awkward situation, a youngish man about town would take himself to a barber. While there he might hint that he had developed strange chancres and ask about treatment. Surviving English evidence suggests that most barber-surgeons recommended a physic containing mercury.[33]

Much less is known about the arrangements made by women, but presumably wives who contracted syphilis from their husbands (or from the live-in servant boy) first turned to a person in the neighborhood they could trust, one of the local midwives. An alert midwife would probably recommend that a pregnant woman abort as soon as possible, knowing that if this were done before the pregnancy was too far advanced she might be able to have children in the future. Yet the availability of trustworthy midwives varied very much from one polity to the next. In many of the German lands, male authority encouraged them to carry on, whereas in England and France authority delighted in destroying their independence. One reason was that town fathers hoped to convert the position of midwife into a career suitable for males.[34] Thus it was highly unlikely that any French male midwife would fall into difficulties of the sort which ruined the career of a female midwife in the Dordogne in 1874. Accused of knowingly passing on her syphilis to ten of her female patients who in turn infected nine husbands and ten children, this woman was found guilty by the court in Brive and sentenced to two years in prison.[35]

Until 1909 when Paul Ehrlich created Salvarsan (a not very effective non-mercury cure), syphilitic gentlemen who were prepared to pay handsomely were often aware that treatments by barber-surgeons were futile. Unwilling to give up hope, they would turn to irregular practitioners who claimed to be able to cure the illness without causing the symptoms which would alert the client's spouse or employer, friends or lovers that he was having a course of mercury treatment.

One of these traders in fear was La Dame Lecadre of Nantes. Typical of thousands of her kind in early nineteenth-century France, she put out an advertisement which claimed that: "having acquired the highest reputation in the treatment of venereal disease, [she] would think that she failed humanity if she did not inform the inhabitants of this commune of her successes in medicine." Lecadre claimed that her remedy did not contain mercury, with its tell-tale symptoms of salivation, loose teeth and falling hair, and that it could be taken by wet-nurses, pregnant women or anyone else, any time, any place. She advised potential clients that they could find her on the first floor opposite the staircase of the Bisson house in the Allée du Boulanger, confident that "the greatest secrecy can be assured."[36] In London, during the same period, a charlatan calling himself Dr Rivers claimed to have a sure cure for the pox. Rivers let it be known that he could be found "at the Golden Ball in Three Kings' Court in Ludgate Hill where he had a light at the door in an evening."[37]

Mercury, by happy coincidence, was named after the Roman god of commerce. As a medication for syphilis it might be rubbed on as a salve, or ingested. This done, the patient was put in a steam bath or covered with heavy blankets. These techniques were based on the humoral theory that a disease poison could be steamed out of the body. Tacked on to this Hellenistic-Arabic theory was the Christian addendum that the agonizing physical pain caused by the treatment, together with its high costs, were a partial propitiation for sin. A course of mercury treatment was regarded as working if a patient's gums decayed and teeth dropped out. Loss of eyelashes, hair and beard were also commonly reported, which was perhaps why in the seventeenth century virile men took to wearing beards and long hair to demonstrate their syphilis-free status, until disease reality—masquerading as fashion—required the use of powdered wigs. Fittingly, the mirrors before which bewigged eighteenth-century gentlemen preened themselves were made of glass coated with mercury.[38]

Changes in Sociability, c. 1480 to c. 1750

By coincidence, the discovery of Europe by *Treponema pallidum* coincided with the winding down of an atypical societal condition—a temporary absence of massive clerical coercion of the sort characteristic of most centuries before our own. During this brief era of openness (which lasted only from the 1450s to the 1490s), town magistrates in Dijon, Augsburg and several hundred other urban places were able to regard their little societies as organic wholes. In a way analogous to the human body, they assumed that each local person had a role appropriate to his or her line of descent, social status, age group and astral influence. As part of their scheme for the well-ordered life, magistrates established special places for sensual pleasures.[39]

A brief survey of mores around 1490 brings us first to a public steam bath. During this golden age, municipally regulated baths attracted the patronage of university scholars, students, respectable artisans and their wives and children. In Geneva, Antwerp or Lyon, on an afternoon a network of married and unmarried friends, male and female, would meet there in the nude to wash, converse and lark about. Since the pools were not fully fenced in, people outside could see what was going on. After 1493, for courting couples the advantages of this system were obvious; a man seen to have infected private parts was clearly not fit to marry. Nor was he fit to patronize a house of prostitution.

On the eve of the syphilis disaster waiting to happen, in scores of towns with populations of more than 4,000–5,000, prostitutes were the pampered inmates of municipal brothels. Following fifteenth-century social theory, these women were kept on hand to provide legitimate outlets for the sexual energies of male apprentices, young newcomers to the town, and journeymen who had yet to finish their craft training. In Dijon and other towns in old Burgundy prostitutes were locally recruited girls from poor families—sometimes gang-raped in their parents' house to set them on their career—known to everyone and a threat to no one. Elsewhere, as in Augsburg and Seville, prostitutes were usually country girls who recruiters knew had no feud-prone family in town to protect them. To ensure that all men knew that the prostitutes were common property available to anyone on request, the girls were required to wear a yellow ribbon, a red beret or other distinguishing mark when they walked about the town. Any girl who showed a clear preference for one client over another would be fined by the brothel keeper. Over time, deductions of this sort might exceed what the girl had earned from servicing four or five men each day.[40]

Yet prostitutes were regarded as part of the civic resources of the town. Writing of the German lands, Lyndal Roper noted that when a great potentate—such as the Emperor Maximilian—and his entourage passed through, custom held that town councillors invite them to spend an evening in the brothel. While in Worms in August 1495 Maximilian told the Reichstag that the new pox was God's punishment for blasphemous cursing; he did not suggest any connection between the sickness and whores. Similarly, in London many quality brothels were on lands in Southwark held by the Bishop of Winchester. In these pleasant haunts foreign ambassadors and other important visitors expected to be entertained at the expense of a great courtier.[41]

Within the community, municipally sponsored loose women had well-defined roles on certain other social occasions, such as the marriage festivities of members of craft guilds. Custom held that prostitutes should capture the groom and then allow his bride to ransom him, symbolizing his passage from reckless youth—and nights out in the brothel—to married respectability.[42]

Though perhaps not entirely aware of it, in an era in which the average marriage lasted less than ten years before death removed one of the partners, in using a brothel young males showed their acceptance of a social system based on gross inequalities in male influence over women. Because of the fortunes elderly patricians might leave their widows—the power of money—

men of advanced age who chose to remarry after their wives had died in childbirth had virtually their pick of young women. Yet the graybeards of forty-five or fifty who might dip into the local pool of marriageable women two or three times realized that it was in their own interest to provide callow youth with centers of sexual sociability where their passions could be spent and, as it were, neutralized. According to these careful calculations, it was not regarded as proper if married men or priests were found patronizing the brothel more than once or twice a year. To ensure that precept bore some relationship with practice, spies among the women reported errant males to the town council.

In the decade immediately before the appearance of the new venereal disease around 1493, the tide began to turn against municipal-sponsored brothels and steam baths. Among the new pressures *not* directly related to venereal diseases was the rapid growth of population in rural areas recovering from the earlier outbreaks of bubonic plague. Younger sons, who had been turned out of the natal villages by parents determined to pass the family farm intact to the eldest boy, took the high road to town to find work. Once there, though initially willing to work for low wages, they often found it hard to make ends meet and sorted out their frustrations in the town whorehouse. Knife fights between low-wage newcomers and resident town youth began to make evenings there less than pleasant.

Uncontrolled immigration also led to increasingly harsh attitudes towards the able-bodied poor begging for alms. Working in combination with other factors, these attitudes enabled reforming friars and clerics to liberate themselves from the naturalistic world-view of self-help by Good Works which lay people had imposed on them earlier. Determined to reassert their authority, they grew more vocal in their denunciations of lust, cupidity and vice.[43]

Adopting only a slightly different tone of criticism, the Humanists, the voices of the secular Renaissance, intensified their campaign to educate a new type of ruler of the sort they mistakenly supposed had been the standard type in the old Roman Empire—literate, historically informed, pious, couth, virtuous and civilized. Though woolly-minded, Humanists could not but notice that several of the courtiers they had in training were being carried off by what was taken to be a sexually transmitted disease. One of the youthful dead was Lorenzo, the Medici Duke of Urbino. When, following the custom, Lorenzo had climbed into his marriage bed in the presence of his friends it had been noticed that he had strange boils and blisters on his legs. His wife Maddalena later died while giving birth to their only child, innocently infected, so the rumor went, by Lorenzo's French disease. Lorenzo himself died in 1519 at the age of twenty-seven.[44]

Thus after July 1495 when Charles VIII's mercenary host broke up and took their infected parts to the four corners of Europe, steam-bath operators and brothel keepers faced growing public awareness of new disease forms, both physical and metaphysical. At the physical level was what Desiderius Erasmus of Rotterdam and his Humanist friends termed the "new plague." Writing in 1526 of the precipitous decline of steam-baths in his part of Europe, Erasmus (then in his early sixties) noted that "Twenty-five years ago, nothing was more fashionable in Brabant, today there are none, the new plague has taught us to avoid them."[45] On the metaphysical level, harried steam-bath operators confronted the notion being spread by medical doctors influenced by the teachings of hegemonic Spain that bathing in water opened the pores in the skin to dangerous airborne things which (or possibly *who*) might cause death or sickness. Out in the countryside, resolutely unwashed peasants had known this all along.

The closure of public steam baths in the 1520s and 1530s on grounds of hygiene (however interpreted) was paralleled by the closure of the municipally regulated brothels. But in this matter, regard for physical health seems to have run second to regard for citizens' spiritual well-being. Beginning in the German lands with Martin Luther in the 1520s and then in France and Switzerland with John Calvin, the Protestant and Catholic reformations in religion broke into full flood.

In vilifying the Old Church in a regional polity they had targeted for takeover, university-educated Protestant reformers often made use of raw sexual imagery. Openly comparing the Pope in Rome to a syphilitic Great Whore of Babylon (as in the German Bible turned out by Martin Luther) the old religion was represented as rotten, corrupt and immoral. To illustrate the point with local examples, preachers denounced priests who had had common recourse to the town brothel despite their vows of chastity. Reformers also chanced to remember that Thomas Aquinas (d. 1274), the greatest of the theologians of the old medieval Church, had approved of public prostitution. St Thomas had likened it to a cesspit in a palace, an essential part of the fittings.[46]

And so the brothels were closed, in part because they did not fit into reformed ideas of what could be tolerated in a properly ordered society and in part, as in Zwickau in March 1526, because "so many young journeymen have been poisoned with the French disease by prostitutes."[47] Once they had shut their brothels town councillors were determined to keep them shut if only to confirm their own righteousness. In Zwickau in 1541, councillors noted that preachers had often accused them of causing poor people to be whipped for moral offenses but only lightly fining rich men who had committed the same offense. Learning that a rich patrician was running a profitable whorehouse on the sly, they meted out exemplary punishment. Herr George Wereman was flogged and forced to reveal his low status brothel-keeping accomplices who—status considerations being what they were—were then sent into exile.[48]

In London, the first part of the offshore island fully exposed to John Calvin's reinterpreted word of God, reformers noted in the early 1550s that the only officially sanctioned brothels were run by the estate management office of the Catholic Bishop of Winchester, Stephen Gardiner. Between 1555 and 1558 the same bishop helped his Catholic queen, Mary Tudor, incinerate more than 300 Protestant martyrs. After Mary's death and the accession of her politique half-sister Elizabeth, vengeful Calvinist reformers redoubled their efforts to reform humankind. They began with brothel keepers and prostitutes. Undeterred by whore-patronizing great courtiers who threatened reprisals, in 1564 London authorities closed down the brothels on the Bishop of Winchester's South Bank estate and a few years later put the special morals court, the Bridewell, into high gear.[49]

Bending itself to the moral tide it had helped bring into being, the Catholic Church after 1563 also cracked down hard on extra-marital sex. In Spain, neighbors were encouraged to bring information to agents of the Inquisition so that offenders could be tracked down and reformed. In Toledo, especially fierce anti-prostitution campaigns were run in 1566–70, 1581–85 and 1601–5. During those years, similar campaigns took place in Seville, the gateway to America.[50]

In summing up the new moral values which touched upon gender differences and the realm of *Treponema pallidum*, let us begin with reformers' ideas about males. If, as university-educated clerics initially held, ordinary laymen could, through introspection, Bible reading and prayer put themselves in possession of all these virtues which women lacked (women being naturally witless), they obviously would have no need for prostitutes or for any alternative forms of sex. From this it clearly followed that after puberty, in the ten or fifteen years before a man was in a financial position to marry, he should remain celibate just as, presumably, Christ had been. First-generation reformers also reinterpreted Holy Scriptures to prove that God intended that *all* men accept the married state as their behavioral norm. Referring to the commandment said to have been handed down at Sinai, "Honor thy father," sons were cautioned to pay heed to parental advice in maintaining moral cleanliness, and when choosing their spouse.[51]

The Catholic Church, not to be outdone by the Protestant heretics from whom it intended to win back the whole of Europe, trimmed its sails to the wind. At the Council of Trent it lent support to greater parental control over the making of marriages. To enforce its authority over parents, the Church used what was essentially a new instrument, the *tête-à-tête* confessional between penitent and priest.[52]

As for women, there was not much in the reformed religion for those who wanted to maintain a separate sphere of their own. In Protestant lands the honorable vocation of celibate nun was abolished and with it the notion that a woman could usefully serve Christ by withdrawing from the company of men, or indeed by serving in any independent capacity whatsoever. In Catholic lands, following the precepts of St Charles Borromeo of Milan, reformers brought women's religious orders under the control of bishops. The same bishops were also coming to control the activities of midwives.

Building on Aristotelian and Platonic ideas that women were morally, mentally and physically inferior to men, Protestant and Catholic Church ideologues (anticipating their nineteenth-century secular successors) held that all daughters of apple-eating Eve were potential prostitutes, and that the women who had fulfilled this potential were the agents chiefly responsible for spreading syphilis.[53] Martin Luther set the tone when he lashed out against "dreadful, shabby, stinking, loathsome and syphilitic [whores] . . . who can give their disease to ten, twenty, thirty and more good people."[54] The idea that males were equally useful syphilis hosts seems never to have entered this reformer's mind.

Following the new ideals of gender, prostitutes were no longer seen as flowers in the crown of a properly governed city as they had been in the early 1490s; instead they were regarded as petty criminals. Yet prostitution continued in being, if for no other reason than that poor girls needed the cash. In big cities, an ordinary prostitute who managed to keep parasitic pimps off her back could earn as much in a night as she might earn in a week as an overworked servant in the household of a respectable burgher.[55] No less importantly, urban prostitution also continued because a male clientele was always on hand. Civil and military authorities had long known that wherever soldiers were billeted, brothels were an easy way to keep them out of worse mischief, such as burning down peasant villages for an afternoon's fun. Brothels also served the needs of young countrymen only recently come to town who, in order to assert their new-found independence, rather liked to do something that their parents and clerics back home would consider nasty and bad.

Thus after the volcanic fires of religious reformation burned themselves out with the winding down of the Thirty Years War in 1648, advanced ideas about moral reformation and the need for constant vigilance against "lust" continued, particularly in the towns. Out in the countryside peasant elders remained selective in choosing what to absorb of town-based teachings and what to ignore. Yet it would seem they rather liked the new-to-towns notion that parents should choose who and when their offspring should marry, especially since it was virtually the same idea that countrymen had long been putting into practice.[56] With this juncture of urban-reformed-new and peasant-elder-old, the way lay open for the bursting forth of a new form of sexual authoritarianism.

The Competition for Control

Starting from small beginnings in Switzerland *c.* 1690–1700, then growing in the 1750s to full maturity in the writings of a Swiss medical doctor who was regarded as one of the flowers of the Enlightenment, the flat-earth/false knowledge of the learned few gave rise to the notion that it was better for a man to turn to a prostitute than to find satisfaction in solitary masturbation.

Detailed information about the consequences of this exposure to syphilis remains somewhat sparse, as well it might, given John Graunt's discovery of the near invisibility of what was a fairly common disease. However, combings from the past suggest that every year thousands of young men desperate for sexual release, but scared out of their wits by what anti-masturbationists said were the terrible consequences of that solitary act, were driven into the arms of prostitutes. Since the disease bacterium could not live more than a few minutes outside a human—whether female prostitute or male client—it follows that by providing a continuing flow of hosts, the anti-masturbation campaign made a major contribution to the maintenance of populations of *Treponema pallidum*. Let us investigate how this situation came into being.

Writing in the Pietist tradition of the 1690s a Swiss minister of religion named Jean Frédéric Osterwald claimed in *The Nature of Uncleanness Considered* that without self-discipline in matters sexual a young person was likely to grow up to be a wastrel of no use to God or man. Castigated in 1710 by an anonymous anti-masturbationist for not actually naming the "uncleanness" of his title, Osterwald was one of many good men concerned about the future of Switzerland now that the Confederation had cut its ties with the German Empire. With this political development, employment opportunities for mercenary soldiers (unwanted village sons) had dropped off. Accordingly, for cleric Osterwald, the only way forward lay in rigid self-discipline and control. Interpreted in terms of sexual behavior, this meant that until such time as a fully mature man entered into late marriage, he should neither masturbate nor engage in any other sort of sexual activity.[57]

Among learned upholders of the Great Tradition, what Osterwald was saying was essentially new. According to a classic text by Galen, in the ancient Greek world naive, innocent young men had been taught how to masturbate by Hermes (the Greek equivalent for the Roman god, Mercury). Influenced in part by this precedent, during the Middle Ages the Christian Church had considered masturbation only a minor transgression. By the sixteenth century, many parents did not regard it as even this. Writing as a specialist in anatomy and sexuality, Gabriel Fallopio (for whom fallopian tubes were named) advised parents to prepare their sons for their adult responsibility to father children by drawing with their hands on the boy's penis until it became strong and long. At the court of Henry IV of France, the king's friends amused themselves by strengthening the manly organ of the infant dauphin in this way. In 1696 Dr Nicolas Venette of La Rochelle, author of the popular sex guide *Tableau de l'amour conjugal*, exemplified gender differences by claiming that an unattended man could empty his sperm sack whenever he chose, whereas a woman was burdened with tired old sexual juices that she could not release on her own.[58]

In establishing how the anti-masturbation campaign came into being (to the greater glory of *Treponema pallidum*) one must not overlook pressures emerging at the village level. Particularly in regions blitzed by Calvinistic teachings, medical irregulars able to speak to local people in their own dialect were quick to appreciate that village elders were keen to demonstrate their own moral worth by searching out the sexual "failings" of the young. Yet in selling throwaway tracts directed against self-abuse (usually attached to a bottle containing some quick cure), wandering irregulars were at a disadvantage compared to established health provisioners. Whatever irregulars wrote before they were moved on was a one-shot affair that locally based medical doctors were unlikely to accept as information worth passing on to their clients. However, the situation would be entirely different if an anti-masturbationist author could legitimately show that he was a medically qualified person of good repute.[59]

In 1710, a "Dr Bekkers," who seems to have been a surgeon of Swiss-German, German or Dutch provenance, published an anonymous tract called, in English, *Onania, Or the Heinous Sin of Self-Pollution And All its Frightful Consequences, in Both Sexes Considered with Spiritual and Physical Advice to those, Who Have Already Injur'd Themselves by This Abominable Practice. And Seasonable Admonition to the Youth of the Nation, (of both Sexes) and Those Whose Tuition They are Under, Whether Parents, Guardians, Masters or Mistresses.*[60] The author cited *The Nature of Uncleanness Considered* by Osterwald in order to criticize him for failing to address masturbation by name.

The "Onania" of the title refers to the Old Testament Book of Genesis, chapter XXXVIII, verse 9 in which Onan either masturbated or withdrew before ejaculation. In an early Middle Eastern setting where God's chosen people were few in number and surrounded on every side by fast-breeding pagan tribes, the act of casting one's sperm on the ground rather than using it to fertilize a Jewish womb could be seen as rebellion against God.

Though "Dr Bekkers" was reluctant to identify himself by name (perhaps fearing that his clientele would regard him as a libertine and take their custom elsewhere), in the English edition he let it be known that he could be contacted at Mr Crouch's London bookstall. For a guinea, he would send contrite masturbators some medicine by return of post. Those who wanted a personal consultation about their problem were advised to report to their nearest surgeon and "open their Case, which if he be a sagacious Man [as all proper barber-surgeons obviously were], may be done with a very few hints."[61] *Onania* proved to be a popular success and went through nineteen editions, each one incorporating more letters purporting to be from contrite masturbators.

In 1756, forty years after "Dr Bekkers" introduced the subject of masturbation into medical discourse, S. A. A. D. Tissot, a fully trained physician and member of the Medico-Physical Society of Basle, announced in a treatise also called *Onania* that men of his rank were now fully competent to pronounce on matters of male sexuality. Aware of scholarly proprieties, Tissot first published his work in Latin. A French translation appeared in 1760 (which ran into difficulties with the French royal censor), followed then by translations into German and Italian. Thereafter, new editions of (to give it its English title) *Onanism: Or a Treatise Upon the Disorders Produced by Masturbation: Or The Dangerous Effects of Secret and Excessive Venery*, were published in rapid succession. Until almost our own time it remained the seminal book in medicalized society's campaign against masturbation. An updated French edition still addressed to parents was published in 1991.[62]

In understanding why Dr Tissot's attack on what he took to be an "unnatural" practice proved so persuasive to literate adults in search of power over others, the historian first turns to the milieu in which it was produced. In France, one element in this milieu was the Mercantilist concern with declining or static population. Here where the number of the king's subjects was growing much more slowly than in rival realms, solitary sexual practices that did not lead to population increase were seen as anti-social. Undoubtedly contributing to the book's popularity as well were recent changes in the structure of the bourgeois family. With the growth of domestic privacy and inward-lookingness, the command structure of the nuclear family required buttressing. In attacking the masturbatory practices of their sons, new-style bourgeois fathers were using a splendid new disciplinary tool.[63] When this tool was fully honed (in the Victorian era), medicalized fathers were advised to show a masturbating son a sharp knife to make it clear that part of the offending penis might be snipped off at his father's whim.[64]

Tissot, in masturbation the creator of full-blown medical authoritarianism, linked two worlds, the not-yet-dead theological and the still only partially formed secular-crusader-medical. Born in 1728 in the French-speaking Pays de Vaud, he was the son of a Calvinist minister and his Geneva-born wife. After studying philosophy at Geneva, young Tissot had deliberately chosen the profession of medicine—he trained at Montpellier—rather than the ministry, claiming that he saw in medicine a way of helping the poor to live better lives. His first paid employment was as a medical doctor to respectable impoverished folk in Lausanne. Later he taught at the University of Pavia where he was instrumental in setting up one of the clinics pinpointed by Michel Foucault as a birthplace of modern medicine.[65]

Tissot's recent biographer sees him as a benevolent paternalist in the best tradition of the Enlightenment.[66] At his most acceptable, Tissot saw his mission as challenging people "to improve their health by a better understanding of hygiene *under the guidance of a physician.*"[67] To this end he published *Avis au peuple sur sa santé* (in English: "Advice to the People in General with Regard to Their Health"). The book was soon translated into twelve other European languages. In it Tissot presented himself as a progressive physician writing for the benefit of country medical practitioners and educated laymen who wanted professional advice when confronted by disease, rather than the old-hat nostrums they would get from charlatans.[68] It seems very likely that because physicians trusted *Advice* and regarded it as a practical up-to-date guide, they were also persuaded to accept the veracity and wisdom of what Tissot said about the horrible consequences of masturbation.

Some idea of the competition which Tissot's *Onanism* faced in his native Switzerland can be gained by looking at a rival anti-masturbation tract published in Lausanne in 1760 by a religiously motivated person who called himself P. du Toit de Mambrini. In *De l'Onanisme: ou discours philosophique et moral sur la luxure artificielle et sur tous les crimes relatifs* de Mambrini cited the scriptural Sodom and Gomorrah and cautioned young people: "do not abandon the invisible conductor of youth. Listen to Jesus your Saviour: for the sake of Christ resist temptation." Using similar scriptural props, he pleaded with parents to discipline their children against masturbation, "this infernal epidemic" which "is *superior in lecherousness* to the simple and natural act of fornication."[69]

For his part, in *Onanism* Tissot as learned physician ignored the religious implications of masturbation. Instead, when setting forth what he claimed were the consequences of solitary sex, he drew heavily on what "Dr Bekkers" had written forty years before. According to that earlier tract, masturbation hindered growth in youth, caused gonorrhea, led to fainting fits and epilepsy and diluted the male seed needed for procreation. If a married man who as a youth had masturbated was able to stir himself to an erection at all, it was likely that the children resulting from this exercise would be so weak that they would be a "Misery to themselves, a Dishonor to the Human Race, and a Scandal to their Parents."[70]

In his capacity as a university-educated medical doctor, about the only really new thing Tissot contributed to the discourse on masturbation was support for the old idea, derived from Hippocrates, that since there was a direct connection between blood supply and sperm supply, masturbation would cut down the richness of blood and lead to "sensible diminution of the powers, of the memory, and even of the understanding . . . the organs of generation are hereby enfeebled [other symptoms would include] bloody urine, loss of appetite, head-aches." From this other horrors would follow.[71]

Soon after the first Latin edition of Tissot's *Onanism* appeared, another Alpine author added his weight to the anti-masturbation campaign. This was Jean Jacques Rousseau, arguably the most influential of the *philosophes*. Among his other activities (fathering children, locking them away in orphanages and forgetting them) Rousseau was interested in defining what constituted "unnatural" sex. In *Emile* (1762), the tract on child-rearing which everyone in the fashionable world read, Rousseau warned tutors in charge of adolescents of the need to

> watch carefully over the young man; he can protect himself from all other foes, but it is for you to protect him against himself. Never leave him night or day, or at least share his room; do not let him go to bed till he is sleepy, and let him rise as soon as he wakes. . . . It would be a dangerous matter if instinct taught your pupil to abuse his senses; if once he acquires this dangerous habit he is ruined. From that time forward, body and soul will be enervated: he will carry to the grave the sad effects of this habit, the most fatal habit which a young man can acquire.[72]

In an early English edition of *Onanism* Tissot quoted Rousseau's admonition word for word. But in a social setting in which professional qualifications were beginning to count, there was a great difference between throwaway remarks about masturbation by a famous literary man and the considered judgment of one of the most "enlightened" medical doctors of the age.[73]

For those prepared to accept the paradigm of pseudo-science within which he worked, Tissot proved that there was a vital difference between solitary sex and heterosexual fornication. In the case of fornication, the mutual pleasure ("joy") this supreme act of sociability gave the two partners restored any damage that might have been done to the blood system for, as he wittily noted, "one inspires what the other perspires." On the other hand, solitary hands-on sex diminished the supply of bodily juices and put nothing back in their place. Following this logic—a dubious path that no modern expert would take—Tissot advised that "masturbation was more pernicious than excesses committed with women."[74] In short, it would seem that for this member of the medical Enlightenment no less than for his scripture-obsessed contemporary in Lausanne (P. du Toit de Mambrini), it was far better to risk hot piss (syphilis) than to masturbate.[75]

More than a century after Tissot had been called to his fathers in 1797, the preference for sex with a prostitute rather than solitary enjoyment was accepted by professional health workers as medically sound. Writing of advice given him in the late 1860s, a man racked with syphilis recalled that:

> The doctor . . . strongly advised me to drop masturbation. He even suggested certain houses where I might meet women of a better class . . . as a lesser evil than the risk of disease in masturbation.[76]

Summarizing what little is known of the situation in Victorian England, Michael Mason concluded that given the near-universal belief that masturbation was both evil and unhealthy "it seems likely that there were many consulting rooms in which relations with prostitutes or mistresses were cheerfully regarded." And as recently as 1920, medical doctor J. Charsley Mackwood claimed that the Moral Purity movement (which was directed against all pre-marital sex) had committed a "crime against humanity" by so frightening young men about the dangers of syphilis that they had taken to the far *more lethal* sport of masturbation.[77]

During the first high tide of Victorian values, England's headmasters, another professional group with authoritarian tendencies, initiated anti-masturbatory campaigns in the public schools (i.e. private schools). Twenty years later—coinciding with the establishment of the first chair in dermatology and syphilology by the French in 1879—the hunt for masturbators in public schools moved into high gear. Thereafter in the changing rooms of the potential rulers of empire, rumors of masturbators being punished by castration, circumcision or by being locked up in lunatic asylums circulated freely. After 1870, with the belated establishment of compulsory schooling at the primary level for all English children, castration rumors began to circulate among working-class boys as well. Then following the near-failure of British manhood in the 1899–1902 Boer War (discussed below), authority figures widened the front of their anti-masturbatory campaign. In the standard Boy Scout handbook used in the first quarter of the twentieth century, Robert Baden-Powell claimed that self-abuse "brings with it weakness of head and heart, and, if persisted in, idiocy and lunacy." It didn't take *much* imagination for a boy to add, following the teachings of the president of the Royal College of Physicians, Jonathan Hutchinson, "and the attention of a surgeon's knife."[78]

In imperialized Egypt in 1882, doctors in the employ of the British occupying force held that masturbation caused trachoma, a serious eye disease that could lead to blindness. Robert Koch, in Alexandria in 1883 to study epidemic cholera, soon put paid to this fantasy. Placing eye pus from a cross-section of trachoma sufferers under a microscope he discovered the Koch–Weeks bacillus to be the causal agent of the disease. Yet it does not seem that the founder of modern medicine made any attempt to overturn the curious notions about masturbation inherited from the Enlightenment. As late as 1899, a medical specialist in the German homeland, Hermann Rohledler, rehearsed "scientific" arguments to prove that masturbation had serious effects on a man's central nervous system.[79]

In his assessment of such things, Michel Foucault wrote of the use of specialized knowledge as part of the mechanisms of power and of "the point where power reaches into the very grain of individuals, touches their bodies, and inserts itself into their actions and attitudes, their discourses, learning processes and everyday lives."[80] This reaching into the very grain of individuals did not happen all at once, but obviously it was well underway by the 1850s and 1860s.

In a recent article entitled "Forbidden by God, Despised by Men: Masturbation, Medical Warnings, Moral Panic and Manhood in Great Britain, 1850–1950," Lesley Hall discusses the ways in which this entrepreneurial campaign affected ordinary men. As her database Hall used the correspondence sent in between 1918 and 1958 by terrified reprobate masturbators to Marie Stopes, author of a bestseller on sexuality. Though these correspondents were self-selected and not necessarily a typical cross-section of British middle- and working-class males, one can assume that they reflected general attitudes. One letter sums up the dilemma confronted by the many men who were keeping populations of *Treponema pallidum* in being: "Before I was married I used to have unions three or four times a night, two or three times a week with different girls in the hope of curing myself [of masturbation] but it was of no use."[81] During these decades *Treponema pallidum* flourished as never before, fed by, among others, terrified masturbators in search of cure.

In Britain before World War I, professional medical thinking was summed up in a review of Iwan Bloch's *The Sexual Life of Our Time in Its Relation to Modern Civilization* which had recently been translated from the German. Here Bloch called for a new openness in the understanding of human sexuality so that young people would not find themselves diseased through ignorance. English medical professionals would have none of this. Writing anonymously in the prestigious *Journal of Tropical Medicine and Hygiene* in 1908, a reviewer concluded:

> That books of this kind do any good when placed in the hands of the public is questionable. The problems to be dealt with are really *how to check masturbation* during the years immediately succeeding puberty, and the means of preventing young men cohabiting with prostitutes. These are really hygienic problems of national and racial importance. In Britain [in supposed contrast with the Kaiser's Germany] we attempt to deal with the first problem by encouraging athletics and athleticism in school and college life. . . . To teach a young man to be proud of his frame and his physical accomplishments is to divert his attention from his sexual functions and to favour a physical state averse to sexual ascendancy. . . . Literature relating to sexual matters is sure of a market, but we have lately debarred it even from our public urinals.

Summing up, the reviewer concluded that Bloch's "*The Sexual Life of Our Times* . . . [is] pernicious literature."[82] Other contributions to the discourse which favored *Treponema pallidum* were lectures like that delivered in the London School of Tropical Medicine in the spring of 1906. This held that:

> The proposal that young persons should be told the meaning and danger of promiscuous intercourse and the *terrible effect of acquired syphilis* was dismissed as impractical, and as wholly inefficacious [*sic*] and undeterrent.[83]

With this, *Treponema pallidum* and a public condemned to ignorance by the medical profession were condemned to be partners for many more years.

Treponema Pallidum *and the Rise of Mass Society*

Just as European anti-masturbation campaigns were grist to the mill of *Treponema pallidum*, so too was the nineteenth-century surge in human numbers. For a world not yet familiar with population explosions the regional burst of growth seen as most alarming was that which happened in England and the Lowlands of Scotland. Here between 1800 and 1850, population doubled. By 1910 it had doubled again to number 40.8 million, four times what it had been in 1800. More typical of West Europe as a whole was the situation in the German lands, where between 1800 and World War I population increased by 240 percent, resulting in a total of 58.5 million. Sweden, with a population of 5.5 million in 1910, had in the course of the previous ninety years grown at a rate similar to that of the German lands to the south.[84]

Also germane to the well-being of *Treponema pallidum* during the century 1815–1914, when inter-European wars were of brief duration and invading soldiers relatively rare, was the percentage of population cutting ties with stable networks of elders and cousins in village communities to become urban dwellers. In the German Empire it was not until 1890 that urbanites finally outnumbered rural people. Yet once the balance was tipped, change was very rapid. By 1914 Berlin had 2.1 million inhabitants, Hamburg 1.1 million and the collection of cities in the Ruhr another million. In Europe overall by 1910 there were thirty-two urban places, each with a population in excess of half a million. If at a guesstimate 10 percent of this urban population harbored *Treponema pallidum* (because of the stigma attached to syphilis, there continued to be massive under-reporting), this totalled 1.3 million cases—a very sizeable disease reservoir indeed.[85]

In a Britain which anticipated by half a century the crash urbanization of Germany (as early as 1851 more than half the British population lived in cities), the social cost of urban drift was particularly high. Because of liberal (free enterprise) ideas about the provision of clean water, sewage disposal and similar basic urban amenities, life-chances for the unskilled rural young drawn to the city were considerably poorer than they were back in the countryside. In the best parts of the "green and pleasant land," the rural south-west, the south and the rural midlands, surveys at mid-century showed a life expectation at birth of around fifty years. In contrast, in highly urbanized Manchester, Newcastle-upon-Tyne, Birmingham, Liverpool, Bristol and inner London, life expectancy was less than thirty-five years. In terms of human perceptions and responses to the threat of venereal disease, this may well have meant that working-class youths who assumed that they would die at an early age from tuberculosis or some other urban disease, saw no reason to trouble with complicated precautions when tempted with pre-marital or extra-marital sex.[86]

Among upper-class Britons who took on board the preachings of Herbert Spencer and later Social Darwinists, figures on life expectancy among the unwashed urban masses were of much less pressing concern than were the periodic reports on army recruitment. During the Crimean War of 1854–56, medical inspectors rejected as physically unfit 42 percent of town-bred recruits; rural rejection rates stood at only 17 percent. During the next half-century, as urbanization and the impact of gentlemanly capitalism proceeded apace, the reported condition of British men deteriorated further.

Between 1893 and 1902 army statistics showed that 34.6 percent of the national total of volunteers were medically unfit. Presaging what many feared would become the future norm, far higher rejection rates were found in major industrial centers than in the countryside. In Manchester (seen as the prototype industrial city) at the beginning of the Boer War in 1899, 66 percent of the volunteers (8,000 out of 12,000) were judged completely unsuitable for service. What gave highly placed observers even greater cause for alarm was that the recruiters, who one might expect to have had some idea of what a healthy Briton looked like, had already accepted as typical specimens of manhood those Mancunian youths whom medical doctors later rejected as "walking invalids." Other statistically based perceptions also suggested a nation in decline. In 1845, 105 out of every 1,000 men were unable to match up to the army's height requirement of five feet six inches. This was bad enough. However, by 1900 there was a fivefold increase in stunted men, with 565 out of every 1,000 failing the army requirement. At a time when the politicians and other agents of the gentlemanly capitalists of London were creating a white-ruled empire on which the sun never set, it seemed obvious that the population of the motherland was undergoing some sort of "racial" decline.

Seen as even worse was the fact that this decline was not a secret known only to the members of the special committee of the Privy Council set up to study racial hygiene. Instead it was part of an all too visible reality which all the world could see. During the Boer War when journalists representing the world press were present in force, tall, hefty Boer farmers faced British enlisted men who were under five feet tall and weighing less than seven stone two pounds (100 pounds). Confronted with this embarrassing display of their pygmy troops, Social Darwinists, eugenicists and publicists of empire spoke more and more openly about national efficiency, manliness and the need for British adolescents to keep their racial tools clean.[87]

In the six decades after 1850 in which intellectuals, school teachers, and yellow press journalists created myths of nationalism to replace earlier localistic loyalties, the political classes of each nation state were determined to confront the threat of syphilis in their own special way. Yet fearing that they might be caught short in confronting a disease about which the medical profession was still in a quandary, each also paid close attention to the venereal disease control measures adopted by its neighbors. Seminal to this interchange were developments in France, the country which since the time of Louis XIV had been the cultural pace-setter of Europe.

In this however there was a paradox. The France that in 1789 had shown all the world how to overthrow a political *ancien régime*, in 1870 still remained a predominantly peasant society. Though there was much tinsel and glitter about its court and capital, it boasted a very modest amount of modern-style (i.e. German) industry. It contained a few large cities—Paris had nearly 3 million people, Lyon and Marseilles a half million each—but not until 1931 did more than half the population live in cities.

At the national level moreover, French planners were troubled by the unwillingness—or inability—of ordinary people to produce children at a rate comparable to that of rival nation states. In 1898, an expert complained that

> other countries double their population at a good rate: Germany in 98 years, Sweden in 82, Denmark in 73, England in 63, Austria in 62, Norway in 51, while in France to double population we must wait for 334 years.[88]

Other sources show that between 1881 and 1911 (when most peasants had finally been converted from localistic dwellers of *pays* into proper, nationalistic, Frenchmen) the average rate of population growth was only about 0.1 percent per annum, compared to 1.2 percent for Germany and 1.1 percent for England and Wales. In other words France was expanding at less than one tenth the rate of its rivals. Though *Treponema pallidum* may have played a role in this (aborted or stillborn babies, mothers sterilized by disease), at the human level it would seem that French adults were unwilling to serve the State by producing large families to serve as cheap labor in textile factories, or after 1830 as settlers in Algeria, or as cannon fodder for dynastic fiascos like the Franco-Prussian War.

In any case, it was in a low-growth France out of step with high-growth rivals that after 1850–60 a distinctively scientific/pseudo-scientific hysteria about syphilis was first expressed. Through the agency of international conferences held in Paris in 1889, in Brussels in 1899 and 1902 and again in Paris in 1919, this French-generated discourse permeated the medical thinking of the Western world.[89]

As the historian Alain Corbin has reminded us, until the mid-1850s, the respectable bourgeoisie of Paris, *tout le monde*, could assume that prostitution (and associated syphilis) was a problem that only affected social groupings other than their own.[90] In this perception, the sort of men whose sexual needs required prostitutes were transients, either urban-based soldiers doing their seven-year stints, or unmarried laborers from outlying provinces who came each season to Paris to work and then returned to their *pays*.

In response to the needs of the armed defenders of the State (the bourgeoisie were notorious for ignoring peasant migrant needs), an institution known as Registration was established in 1802. Based in cities with barracks-housed soldiers, the scheme permitted police medics (usually males) to inspect the bodies of prostitutes (females) using a speculum, popularly known as the State Penis, to determine whether they had syphilis. The scheme worked to the satisfaction of the political masters during the first half of the century.

Then as a result of Second Empire prosperity, more and more rural migrants stayed on to become Parisians and brought their village sweethearts and wives with them. Fashioning themselves into Parisians who followed a narrowly correct artisan or *petit bourgeois* life-style, these new city-dwellers confined their sexuality to marriage, using *coitus interruptus*, abortion or midwives' teas to keep things under control. This conservative behavioral pattern gave no cause for hysteria about syphilis.

As a result of this and of the "Haussmannization" of Paris and other city centers in the 1860s, registered prostitutes lost much of their clientele at the lower end of the social spectrum. Public buildings and spaces had replaced the tight-packed medieval maze of streets, dead-end alleys, cheap rooming houses and tenements in which migrants and workers had formerly lived. Responding to this gentrification, wily prostitutes adjusted their marketing techniques to attract the bourgeois paterfamilias. Bourgeois males proved willing. Breaking with the custom of keeping only a wife for motherhood and a mistress or two for sex, in increasing numbers they took to finding casual pleasure with jazzed-up young working-class prostitutes.

Spot checks in brothels showed that this new clientele seldom used the English-designed protective rubber condoms which had been invented in the 1840s, but then, neither did working-class males. Both instead continued to believe that douching with water immediately after coitus would kill off any syphilis.[91] Not until German scientists at the Berlin Academy discovered the bacterial causal agent of the disease in 1905 was the futility of post-coital washing recognized by specialists. But because of the medical conspiracy of silence about disgusting venereal disease, this knowledge was for long kept hidden from the general public.

In the mid-1870s, after the German military had destroyed the French Second Empire and sat on the sidelines while bourgeois Versailles tore working-class Paris apart (graphically described by Emile Zola), bourgeois moral entrepreneurs began to mold prostitution and syphilis together into a coherent ideology of anguish. In this, the leader was Alfred Fournier, soon to be appointed to the first chair of syphilology at the Hôpital Saint Louis. Using the professional jargon of the Clinic—which nineteenth-century patriots and, in our own time, Foucault held made France the medical center of the world—Fournier claimed that the third stage of syphilis caused total collapse of the nervous system and with it, insanity. Bursting with the pride of flat-earth science he asserted that:

> It emerges from recent research that syphilis can, because of its hereditary consequences, debase and corrupt the species by producing inferior, decadent, dystrophic and deficient beings. Yes, deficient, they can be physically

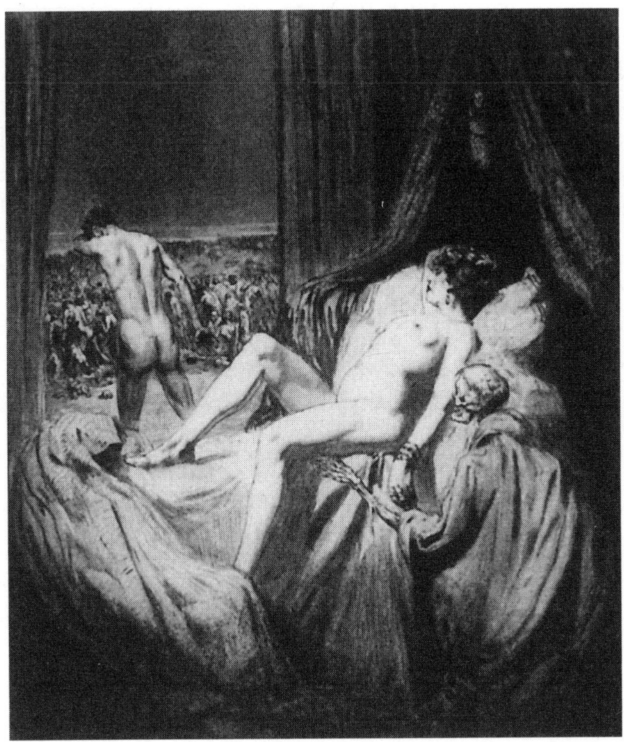

12. Sin, syphilis and skeletons. Nineteenth-century watercolor by R. Cooper.

> deficient . . . or they can be mentally deficient, being, according to the degree of their intellectual debasement, retarded, simple-minded, unbalanced, insane, imbecilic or idiotic.[92]

Accepted across the Channel by experts such as Dr S. A. K. Strahan (who doubled as a barrister at law) as "one of the greatest authorities upon syphilis which the World at present possesses," Alfred Fournier was taken to have proved that:

> Aided by drunkenness, poverty and squalor, syphilis is largely responsible for that residuum of humanity to be found in the dark places of our great centres of population, from which are recruited the consumptive, the scrofulous, the epileptic, the prostitute, the idiot, the habitual drunkard, the instinctive criminal, and the insane.[93]

By 1905, Fournier's son and successor as purveyor of false knowledge claimed that *all* the dread diseases to which children and adults were prone—chronic masturbation, delirium tremens and tuberculosis—might have been inherited from a syphilitic ancestor *several generations back*. Since the Fournier ideology held that syphilis was carried in a man's sperm, medical convention now recommended that before a woman married she should study her intended spouse's family photographs and visit living family members. Her purpose was to discover whether any of them had the hollowed-out upper incisor teeth that Jonathan Hutchinson identified as a certain indicator of syphilis, along with deafness, bodily deformities or mental problems. If any living or dead family member showed evidence of these, medical wisdom held that they had been caused by hereditary syphilis. A family carrying this was tainted and, if allowed to breed, would further degenerate the racial stock of France.[94]

At a time when anarchists and trade unionists were staging general strikes (1891), throwing bombs into the Chambre des Deputies (1893) and assassinating the President of the Republic (Sadi Carnot, in 1894), medicalized ideologues held that all prostitutes were vindictive descendants of former serfs and slaves who, by purposely infecting bourgeois and aristocratic males with syphilis, were avenging the wrongs done to their kind since the time of Clovis (*fl.* 496 CE). Picking up on ideas generated on the other side of the Alps by Professor Cesare Lombroso, holder in the 1880s of the chair of legal medicine at the University of Turin, medicalized moral entrepreneurs held that the prostitute was *ipso facto* the product of a debased race—an atavistic throwback to earlier primitive human types. Cut out by her tainted inheritance to be a prostitute and by temperament unwilling to do any honest work, her arms and shoulders were stronger than an ordinary woman's, her voice deep, her feet prehensile. Putting the bourgeois male and debased prostitute together in an act of unprotected sex would lead to the creation of a race of degenerate masturbators, syphilitics and alcoholics who would spell the end of civilization.[95]

Just to compound the anxiety, and with it the security of their position, French medical doctors steadfastly insisted on maintaining the confidentiality of consultations with clients. Their convention held that a potential husband's medical doctor should never tell his intended bride's father, brother or guardian that the man was syphilitic. Though the doctor was permitted to warn the youth that he should—for the sake of his bride—delay marriage for the four years it supposedly took for a mercury treatment to take full effect, the profession refused to seek legal means to prevent young men from infecting young women.

Making matters even worse was the bourgeois convention that one never talked about sexual matters before a lady. Studies of the 11,000 letters exchanged among members of the Boileau family between 1873 and 1920 found that sexuality was not once mentioned openly. This leads one to conclude that if syphilis was the secret plague between 1493 and 1920, the convention that it should not be discussed in polite society was the Great Conspiracy. Of this, the only beneficiary was *Treponema pallidum*.[96]

In defiance of bourgeois respectability, some French intellectuals purposely spread their diseased sexuality abroad. In 1877—accepting the Fournier dictum that third-stage syphilis madness would lead a creative writer to the full flower of his genius—the Norman short story writer Guy de Maupassant joyfully bragged that he had finally succeeded in catching syphilis rather than merely gonorrhea. Thereafter he pursued prostitutes with renewed vigor, laughing in their faces when after copulation he told them he had just committed them to a life of syphilitic misery. Maupassant died in a madhouse in 1893. Another syphilitic writer was Gustave Flaubert (b. 1821) author of *Madam Bovary* and *The Temptation of Saint Anthony: Or, A Revelation of the Soul.* Dashingly handsome in the Norman way, Flaubert began his sexual adventures late in November 1849 in a back-street dive just behind the Hotel Orient in Cairo, about a mile from where *Epidemics and History* is being written. While doing field research for his hatchet job on the father of western monasticism (St Anthony), Flaubert brazenly infected unknown numbers of young Middle Easterners with syphilis. Intellectuals like him, working in unacknowledged alliance with power/false knowledge medical doctors at the Hôpital Saint-Louis in Paris, enabled *Treponema pallidum* to flourish as never before.[97]

Reflecting on this dire situation from the perspective of the Cairo Conference on Tropical Medicine in 1928, Dr Payenneville of Rouen (chief city of the province that had spawned Flaubert and Maupassant) suggested that the histrionics of Drs Fournier *père et fils* had backfired. According to Payenneville, as a result of their self-congratulatory campaigns, the French government had declined to create a responsible central agency charged with bringing syphilis under control. The doctor added that ordinary lay people's response to what they perceived as medical men's power/false knowledge was also adding to the sum of human misery. Rather than tangle with professionals who claimed to know everything, people of all classes suffering from syphilis commonly resorted to charlatans.[98] By finally bringing these sociological truths out into the open, Dr Payenneville helped lay the groundwork for the development of positive policies for the control of syphilis.

Another avenue was through legislation. Seen by major world powers as unenforceable, this was occasionally used in peripheral polities. For instance, in a Norway smarting under its subordination to Sweden and determined to build up patriot numbers, in the 1860s legislative authority permitted magistrates to jail people of either sex for three years if they knowingly infected a partner with syphilis. And in the North American state on the other side of the Atlantic in which Norwegian immigrants were particularly numerous in the 1880s and 1890s, men or women who knowingly transmitted syphilis were liable to a fine of $2,000 and a year's imprisonment. This Minnesota assessment was the highest known anywhere in the federal union, and if collected, would have been more than the annual earnings of a general carpenter like my Minnesota immigrant

Norwegian grandfather (1855–1920). In two other peripheral regions, the Swiss cantons of Tessin and Schaffhaus, magistrates were authorized to throw people into prison for three months if they knowingly infected an innocent party.[99] In these Swiss cantons, just as in Norway and Minnesota, authority worked on the assumption that it would be possible, through legislation, to suppress pre-marital and extra-marital sex, and thus to re-establish "the golden age of innocence" in which as Fournier of Paris had put it, "the days of syphilis would be numbered." Despite its utopian flavor, this argument did at least weaken the hold of the old dual standard, by insisting that erring men and erring women be punished in the same way.[100]

In her celebration of eighteenth- and early nineteenth- century Britons, Linda Colley confessed that Great Britain's restrictions on women were harsher than those found in most other parts of the world. "Stripped by marriage of a separate identity and autonomous property, a woman could not by definition be a citizen and could never look to possess political rights."[101] Yet this condition would not endure much longer. In the 1860s, determined to do something about the enforcement of venereal-disease controls among prostitutes, a number of Queen Victoria's genteel subjects violently hurled themselves onto the political stage.

At that time, it was obvious to the official British mind (male) that the effective cause of epidemic syphilis lay in female prostitutes. No one knew how many there were. Estimates for London alone run anywhere between 5,500 and 80,000. Low estimates counted only full-timers known to the police while the high ones included part-timers (clandestine prostitutes). Yet uncertainty about numbers did not prevent any gentleman walking about St Paul's Cathedral or along any principal thoroughfare in Westminster on an evening from being physically jostled by some sort of prostitute. In 1864, worried about the threat loose women posed to British military might (with a VD rate of around 369 per 1,000 servicemen [!]), the government instituted the first of its two Contagious Diseases Acts.[102]

According to this Act, following the lead of the French and Belgians, prostitutes in named English garrison towns were required to register with the police. The stipulated towns included Portsmouth (navy), Woolwich and Aldershot (army), and, after the second act was passed in 1869, in the cathedral towns of Canterbury and Winchester. Conspicuously absent was London, with its listless, loitering aristocrats and statesmen hovering around barracks and palace compounds. Within a ten-mile radius of the centers of the stipulated towns, police moral squads were empowered to arrest any woman found suspiciously waiting about and to have her inspected with a State Penis. In class-bound Britain, these loitering woman were nearly always from the lower classes. Women who refused to undergo this humiliating and—though no one then knew about germs—grossly unsanitary test were assumed to be diseased and were carted off to lock hospitals (special purpose quarantine stations); there they were put to work laundering other people's bed sheets. In London where the Lock system did not pertain, good-looking prostitutes were in danger of being brought into mission hostels by compulsive do-gooders such as William Ewart Gladstone, the liberal Prime Minister who in 1882 presided over the rape of Egypt.[103]

Genteel women in search of a cause soon cottoned on to the sexist, class-determined nature of 1864–69 style Registration. Drawing on their mothers' experiences in the anti-slavery campaigns between the 1780s and 1833 and the Anti-Corn Law League of 1838–46, they organized a campaign to force Parliament to abolish Registration. From its inception in 1869, leadership of the campaign fell to Josephine Butler, a woman of means born in 1828 in Dilston, Northumberland. For Butler and her kind, it was obvious that women left to their own devices did not need sex at all and that prostitution was caused entirely by male lust. And given that a sex-crazed male clientele was always on hand, women might slip into prostitution when they had no other way to make a living. There was a simple Butlerian solution: create a world in which working-class women were allowed to find honest jobs with fair pay. Further Butler dogma held that once married and contemplating motherhood, a *proper* woman regarded sexual congress with her husband as a burdensome duty to be endured, not as an experience to be enjoyed. Winding up her standard lecture, Butler let packed halls and the world know that the only reason why prostitution continued to exist was that Members of Parliament, the judiciary, the morals police and medical doctors were party to a Great Conspiracy against working-class girls and against womankind in general. Proof of this conspiracy lay in the Contagious Diseases Acts.

Heir of the universalizing truths of the Enlightenment, Butler rallied her troops of both sexes by trumpeting the cause of "deliver[ing] *the World* from the wound of legalized prostitution."[104] In the course of the bitterly fought campaign, which in 1885 ultimately led to the repeal of regulated prostitution, the British feminist cause was born. In 1913, the central message of this cause as it then stood was summed up by Christabel Pankhurst as: "Votes for Women, Chastity for Men." Another Pankhurst dictum was that "[syphilis] is directly due to man's defiance of the laws of nature."[105]

The bill which repealed Registration in 1885 also contained clauses which ended legal tolerance of pornography and homosexuality. Once it became a statute, its immediate impact was to encourage the rise of social purity movements. Calling for the repression of all forms of sexuality, openly enjoyed, participating groups included the White Cross Societies, the National Council of Public Morals, the Moral Reform Union, the Boys' League of Honour and local vigilance societies. After 1901 the cause was taken up by the Free Church Council. In the form propagated by the FCC social purity combined revivalism for Christ and sexlessness for youth in a way reminiscent of the preachings of P. du Toit de Mambrini of Lausanne in 1760.[106]

Feeding into the ideology of social purity were also several strands of subjective, *secular* medical thought. Within the public health sector, liberals such as Arthur Newsholme, medical officer of health at Brighton between 1888 and 1908, held that syphilis was spread almost exclusively by "sexually immoral persons . . . enemies of society who cannot be tolerated." Like others in the Gladstonian tradition, Newsholme (later knighted and made a leading member of the Ministry of Health) believed that the only way forward against syphilis was to encourage "moral" and "ethical evolution" away from "barbarism" towards "civilization."[107] It is obvious that these sentiments were light years away from the truly scientific, objective observations of medical doctors like Dr Payenneville, conference participant at Cairo in 1928.

As Charles Darwin had taught, for "evolutionary" processes to continue among any sort of creatures, including humans, heterosexual congress remained essential.[108] In light of current knowledge about how syphilis is spread, we now know that the only effective barrier to the transfer of *Treponema pallidum* during penetration by the male organ is an intact rubber condom. To be effective agents of disease control, condoms had to be widely available, which in practical terms meant they had to be both cheap and socially acceptable, with medical doctors and Government strongly encouraging their use. Unfortunately, in the years before World War I, neither criterion was met.

This brings us to the third party who would need to be involved in any condom scheme: producers/suppliers. Though this issue has yet to be investigated in detail, it would seem that negative attitudes again won hands down. Using modern analogies, one can assume that in sorting out the marketing of their full range of products, B. F. Goodrich, Dunlop and other rubber companies found that profits from *one* pair of rubber bicycle tires or from two pairs of automobile tires were larger by far than profits from several score packets of condoms. The principle of bottom-line cost accountancy being as important then as it is now (as Congolese rubber harvesters facing extinction in the heart of darkest Africa had reason to know), it seems that rubber companies decided that it was not worth their while to attempt to educate the public and the medical establishment in the role of condoms in preventing disease. Taking the road of least resistance and of highest profit, they conducted their civilian marketing campaigns accordingly.[109]

Brand-name vehicle tires were a part of the distinctively modern context in which opportunities for *Treponema pallidum* to propagate were likely to arise. While on their bicycles (in the 1890s) or in an automobile (in the early teens of the twentieth century) young people would find themselves together in quiet, isolated places, blissfully ignorant of the life-preserving techniques useful in tight situations. In such matters, medical doctors still offered no counsel.

For her part, Marie Stopes, in 1918 virgin author of a widely acclaimed book, *Married Love: A New Contribution to the Solution of Sex Difficulties*, effectively ignored the existence of condoms. Stopes's ideology of "joy," held that decent people would confine their sexuality to marriage. She also held that a loving husband would do nothing to impede the flow of his sperm into his wife's vagina. The one birth-control practice Stopes actually named, so as to discourage its use, was *coitus interruptus*. This technique of course had absolutely no impact at all on continuing high rates of syphilis infection, since it was the contaminating juices coming from sores *on* the man's penis rather than the sperm he ejaculated from the aperture at its head that spread the disease. Other Stopes dicta were that

> It should never be forgotten that without the discipline of control there is no lasting delight in erotic feeling. The fullest delight, even in a purely physical sense, can *only* be attained by those who curb and direct their natural impulses. . . . Only those actions are worthy which lead the race onwards to a higher and fuller completion and the perfecting of its powers.[110]

In the 1920s, the years immediately after the holocaust of World War I—in which 10 million European males were machine-gunned or otherwise exterminated—Marie Stopes's book was regarded as the only sensible sexual advice literature suitable for decent persons. Given the extent of its availability and influence upon the lay reading public, it was tragic that Stopes did not mention condoms or the need to prevent the transmission of syphilis. Other moral campaigners less enlightened than Stopes (relative to the times) were openly hostile to "french letters," seeing in them a gratuitous encouragement to vice. In this, the enfranchised populace, on which the fate of elected ministries ultimately depended, seemed to agree. As late as 1923, the British government intervened on the grounds of obscenity to prevent women activists from distributing pamphlets containing information about contraceptive devices including the condoms which would have prevented the spread of syphilis.

In retrospect, it is now known that Government was in fact back-tracking on what had been a very real earlier advance. During World War I, when it had been obvious that the fate of Britain hinged on keeping its military forces in fighting trim, the army had included condoms in every soldier's basic kit. Yet with the return of the proprieties of peace, and knowing that every five years (or less) it had to face the British voter, Government again adopted the politically safe stance of social purity. This movement had come into being two generations earlier.

In Britain, the triumph of what Ronald Hyam terms "neurotic puritanism" had coincided with the full ripening of working-class consciousness in the 1890s.[111] Here "manliness" consisted of having a job that paid well enough to allow a man to keep a wife at home employed in "separate sphere" tasks as mother and housekeeper. Terrified by the middle-class anti-masturbation propaganda they had absorbed in school changing rooms and playgrounds during their early adolescence after 1870, but slow to adopt middle-class ideas about limiting family size, most English working-class males found companionship with their mates at the pub. Binges there tended to become nightly affairs during their wives' frequent pregnancies or while their wives were recovering from an abortion—the favored working-class form of birth control. After a five-and-a-half day working week, taking his ease on Saturday afternoons, Dad and his mates would go off to Association Football or some other spectator sport. Then, befuddled with drink, they would end up in a whorehouse, grist to the mill of *Treponema pallidum*.[112]

Wherever working-class Mum ruled an English household, sons with spunk were seldom found at home. In school they learned nothing about protecting themselves against syphilis and as school-leavers still ignorant of the basic facts of life, were good candidates for a bout of pox. When they showed the initial symptoms, they, like their fathers, were likely to turn to "ignorant vultures who . . . feed and grow fat on the weak, the credulous, and the ignorant"—the patent medicine dealers, the charlatans and medical hacks.[113]

In the German lands, women's consciousness of womanliness took forms quite different than those found in Britain. Here where two-job families were common, German feminists were particularly concerned about the provision of crèches for working mothers. Typically in *fin-de-siècle* Vienna, 40 percent of the women had full-time jobs and an additional 40 percent were in part-time employment. Though it is difficult to prove—syphilis was everywhere a stigmatizing disease to which no one readily confessed—it would appear that German husbands, teenage sons and daughters were less likely than their English counterparts to be driven out of the house by nagging wives and mothers into the arms of partners in casual sex bearing *Treponema pallidum*. This supposition is in line with the linkage the German pioneer sociologist, Max Weber, drew between meaningful employment and assessments of self-worth.[114]

It would seem too that the now unified German state, looking over its shoulder at the pathetic efforts of France in the wake of its military defeat in 1870, recognized that the syphilis scourge was a challenge which any *Kultur* that regarded itself as modern must confront head on by ditching the old head-in-sand ostrich approach. In any case, it was German experts—Fritz Schaudinn and Erich Hoffmann—who in 1905 first discovered the causal agent of syphilis. In the next year, another German, August Paul von Wassermann, applied practical science to a pressing social need by devising a test for non-visible syphilis. The creation of the Wassermann test was followed in 1909 by Paul Ehrlich's (another German) discovery of Salvarsan, a sometimes effective arsphenamine which had none of the terrible side effects of the mercury treatment used by both charlatans and medical doctors since 1493.[115]

In the course of and immediately after World War I, European governments decided to use Salvarsan and the Wassermann test to prevent what French experts warned would be the further degeneration of the white race through hereditary syphilis. With the coming of peace in 1918, at government level there was some discussion about what to do next. The alternatives were seen as (1) setting up massive education campaigns about condoms (an idea which obviously would infuriate social purity campaigners); and (2) adopting a curative program for the disease—which only an enlightened few realized it was no longer necessary to contract in the first place. It was the second course which won through.

According to theory, these new clinics were to provide all comers with free, confidential care. In practice, the real test was the sort of treatment and medical response "all comers" actually received. In such matters the positive pace-setter was the kingdom of Belgium (half of whose cities had been levelled by the German war machine). Serving a population of fewer than 8 million, by 1923 Authority had established some 400 clinics, roughly one per 20,000 of the population. The Belgian clinics were required to function at times of the week and in a manner that suited the practical needs of clients rather than the convenience of medical doctors, who were accustomed to clinical work schedules running from 9 a.m. to 5 p.m. By the 1930s, Belgium's enlightened policy was contributing significantly to a marked local decline in the incidence of syphilis.[116]

Token progress in this direction was made in England. Here before 1917 no formal medical provision for VD treatment had existed for the bulk of the population, those civilians dependent upon local health authorities or the Poor Law. However, following the shift in government policy which was intended to make England a "home fit for heroes," a network of VD clinics was established. By 1920, 190 state-supervised treatment centers were in operation, roughly one for every 200,000 people. Yet difficulties remained. As David Evans has recently shown, in addition to the inadequacy of provision for women (men patients outnumbered women by 3.5 to 1), English venereal disease doctors, nurses and clinic staff generally regarded their patients as depraved sexual offenders. This attitude among carers, together with the scruffy squalidness of most clinics, tended to put patients off. Though a series of treatments with Salvarsan required eight separate visits, fewer than 8 percent of the patients who reported for initial treatment ever bothered to return. Of the 92 percent who stayed away, some few may have enjoyed remission from the disease for no known medical reason but most continued to be infective. Thus, in England, with less than a tenth the number of clinics per capita found in Belgium, and with the dominance of the social purity ethic in those few that actually did exist, the syphilis situation remained explosive.[117]

North of the border in Scotland, where some clinics were established, the immediate post-war situation was marginally different. Here a cadre of surgeons and clinicians eager to serve as pioneers of medicalization *à la mode moderne* persuaded members of the UK Parliament (in Westminster) to introduce a bill for compulsory notification of VD. Within Scotland opposition to the bill came from social purity groups, concerned that it made no mention of moral reformation, and from doctors in private practice worried about creeping statism. In the end the bill was killed on its second reading in the Commons on the initiative of a man not known for his skills in recognizing potential for disaster when it stared him in the face, Prime Minister Neville Chamberlain.[118]

If medicalization proceeded slowly in the English and Scottish kingdoms, progress was even slower in the French republic. At a time when birth rates continued to be low, effective syphilis control was hampered by the lack of mutual trust between young urban working-class people and the graybeards in command of the nation state; it was these old men who had brought France near to defeat in world war, all the while insisting on citizen discipline. Though the Third Republic did establish some free syphilis clinics, at the rate of one clinic for every 200,000 citizens, this was far short of the number needed to bring the country into line with exemplary Belgium.[119] Yet as might be expected, in such matters there was a special French way.

In the absence of full-scale commitment to *medical* care for the masses, French inter-war authority resorted to high-profile scare campaigns that stressed the virtues of abstinence from sex rather than how much fun sex might be if one used a condom. These jazzed-up social purity campaigns gobbled up hugh budgets, but probably did little to contain syphilis. Quétel quotes alarmist figures put out by the Ministry of Health in 1925 which claimed that one French person in ten was syphilitic and that 80,000 were killed by syphilis annually; 20,000 of these reputed victims were innocent children. To drive its anti-sex awareness message home, the government patronized the popular press, radio broadcasters, film stars, actors and wall-postering companies.

Financially rewarding though all this was for media and entertainment types, it was not calculated to encourage ordinary young women and men to touch, to kiss, to make love, to marry or to have children. Neither did it help persuade them to trust Authority. Instead, after dusk in Paris, bored young men not satisfied with abstaining from masturbating at home (least they join the ranks of the masturbatory mad), often took themselves off to dark spots in the Bois de Boulogne to find sex with people they need never see again. There were similar haunts in most provincial towns. All this was continuing grist for the mill of *Treponema pallidum*.[120]

One policy alternative open to fully authoritarian regimes was established in Adolf Hitler's Germany after 1935. Under the Nazis, preparatory to marriage both parties were required to undergo a Wassermann test. Either party, if found to have syphilis, would be sterilized. People bearing the traits of inherited syphilis (earlier defined by the Fourniers *père et fils*) were sent off to euthanasia camps. To the same destination was sent anybody who knowingly infected others with syphilis. In the interests of further moral reformation, the brothels of Berlin and Hamburg which had given the Weimar Republic its tinselly sparkle were ruthlessly closed down. In moves somewhat more life-enhancing, wives were encouraged to give up their professional careers and remain at home to breed tow-headed children for the Fatherland. Updating Jean Frédéric Osterwald's ideology of self-discipline, the new young were enjoined to take long walks and cold showers when not keeping their animal passions under control by reading Immanuel Kant and the Stoics. Meanwhile fewer and fewer people with Hutchinson's notched incisor teeth, collapsed noses or other tell-tale characteristics of a syphilitic seemed to be about.[121]

In a West Europe blighted by the coming of the second global war, the survival prospects of *Treponema pallidum* were little altered until the mid-1940s. Then all at once penicillin, the one-shot fix against syphilis, became widely available. So too did rubber prophylactics, following their introduction and widespread use among World War II servicemen. By the 1950s, the two interventions working in tandem—condoms to prevent, penicillin to cure—encouraged a now fully scientific medical profession to think that syphilis might be eradicated. Unfortunately (for humankind) the disease which had first mutated itself into being within European hosts was not to be conquered so easily. After around 1958, the decline bottomed out, and incidence again began to rise. As of this writing, within its European homeland, *Treponema pallidum* still lives.[122]

Syphilis and "Syphilis" in China, c. *1860 to 1965*

Historical accounts of syphilis and Construct syphilis in China until the year 1965 hinge on two variables. The first concerns *perceptions* of the incidence of venereal syphilis on the one hand and of yaws and endemic syphilis (bejel) on the other. Actual incidences of any of these diseases are, of course, unknown and unknowable. Much more accurate information however is available about the second variable. This I take to be the rise and peaking of negative western attitudes about China; in short, Sinophobia.[123]

In western-language reports—in which nothing is quite what it appears to be—interest in Chinese syphilis began soon after the Taiping Rebellion/ Revolution of 1850–64 left 20 million Chinese dead. Riding on the shirt tails of the armies which had proved that western weapons were infinitely superior to Chinese, ideologically motivated missionaries and medical doctors set up compounds in treaty ports along the coasts and along inland rivers. Many of these enclaves remained in western hands until the Communist takeover in 1949.[124]

For "respectable" Europeans in China after 1860 (thus not counting sailors who deserted their ships and "went native"), omnipresent "venereal syphilis" was a distinguishing mark of the Chinese "Other." Given the obvious weaknesses of the old order—the prevalence of warlordism in the provinces and the absence of a central authority enjoying the Mandate of Heaven—European attitudes could not but affect the way in which future-orientated Chinese medical personnel regarded their own society and their own traditions.

Ironically, until around 1850, *Treponema pallidum* had excited far fewer tensions in China than it did in Europe. Arriving in the bodies of Europeans coming in by sea to Canton in 1504, it had found itself in a nearly 2,000-year-old polity which encompassed a quarter of humankind. For a century or so after "plum-tree poison" came on the scene, the Celestial Kingdom continued in reasonable health. At the central and local levels, government was in the hands of Mandarins, a non-hereditary male bureaucracy who had been trained in the Confucian ethical tradition. This ethic gave high priority to stability, order, cohesion, respect for the ancestors and for the living (male) head of the family. Yet it was only one of three ethical systems; the second, Buddhism, need not detain us here. The third, Taoism, was of considerable importance since most Chinese medical practitioners were adherents either wholly or in part.[125]

Taoism was concerned with enhancing Man's control over Nature in all its many forms. Its devotees included bridge builders, artists, craftsmen and creative professionals as well as medical doctors. Taoists were proud of their ability to work with their hands and, in terms of social esteem, were members of the middle strata. Ranking above them were the Mandarins (literati who entered their high-status jobs by passing rigorous examinations) and the producers of food, the peasantry. Below them were lowly soldiers. Chinese merchants (based largely in the cities of the South) were also seen as low-status beings who produced nothing for the common good but only sold for their own profit what better men had made. Since the majority of Europeans in the treaty ports after 1860 were either soldiers or vendors of something, their already strong antipathy to "John Chinaman" was, to say the least, exacerbated by the low status of their local counterparts.

Young Chinese males intending to become Taoist health provisioners trained under a senior practitioner, very often living with him in his house. Apprentices learned that if different cures cleared the same disease, they should use the one most fitted to local circumstances. Characteristic of Taoist concern with the health of the body and of the sexual glands was a written injunction that boys from the age of fourteen on should ejaculate twice daily (no hang-ups about masturbation here).[126] After *Treponema pallidum* arrived at Canton and began to spread among townspeople, Taoists talked in militant terms of bodily defenses, fortifications and bullets. Not having any magic bullets themselves, their treatments included mercury and possibly arsephenamines and were just as effective as any treatment European missionary doctors had at hand.

With their ingrained habits of applied empiricism, Taoist practitioners were free of any notion of an ultimate, unitary truth.[127] In another, more just world than planet earth, pluralistic, pragmatic Taoists would have come into direct communication with Sir Francis Bacon while he was creating his great empiricist system the *Instauratio Magna* (The Great Instauration). As it was, the seventeenth-century Lord Chancellor knew nothing of the Taoists, and they nothing of him.

In the decades after 1700, for reasons having more to do with moral politics than with medicine, leading Taoist practitioners were blighted by the sterile, yin–yang opposites of Confucian teaching. Paul Unshuld uses the telling analogy of a great tree whose roots have been cut. Though the potential for new life was gone, the wood in the trunk and branches continued in being, serving useful purposes.[128]

Frank Dikötto has drawn attention to the special contribution made by the discourse of race in the medicalization of China. Typical of the discourse was a statement sent out of Hong Kong in 1887 by Patrick Manson, the man who went on to become principal founder of the School of Tropical Medicine in the capital city of the British Empire. According to him:

> Those who have been, even but a short time, in the country, know what a wretched thing native medical practice is. And no wonder. There is no educational system. It is chosen more as a trade. A man buys two or three books and begins to practice. It is possible that here and there may be a man of great natural talent who may know something and may at times do good. But the body of the profession, if we may dignify it with such a name, are as ignorant as they are dishonest.[129]

Four decades after Manson penned this scathing indictment of Chinese medicine, Sir Donald MacAlister, MD, president of the General Council of Medical Education of the UK, had this to say:

> A hundred years ago no human enterprise could have seemed more hopeless than the physical and spiritual transformation of China. Millions were in soul and body sick until death; but the science of healing was unknown, while its native practice was discredited, and indeed discreditable.[130]

But writing in 1921, MacAlister was encouraged to find that things were looking up now that Chinese students were coming forward to attend western medical schools of the sort which Patrick Manson had established in Hong Kong.

However, when it came to syphilis, Chinese interns and trainees in these medical schools found their western mentors an embarrassment. Impervious to the idea of cultural pluralism (born in late eighteenth-century Prussia), the self-selected western medical personnel who went out to China had *known* before they set out that venereal syphilis was eating into the life-blood of the Chinese people. In fact, what they were perceiving through their western cultural filters was Construct syphilis.[131]

Living in 1921 under the revolutionary Chinese regime that had succeeded the Celestial Kingdom, the western medic W. W. Peters advised readers of a leading journal that statistical studies had convincingly proven that venereal syphilis was China's leading cause of death. Other studies undertaken in the 1930s claimed that there were some 30 or 35 million syphilitics in rural and urban China, getting on for 10 percent of the population. Taking these figures at face value, a modern writer could claim that "VD in China represented a much more serious problem than in the West in the same period."[132] Yet as we know, in any statistical survey, the ideological compulsions behind the collection of the data are of real significance.

As Joseph Needham pointed out many years ago, western concepts of sin and guilt were conspicuously absent from the great ethical systems of China. Working within the rules provided by these systems, 10 percent of the families were headed by polygamous males.[133] Finding the implications of this conjunction of sinlessness and polygamy troubling, western missionaries decided to strike directly at the point where the life forces of the Chinese present (sexual congress) created the Chinese of the future. Borne up by news that social purity movements back home in Europe and North America were having considerable success in banning all forms of sexuality outside of monogamous marriage, western missionaries decided to tackle what they saw as a key element in the Chinese world, namely female prostitution.[134]

In China, as in mid-fifteenth-century Europe, prostitution was seen as an acceptable way for a poor girl to make a living. Sent by her rural parents to a town in the expectation that she would maintain them with the money she sent home, a young woman in service might become a courtesan skilled in singing, dancing and vaginal maneuvers and appear in the entourage of a high dignitary of state. Less talented girls might end up as common prostitutes under the control of a manager. Yet even these humble prostitutes knew that they would have an honorable retirement. In China, no stigma was attached to the profession.

Typical of the European response to what was in western eyes "the slavery of prostitution" was a petition which Mrs C. B. L. Haslewood, wife of a British naval officer stationed in Hong Kong, sent to the Colonial Office in 1919. Her diatribe was written at a time when 20 million peasants in the north of China were starving, following a drought and continuing lawlessness in the countryside. Under these circumstances, as any sensible Chinese person would have been able to point out, peasants fortunate enough to have daughters to send as prostitutes to southern cities might, through remittances sent home, just manage to survive. The others would starve to death. Perhaps aware of the complexities of the situation, Colonial Office mandarins in London made soothing noises to Mrs Haslewood, but did nothing. They were probably also taking into account that the Chinese central government had joined the Allied war effort against the German Kaiser and was, in formal terms, an ally.[135]

In early post World-War-I Shanghai, working under the auspices of the British, American and French "concession," well-intentioned western doctors set themselves the task of determining the incidence of syphilis among Chinese social groupings, using the new Wassermann test. At that time, even in advanced European countries, there was much confusion about what Wassermann testing could achieve. Writing of Scotland in 1927, an official complained of "the technical inefficiency, the slip-shod methods, the antiquated notions, the degree of ignorance" of most medical doctors with respect to syphilis [and testing].[136] Indeed as recently as 1993, WHO experts agreed that yaws, endemic syphilis and pinta "are characterized by a positive serologic test that *cannot be distinguished* from the positive test caused by *venereal syphilis.*"[137] Of course in the early 1920s, this lack of differentiation among the treponema diseases could not be generally or publicly admitted, for that would question the pretensions to scientism, the quality most distinctive of western medicine, and indeed of the West's own image of itself. Another unacknowledged difficulty facing the inter-war Shanghai Wassermann testing program was that much of the actual work was done by culturally sensitive Chinese interns.

The results were interesting for reasons which have little to do with "scientific medicine," but which nicely demonstrate how important it is to take disease constructs into account. In the Shanghai test, high rates of venereal syphilis were found among soldiers and merchants, middling rates among craftsmen, pedlars and artisans, and low rates among teachers, clerks, professionals and students. Not by coincidence this ranking was identical with the pecking order of rank, respect and esteem in classical Chinese society. People in the most honorable niches—learned professionals and students—*necessarily* (as managed by Chinese interns) had a far lower incidence of what westerners taught was a shameful disease than did members of the lowest social orders: merchants and soldiers. Unaware of the fundamental social conventions of the country in which they lived, the Shanghai mission doctors never cottoned on to what was happening.[138]

At a time when the Chinese political nation was on the verge of dissolution and the tap root of its culture had been cut, young Chinese medical doctors such as Sun Yat-Sen (instrumental in 1911–12 in overthrowing the ruling dynasty and replacing it with a republic) recognized the urgent need for root and branch modernization to prevent China from being entirely gobbled up by Europe, America or Japan. Among other areas of thought which the intelligentsia decided needed urgent attention were attitudes towards disease. So it was that in the 1930s, the Communists (then the wave of the future) recognized and accepted syphilis as *the* disease which best symbolized Chinese decadence, moral inferiority and subservience to the West.[139]

Soon after they seized power in 1949 the Communists followed this argument to its logical conclusion and undertook a syphilis eradication campaign. They began with urban brothel keepers. Branded as "scoundrels, drug peddlers or gangsters [they] were dealt with directly by the angry masses [of the risen people of China]."[140] After this purge was underway, cadres of government inspectors circulated through the countryside areas and the inner provinces with printed forms politely asking everyone to answer questions about recent skin infections, chancres, sores and the like. Illiterates who might have trouble with the form were told to ask their literate neighbors to help them fill it out.

And so, under the guise of identifying syphilitics, feuds between neighbors that had been festering for generations were decisively settled in favor of the literate. What was done was to mis-identify as venereal syphilis what in Mongolia and other inner areas was probably endemic syphilis (non-sexually transmitted) and in coastal areas probably yaws (also non-sexual). During the great clean-up of what was in fact largely Construct syphilis, the official Communist party line was that enormous quantities of penicillin were used in treating and curing patients. Going further, the Party claimed that production of penicillin was so successful that China was able to export a surplus to less well provided parts of Asia. By 1964, with vast stores of surplus penicillin still on hand, the Communist government was able to boast that "active venereal disease has been completely eradicated from most areas and completely controlled throughout China."[141]

In the context of a People's Republic determined to wipe away what it perceived as the decadence of the past by a single great purge, it seems likely that in order to die from venereal syphilis during the campaign it was not at all necessary to be infected with *Treponema pallidum*. Instead it was quite enough to have earned a reputation among the cadres as being an anti-social troublemaker, in other words, a Construct syphilitic. Twenty-five years after the kill or cure campaign ended, people from the outside world began to learn of brimming graveyards along the road between Beijing and the airport.

In the official Chinese interpretation of what happened in 1964 ("syphilis has been completely eradicated"), what was important was that the "plum-tree poison" which had first been brought in by the West and then used by the West as the symbol of Chinese animal sexuality had been banished by the Chinese themselves from the Chinese earth. After its eradication—by whatever means—all mention of venereal syphilis was removed from medical students' texts. Within the People's Republic, study of syphilis had become irrelevant.[142] As of 1965, it was only beyond the fringes of civilization where Others dwelt—in Europe, America, Africa—that stigmatizing syphilis continued its destructive reign.[143]

5 Cholera and Civilization: Great Britain and India, 1817 to 1920

The greater part of the world has, properly speaking, no history, because the despotism of Custom is complete. This is the case over the whole East.

John Stuart Mill, *On Liberty*, 1859

Introduction

Cholera emerged in epidemic form in India in 1817, and after an initial false start, arrived in Britain in 1831. Coinciding with these happenings, the private trading firm known as the East India Company (which had conquered Bengal in 1757) undertook further diplomatic and military maneuvers to bring the remaining provinces of the subcontinent under its sway. In this it was uncommonly successful. Thus came into being a situation in which a *single* London and Home Counties based ruling elite was in command of two very different, cholera-stressed societies.

In the course of the nineteenth century, Britain lost an estimated 130,000 of its resident subject people to five cholera epidemics, each of which, after 1848, claimed fewer and fewer lives. During the same century and first quarter of the next, India lost in excess of 25 million of its people to the same disease. Even more striking was the fact that while England's cholera mortality rates moved steadily downwards, those of nineteenth-century India dramatically increased. In 1900, the most disastrous of the years for which statistics had been kept, cholera claimed the lives of upward of 800,000 people, 163,889 in the single provence of Bombay.[1] These vastly different totals of cholera dead, relatively small in Britain, absolutely enormous in India, can in part be laid to the accidents of chance. Yet the role of human agency cannot be ignored. Indeed, as I see it, it is central to the whole issue.[2]

As almost every school-leaver should know, the Prussian bacteriologist Robert Koch completed his investigations into the nature of the bacterial causal agent of cholera (the comma bacillus) in water-tanks in Calcutta in 1884. With the discovery of the role played by the human gut in the life-cycle of the *Vibrio cholerae*, and confirmation of the vital importance of water in the transmission of cholera through infective human wastes, the way was clear—in theory—for containment and control of the scourge. At the micro-level, all that needed to be done was to isolate affected patients and every bit of the fecal matter, vomit, urine or sweat they expelled. These tasks could easily be performed by illiterate locally born health provisioners under the general supervision of competent medical authorities, provided of course there was mutual trust. Unfortunately, as we will see, in British India, until well beyond the third decade of the twentieth century, none of the preconditions necessary for the containment of cholera was present, in the form either of personnel or of mindsets.

Writing in 1994 about the role of ideology in the making of the Raj, Thomas Metcalf affirmed that "As a people . . . the British have always eschewed grand . . . theories in favor of ones perceived to be derived from empirical observation, and from John Locke onward, they insisted upon the value of experimental modes of understanding." Recognition of this was hardly new. In 1889, a decade before India's worst cholera crisis, a perceptive English-educated outsider resident in the kingdom bewailed "our monstrous worship of facts."[3]

Throughout the cholera era, the idolatry of facts was tenaciously maintained by those politicians and puppets of the gentlemanly capitalists of London who were directly concerned with the Development of India. For our purposes it must be pointed out that worshippers also included many—perhaps most—upper-echelon officials in the Indian Medical Service (IMS). During any crises which threatened or actually involved cholera, their invariable response was based on the "facts" and "scientific truths," which, as I see it, were better suited to the requirements of Development than to human control over the disease environment.[4]

Whether openly admitted or not, Development itself was intended solely as a means of providing London with an uninterrupted flow of dividend returns on capital investment. Impacting most heavily on the ability of cholera to slaughter millions were gentlemanly capitalists' very substantial investments in irrigation, in railways and port facilities and, equally decisively, the near absence of investment in public health.[5]

Writing a generation ago, Charles Rosenberg suggested that cholera was "a tool for social and economic analysis" of nineteenth-century Europe. More recently, Bill Luckin has written of the need for rigorous contextualization in establishing the "epidemiological past" of earlier disease crises. Equally germane is the novel written by a former British colonial officer in Asia, George Orwell. In *Nineteen Eighty-Four*, Orwell makes the immensely valuable point that whoever controls the present, controls the writing of the history of what went on before, and that this reconstructed "historic" past legitimizes the rulers currently in power.[6]

In this chapter I intend to treat cholera as a phenomenon in its own right and to clear away the cultural accretions it has acquired in the years since 1817. After briefly looking at the peculiarities of the illness, my course will be to examine its early years in India and then to bring it across to England.

Within the rapidly changing context of that island society, I will discuss some of the secular responses cholera engendered during the period—ending around 1855—when it was last seen as a clear and present threat. Included among these responses was the water-borne theory arrived at by John Snow in his famous demonstrations at the Broad Street pump.

In 1849, Snow, a York-born anesthetist who had worked with cholera victims in the coal mines outside Newcastle-upon-Tyne during Great Britain's first epidemic (1831–32), conducted empirical research which led him to suggest that cholera was spread through contaminated water. Writing in 1854 Snow made a point of mocking the Indian Medical Service's contention that cholera generally targeted only those who were predisposed to catch it. As he put it, "The alleged predisposition was nothing visible or evident: like the elephant which supports the world, according to Hindoo mythology, it was merely invented to remove a difficulty."[7] Not all medical doctors, even in England, were prepared to jump on Snow's bandwagon. Reluctance was perhaps related to a social accident: unlike gentlemen of the better sort, Snow was not the product of a public school. Then too his medical degree was from London's University College (the "godless" institution established by Jeremy Bentham) rather than from a "proper" university. Notwithstanding, after the middle 1850s most doctors in England were at least prepared to consider Snow's as *one* of *several* theories which might prove useful in controlling cholera.

In the event, gentlemanly capitalists and their medical supporters in India did not see Snow's explanation as particularly well suited to their own needs. I analyze some reasons for this in the final section of the chapter. There, we re-enter India in the wake of British suppression of the Rebellion of 1857–58 (formerly termed the "Mutiny"). Soon after this event gentlemanly capitalists decided to forge ahead with investment in infrastructure on a scale unprecedented in the past. Following this, cholera mortalities soared.

Cholera as Disease

Today when cholera is all but unknown in Western Europe, health provisioners from economically advanced lands frequently revert to inherited attitudes and assume that its presence in a non-western country betokens needless poverty that an appropriate dose of moralizing might put right. Far more helpful is the 1990s morally neutral position which in basic outline was established by Robert Koch in 1883 (when he studied cholera in Alexandria) and 1884 (when he completed his studies in Calcutta). This modern understanding holds that cholera is caused by a water-borne bacterium of the genus vibrio which is usually ingested into the human gut by the swallowing of water containing cholera-infected human fecal matter. Eating shellfish, lobsters, oysters, melons, strawberries, vegetables, or other victuals which contain quantities of fecal-infected water or any food on which flies have dropped infected human feces can also bring the vibrio into a potential victim's system. Another chain of transmission might be through the ingestion of a victim's sweat by the wearing of his/her imperfectly cleaned clothes and bringing the end of a sleeve to the mouth. Another might be by carelessly swallowing drops of the lethal water used in laundering cholera-soiled bedsheets.[8]

Modern etiological understandings pinpoint a number of variables. One is that cholera is age selective: a disproportionate number of its victims were adult men and women in the prime of life, many of them wage earners and parents of young children. Also of interest were the differentials in death rates among diverse socio-economic groups. Given that no human had any long-term immunity analogous to that provided by a mild case of smallpox (which gave lifelong protection against reinfection), for cholera the differential hinged on the general state of a person's health. It appears that the stomachs and intestines of robust, healthy people—for example soldiers at the time of recruitment—secrete acids and alkali which counteract the *Vibrio cholerae* and prevent the exposed host from coming down sick. Ability to secrete these protective substances is reduced if an exposed host is suffering from starvation as in time of famine, is carrying a load of intestinal worms, is generally sick and run down, or is suffering severe mental depression.[9]

In this matter of "state of mind" and physical condition, it is important to be explicit about my approach. The bedrock of my understanding rests on the simple principle that the modern cholera paradigm—positing a *bacteriological* cause triggering a normal bodily response—is a holistic unity. Given this elementary truth—paradigm as coherent whole—it is no longer valid to follow the time-honored Whig practice of extracting bits and pieces of pre-Kochian understandings and then, finding that some of them seem similar to some elements of the new Kochian model, to say—ah! these medical pioneers were on the right track after all! It will be recalled that the overall Whig schema posited the incremental growth of medical knowledge, each generation adding its own contribution to those of its predecessors who in turn built on the work of the ancient founders. However, as Michael Neve, Vivian Nutton and others have recently shown, this old methodology is no longer seen as a useful tool in moving forward with the recreation of the medical past as it really was.[10]

More fruitful is recognition of the obvious point that physicians and other health professionals necessarily act in accord with what they learned during their formal education rather than on the basis of information discovered some ten or fifteen years later on. In practical terms this meant that most nineteenth-century ideas about cholera were based on the nineteenth century's rather muddled Galenic understandings. These consisted of two elements: great sweeps of moralization tacked onto ideas from Galen. Depending on the attitude of the particular writer, it was often a moot point whether moral meanings—of the sort found in the annual report submitted to the UK Parliament on the "*Moral* and Material *Progress* of India"—outweighed straightforward Galenic elements.

One core Galenic concept we met earlier (p. 13 and fn. 23) was the Non-Natural mental state known as melancholy or depression. Melancholy and the behavioral patterns accompanying it were seen either as *predisposing* the victim to a pestilential disease or as its effective cause.[11] Thus, in 1887, in reporting factors that led to death during a cholera epidemic, the special scientific adviser to the sanitary commissioner with the government of India attested that "everyday experience" showed the "fatal action" of fear and grief. Similarly, in writing up his report for the year 1898 (fourteen years after Koch), Dr Weir, the health officer for Bombay, showed his continuing faith in the old idea by claiming that "a hopeful disposition" was "most unfavorable" to the growth of disease in human beings.[12]

The other Non-Natural was the notion of "environment." In physical terms this infinitely flexible "environment" consisted of the meteorological phenomena governing the amount of rainfall, wind direction and the like, as well as the state of the air, the amount of dust it bore, the quality of local soils, the quality of local waters, and the level of sub-surface waters. Following the teachings of Newton, and at only a slight remove, the teachings of the Philosopher (Aristotle), it was thought that all these Non-Natural "environmental" factors fit into a cyclic pattern which only painstaking analysis of a long series of detailed statistical records would finally reveal. It was also thought that the end result of this "scientific" analysis and determination of pattern would permit action to be taken before disease threats actually manifested themselves as epidemics. In India, this line of reasoning worked in alliance with the dictates of an influential one-time member of the English General Board of Health (Edwin Chadwick, still giving public lectures in 1877) to provide the theoretical underpinning of long-standing IMS beliefs. In a nutshell, these held that each region of India had its own distinctive disease environment. It was these "local causes" which alone produced the horrendous epidemics of lethal disease to which the Indian subcontinent seemed so prone.[13]

It is now known that *Vibrio cholerae* can live for several days in tanks of water such as those carried aboard a ship or railway carriage, and up to two weeks in the warm water within the hump of a camel engaged in, for example, the carrying trade working out of Afghanistan northward to Russia or westward to Persia and Iraq. This was the route cholera travelled when it left India for points north in the 1820s. For variable periods of time the vibrio can also live in the guts of a human carrier who has *no* apparent symptoms, but who excretes cholera-infected feces. Modern studies in regions with endemic cholera have found that even a small number of long-term carriers who give every appearance of being in perfect health is enough to keep the disease in being.

To account for the movement of cholera, the modern understanding is that it follows land-based lines of human movement (roads and footpaths). It also follows waterways which might be used as sources of drinking water and which contain human excrement. These suspect sources include canals, drainage ditches, rivers and harbors, water pipes, public pumps, ponds and wells. Nowadays of course the vibrio can also be transported by airplanes, as for example in 1991 when it travelled from its base in Peru to the United States on an Argentine airliner.[14] Before the cholera and water relationship was hypothesized by John Snow, then effectively confirmed by Koch's microscopic tests in 1884, part of the shock effect of any epidemic was the logic-defying way it moved about. In northern England late in 1831, in the Île de France in the spring of 1832 and in Castile in 1834, observers remarked on cholera's crazy-quilt patterning, striking every third or fourth house along a street, skipping half a mile to hit another street, then alighting on villages usually seen as out of the way, remote, and in the old days of bubonic plague, safe.[15]

Some work has been done in reconstructing local patterns of transmission. For France, during the epidemics of 1832 and 1848–49, it has been found that wet-nurses tending Paris-born infants carried cholera back to home villages within a radius of twenty or thirty kilometers of the capital. Half a century later, it was refugees fleeing from a cholera outbreak in Provence who brought the scourge to Naples. Other reconstructions have shown that during imperializing processes in the early 1830s, French soldiers carried cholera to Algeria. Similarly in 1853–54 troops recruited in the north of France for Crimean War duty against the Tsar of Russia carried the disease with them to Marseilles and then to lands facing the Black Sea. Ironically, this deadly gift from the West manifested itself in the death of civilians living not far from the place where in 1347 the bubonic plague bacillus had boarded the Genoese merchant ships that later took it to the Mamluk lands.[16]

Though educated Europeans in the post-Napoleonic era were acutely conscious of the importance of statistics, detailed patterns of cholera mortality remain obscure. Reflecting social stigma, sufferers were either under-reported or over-reported.[17] In an era when accurate disease identification was still in its infancy and it was thought that cholera specially targeted rough, reckless persons from the lower social orders, anyone of that description who died of some not very clear cause during an epidemic might in good faith be entered as having died of cholera. Short of examining the fecal matter of the deceased under a microscope to see if it contained *Vibrio cholerae* (before Koch in 1884 this technique was practically unknown), in doubtful cases there was no sure way of knowing what the actual cause of death had been.

Skewing figures in order to maintain the repute of the dead was relatively easy if the patient had been allowed to die at home instead of being carried off to a special cholera hospital where death from cholera or from pneumonia, typhus or starvation was nearly certain. Under a home-care regime, death rates might be marginally lower as a result of sympathetic nursing using cold compresses on the brow and oil and chalk rubbed into the body. Sensible home-carers knew that any medical doctor who insisted on bleeding cholera victims to relieve what he perceived as the "exciting causes" of "fever"—the standard approved technique—had to be kept well away from the patient, since *that* cure was even more lethal than the disease. Another advantage of home care was that it greatly reduced the possibility of confusing a deep coma with death and with it, the loved one's premature burial or premature cutting-up in one of Britain's new anatomy schools founded to give medical apprentices from the respectable classes a start on their careers.[18]

In 1832, cases of families fleeing in the face of death and leaving cholera victims to the mercies of clean-up crews were recorded in Bilston near Wolverhampton and in the Scottish border town of Dumfries. On a per capita basis, these two villages were among the worst affected in Britain. On the Continent, in the scattered villages and towns of the Luxembourg province of Belgium in 1866, cholera cadavers also lay unattended, awaiting the attentions of privately hired clean-up squads or dogs.[19] A decade later, writing of the situation in the presidency of Madras during the cholera epidemic and famine of 1877–78, the sanitation officer reported that "it was not uncommon for district officers in their tours across country to come upon numerous dead bodies and skeletons in the course of a morning's ride." Here it was obvious that dogs and other scavengers had been eating their fill.[20]

Dying from cholera—*mort de chien*, dog's death, or the blue terror—was one of the most ghastly experiences a disease could inflict on a human being. More or less healthy persons going about their ordinary affairs were suddenly struck as if by a hammer blow on the head. The initial shock was followed by vomiting and uncontrolled voiding of rice-water stools which leached the body dry of fluids. When dehydration was reaching a critical stage, cramps convulsed every muscle in the body, causing victims to writhe and scream with pain. Perhaps young and attractive in the morning, by nightfall they had become shrivelled wrecks with darkened bluish skin, sunken eyes and protruding teeth. Even worse, until almost the very end, victims might be aware of the terrible things happening to their fecal-stained, dehydrated bodies. Yet physical degradation did not cease with death. For an hour or so after the spirit of life was extinguished, the legs and arms of the body continued to thrash about, leading those hovering nearby to hope that the corpse was not really dead. Occasionally these doubts were justified. Among the common people of England, the fear that carrion removal squads would haul one off while still alive was matched only by the anxiety about who cholera would alight on next. Amongst the stricken, mortality rates averaged around 50 percent. Among victims who survived, permanent scarring, crippling or speech impediment was common.[21]

Cholera in India to c. 1857

In August 1891, Surgeon-Major Thomson of the Bengal Medical Service, B. Rake, G. Buckmaster, and other members of a government commission reported that in assessing the state of the health of the people of India they had found it convenient to note local tolls from cholera. They argued that:

> It may be assumed that where cholera is worst the hygiene and physical powers of the people are lowest. . . . cholera may be assumed to be a better test of the health and wealth of a region than the decennial rate of mortality which at best must always be an uncertain quantity for a vast country like India, and therefore quite inadequate as a standard of healthiness.[22]

This use of cholera statistics as a barometer of public health reflected educated Britons' long-standing perception of India as the homeland of a disease which directly threatened the well-being of populations in the West. Giving voice to this in 1872, an up-and-coming statistician named W. W. Hunter reminded his readers that

> One of man's most deadly enemies [the cholera morbus, remains] ever ready to rush out upon the world, to devastate households, to sack cities, and to mark its line of march by a broad black track across three continents . . . [striking down] thousands of the most talented and the most beautiful of our age in Vienna, London, or Washington.[23]

As Hunter should have realized, claims of this sort had serious political implications. Thus at the International Congress on Hygiene held in Vienna in 1887, most non-British delegates were fully convinced that Indian-based cholera was a standing threat to the West. Yet given that Britain was the world's greatest naval power, the Congress was not in a position to force it to adopt rigid quarantine on all ships leaving Bombay, Calcutta and other notoriously infected Indian ports.[24]

Partially masked by the runaway population growth of Calcutta (by 1820, with 350,000 people, the second largest urban place in the Empire), until after World War I India was characterized by *near population stagnation.* In the central and western regions (including Bombay) in the decades of 1891–1901 and 1911–21, there was actually population decline. In the northern region including the Punjab, the province whence Britain would recruit most of her Sepoy troops after the Revolt of 1857, in the decade 1891–1901 average life expectancy at birth for boys was 17.5 years and for girls 23.1. In the decade 1911–21, female life expectancy dropped to 20.3. In 1891 India had a population of around 150 million. According to a recent estimate, when Charles, first Marquis Cornwallis arrived in 1786 to take up the post of governor-general, the subcontinent had contained several million *more* inhabitants than it did a hundred years later.[25]

In seeing how this came to pass, one can begin with mindsets, and in particular with the mindset brought into being by the scheming young follower of Jeremy Bentham, acid-tongued James Mill (1773–1836). Born in a Scottish village and educated at Edinburgh University, James Mill hit upon the idea of writing a definitive philosophical history of India. Once completed, his *History of India* earned him a lifetime post as secretary of the East India Company (EIC), a position in which he was succeeded by his famous son, John Stuart Mill. A principal theme of the *History* was that Indian society had remained unchanged since remote antiquity. Serving as required reading for all EIC and later British government employees going out to India, it was doubtless a reason why in official reports coming out of India the phrase "customs dating from time immemorial" was so frequently used. Translated into general policy, this code-phrase meant that Indians themselves were intellectually somnolent, decadent, and stood in urgent need of the moral uplift which the conquering British alone could provide.[26]

In relation to the type of British action that might be required in time of cholera, the Millian construct served to legitimize no action at all. The relevant premise was that Indian villagers were filthy, preferred to be filthy, and had been filthy time of out mind. As Dr J. M. Coates, Bengal sanitary officer put it in 1877, "[the general body of the people] do not believe in the value of pure air and water . . . and are . . . content to abide by the habits of their ancestors, and if they suffer and die, they attribute the contingency to fate."[27]

To gain an objective understanding of the role of the British in depriving India of its history (following James and J. S. Mill), and of the process of converting what seems to have been merely a local disease, endemic in Bengal, into a chronic India-wide problem, it is useful to sketch out the actual history of pre- and early conquest India. As reconstructed in the last fifteen years by Indian and English revisionist historians, pre-British seventeenth- and eighteenth-century India was well on the way toward becoming a fully commercialized society which owed nothing to the Development processes then going on in Europe.[28] Located at the fulcrum of great trading networks stretching from north China in the east and to the Red Sea and Egypt in the west, Indian overseas trading firms built and owned their own purpose-built ocean-going ships and used complex financial devices such as promissory notes to keep the wheels of commerce in motion. Supplementing overseas trade in every sort of product known in the West plus hundreds more was a fine grid of internal commodity exchange which involved the transport of basic and luxury goods to every corner of the subcontinent on huge convoys of pack bullock. On the west coast, feeding into this network were thousands of ateliers producing the fine and all-purpose woven cloth which made this region one of the great workshops of the world.[29]

Central to Indian social ordering, and around 1740 still seemingly immune to changes brought about by rapid commercialization, was the notion that the ultimate reason why an Indian landowner or merchant collected wealth was to recycle it into socially worthy causes. Motivated by this altruistic impulse, merchants, bankers, government officials and others whom we would regard as "modern" all contributed to the maintenance of social service facilities. These included temple complexes which invested in training colleges, scholarly libraries, roadside fountains, hostels for travellers, and in the South around Madras, hundreds of tank wells for irrigation during the dry season. Moreover, in time of dearth, convention held that great landlords should restrain the greedy impulses of traders in basic foodstuffs and take steps to insure that food was distributed to the poor at pre-dearth prices. The effect of this was to encourage the poor to stay in or near their natal villages, rather than rushing off to some great city in a vain search for food. We will have occasion later to assess the effects on public health of the cancellation of this policy by the British.[30]

In pre-British times, before notions of caste solidified, there was great diversity in the layering of society. Geographical and social mobility worked against any hard and fast notions of hereditary status and countered the tendency for occupations to descend from fathers to sons. In Bengal and South India, among people who recognized themselves as Hindus there were a few thousand elderly scholars (the Brahmins) who, after tiring of youthful passions, spent their time recopying and studying ancient Sanskrit texts. Paralleling them in the world of Islam were aging scholars who passed their days studying sacred Arabic writings. Both intellectual elites had firm ideas about which concepts of purity and pollution established the proprieties of behavior. Unfortunately, British Orientalists (students of Eastern culture) quite mistakenly assumed that these rather incoherent, rarified ideals were normative for society as a whole.[31]

In actuality, in pre-British days these elitist ideas were virtually unknown to ordinary semi-settled rural people and the semi-nomadic tribal peoples of the west and far north. Instead, what governed these people's day-to-day activities were each group's local customs. In time of crisis unwritten customs might require that the community be brought together as a moral whole by propitiating local deities with special forms of ritual behavior and sacrifices. Yet because of the great diversity of India's social groupings—which could be numbered in their hundreds—any quasi-anthropological attempt to generalize from one or two local examples runs the risk of caricaturing the reality of India. In colonial hands in time of cholera the habit of assuming that all Indians fit into a single stereotype, a subaltern "Other," was highly damaging and mischievous.

Pre-British India was ruled by Mughal emperors (descendants of Babur, d. 1530). These rulers regarded western traders as troublesome interlopers who had nothing to sell which any Indian might want other than the useful stores of silver the Westerners left behind. However, with the decay of

Mughal power beginning in the late seventeenth century and the emergence of princes vying with each other to build up small, efficiently organized localized states—such as the Marathas Confederation and Mysore under Haidar Ali and Tipu Sultan—western silver (much of it American in origin) came to play an increasingly important role in determining local balances of power. Silver was needed to pay mercenary soldiers, as well as the Indian, Persian or Turkish artisans who turned out artillery pieces and other requisites of modern war. Silver was also needed to pay the owners of the bulk-transport-hauling bullocks used in the continent-wide provisioning system as well as the managers of the tens of thousands of elephants that served in battle as the equivalent of modern tanks.

As for the English, before 1765 they had depended almost entirely on New World specie to buy their way into India (it was for this that indigenous miners in smallpox-riddled Mexico and Peru worked, sickened and died). Imported silver was used to subsidize English traders so that they could undercut the prices charged by their Indian or Middle Eastern rivals at the great port at Surat in commodity exchange with traders crossing the seas to China, or to south-east Asia, or to Egypt. Once underway, the process moved ahead swiftly: by 1750 indigenous mercantile enterprises in Surat were falling into serious decline. By 1820 they had been supplanted entirely by the British-controlled emporium at Bombay just down the coast.

New World specie was also used to construct the English-officered Sepoy military force which by 1798 had become one of the world's largest armies. Troops were recruited from Bihar and elsewhere in northern India, special care being taken to pay them regularly and at a slightly higher rate than they would receive from an Indian princely employer.[32]

Contributing to the collapse of centralized Mughal power, between 1742 and 1751 Maratha cavalry from west-central India raided deep into the Mughal Bengali heartland, putting village farming populations to flight and utterly disrupting the transport of Bengali grain and rice south to Tamil-land. In 1757, adding to the general chaos was the conquest of Bengal by East India Company troop commander Robert Clive. Like an imperial Roman conqueror of old, after his victory at Plassey Clive pressured local tax collectors to bring in revenues. In 1765 the EIC formally assumed the fiscal administration (*diwani*) of the provinces of Bengal, Bihar and Orissa.[33]

This was the general situation in 1769 when the rains failed, leading to the great famine of 1769–70 in which an estimated 10 million people, a quarter of the Bengali population, died. Writing of the crisis, a Dutch naval commander who was in the area claimed that:

> This famine arose in part from the bad rice harvest of the preceding year; *but it must be attributed principally to the monopoly the English had over the last harvest of this commodity, which they kept at such a high price* that most of the unfortunate inhabitants . . . found themselves powerless

> to buy the tenth part of what they needed to live. . . . To this scourge was added smallpox, which spread among persons of all ages and of which they died in great numbers.[34]

Thus from the very beginning of their 190 years in India, the British set the pattern of rule though violence, intimidation and coercion which they would follow to the end of their stay.[35]

Epidemic cholera as a continent-wide phenomenon seems first to have appeared in 1817, beginning with outbreaks in Jessore in Bengal, and later that year, in central India in the East India Company army being led by Lord Moira, Marquis of Hastings, against an alliance of Marathas forces and Pindaris (roving bands of unemployed mercenary soldiers).[36] On 13 November Hastings noted in his diary:

> Camp Talgong. The dreadful epidemic disorder which has been causing such ravages in Calcutta and in the southern provinces, has broken out in camp. It is a species of cholera morbus, which appears to seize the individual without his having had any previous sensations of the malady. If immediate relief is not at hand, the person to a certainty dies within four or five hours.

Hastings's diary entry from two days later reads: "The march [across the Pohooj River] was terrible for the number of poor creatures falling under the sudden attacks of this dreadful infliction . . . 500 have died since sunset yesterday."[37] Writing of this all-India epidemic, a World Health Organization historian noted that it had been preceded by famine: "the year 1815 and still more that of 1817 had been marked by extremely heavy rains followed by disastrous floods and harvest failures."[38]

In 1825 (four years before cholera moved out of India to strike Tsarist Russia and the Habsburg lands before moving on to the kingdoms of England and France), Dr Annesley, an English medical doctor who had served for twenty-five years in India, wrote to friends in London about what he had discovered of the history of cholera from "those acquainted with the writings of the Hindoos." These investigations led Annesley to conclude: "That we have *no* proof of the prevalence of cholera in India, as a wide spreading epidemic in former times." Though he knew that localized outbreaks of a disease like cholera had been reported by Portuguese, French and English traders in Indian ports in various years before 1817, Annesley was in effect suggesting that the cholera epidemic currently rampaging throughout most of Asia was a new phenomenon.[39]

However, back in England at the recently established East India Company college at Haileybury, the younger generation of John Company servants being trained in James Mill's invented history of India (published in 1817) learned that India had been physically and morally corrupt time out of mind. Confronted with this powerful mindset, Annesley's sensible suggestion that "wide spreading epidemic" cholera was a new phenomenon was set aside. Superseding it was the assumption that epidemic cholera had *always* been common throughout the whole of India even though before 1817 white men had not been there to record it.[40]

As we have seen, in the Kochian understanding cholera as actual disease does best among people who are mentally depressed because their life-worlds have been shattered, or because they are physically malnourished or suffering directly from famine. These prerequisites were all provided in the run-up to the major epidemic of 1817. The leaders of those who caused mental depression included the first governor-general Charles, the Marquis Cornwallis, his companions and their immediate successors. These "true Britons" all sprang from English/Irish/Scottish families who back home were using the techniques of Agrarian Patriotism to debase country people in the lower social orders through the destruction of their customary rights by enclosure, rack-renting and mass eviction. When confronted with the strange alien land that was India, these true Britons had no compunction about destroying communitarian patterns there as well.[41]

Described by his biographer in the *Dictionary of National Biography* as not being "a man of startling genius," Charles Cornwallis, Old Etonian, Governor-General of India after 1786 immensely furthered the destruction of the tissue of Indian society. Soon after arriving, he imposed western ideas of morality by banning company employment of half-castes, the result of the unregulated sex life of the companions of Robert Clive. Thus even before the wives of Company servants of the officer class were encouraged to come out to join their husbands in the 1820s, the relationship between true Britons and subject people was characterized on the British side by deliberately affected racial separatism. For Indians of quality who were prepared to collaborate with the British conquerers and to learn their ways, this policy was demoralizing.[42]

Since true Briton officers regarded ordinary British Company soldiers as little better than the sweepings of gaols (in 1817 Hastings termed them "creatures"), men of that sort were still permitted to satisfy their sexual urges with Indian prostitutes. Whenever a British army moved out, it was accompanied by hordes of camp followers who in fleeing back to their villages to escape death by cholera would bring the cholera morbus with them. In a comment on this situation during the Indian-wide epidemic of 1817–23 it was claimed that:

> it was the Pindaries [*sic*] moving from place to place and the British troops *and their vast horde of camp-followers following them*, which aided materially in spreading and keeping up the epidemic, which lasted *just so long* as those movements continued.[43]

Cutting particularly deep into the grain of Indian social structures was Cornwallis's Permanent Land Settlement and associated legal reforms of

1793. Arising from these were a new sort of *zamindars* who were responsible for paying taxes for "their" landed estates, on pain of forfeiture. Pre-Cornwallis *zamindars* had had no proprietary rights but merely served the Mughal as revenue collectors for stipulated territories. In creating the new kind of *zamindar* Cornwallis brought into being a category of people he believed would serve in much the same capacity as the local gentry of Suffolk or Kent in pressing forward with the destruction of customary use-rights and establishing wage labor as the normal rural pattern. In the event, this exercise in the creation of legally enforceable rights in land where none had existed before led to a considerable turnover of Hindu big men, as those compelled to sell were replaced by new Hindi collaborators (*bhadralok*). Emerging from this by the 1820s were *bhadralok* absentee *rentiers* driven by the suddenly fashionable British ideology of possessive individualism. More often than not these "new men" forgot that the proper purpose of wealth was to further social betterment schemes: hospitals, schools, roadside fountains. In time of famine, men of their sort would not be inconvenienced by British refusal to control the export of grain—the commodity on which life itself depended—*out of* areas of grain scarcity *towards* other areas which would pay a higher price.[44]

Cornwallis's land revenue and *zamindar* policies were only one contribution to the massive transformation of the social composition and ecology of India. Following the terms of the legal code he introduced in 1793, all weavers and artisans were placed under contract to the East India Company and prohibited from supplying independent merchant dealers. Goaded by English tax collectors to pay up but given sub-starvation wages by the monopolistic EIC, hundreds of spinners and weavers gave up work and fled to their native villages where they sank into the residuum of the desperate poor. According to historian J. E. Wills, by the late 1790s the deterioration of the quality and quantity of fine Indian cotton cloth had become generally apparent.[45]

Writing of the situation a quarter of a century later, the French Orientalist Abbé Dubois claimed that Europe had depended on India for fine cloths "*from time immemorial*" but that now they had become redundant, victims of advanced British cloth-making technology. He went on to say that:

> This collapse in the cotton industry has indirectly . . . [stopped] the circulation of money, and the cultivators can no longer count on the manufacturers . . . to buy up their surplus grain. . . . This has led the cultivators to the hard necessity of relinquishing their grain to them, and thus becoming the prey of remorseless usurers.[46]

The successor to Cornwallis was the Old Etonian, Richard, Marquis Wellesley. The marquis and his brothers Henry and Arthur (the later Duke of Wellington) let themselves be persuaded by William Jones, H. T. Colebrooke and other Orientalists that warring Indian princes' efforts to build small-scale successor states to replace the over-extended Mughal Empire were perverting the "ancient constitution" of India. That this "ancient constitution" was a mythic construct knocked together by eccentric Brahmins for western Orientalists in no way diminished its effectiveness as a rationale for British conquest.[47] Relying on it and on public school teachings about imperial Roman precedents of "salutary terror," the brothers Wellesley warred on Indian princely separatists and, after their surrender, slaughtered their commanding officers in cold blood.[48]

The brothers' sense of urgency was strengthened by their fear that agents of the French Revolution of 1789 might infiltrate India and in alliance with rebels (seen as criminal gangs) bring down the British fiscal-military regime. Rather unwisely, Tipu Sultan of Mysore played along with this by planting a Liberty Tree and calling his friends Citizen X or Y. This stance brought on him the full force of the Wellesley military and, with it, defeat in battle and an inglorious death (in 1799). Yet before this denouement, the Mysore rulers had established policy precedents—for their regional state—which anticipated much of what the British would soon do in India as a whole. In a nutshell, princely Mysore policy was to bring the full weight of a regional state to bear on the life of all cultivators by forcing them to settle down so that they could be taxed, judged and otherwise kept under bureaucratic supervision.[49] Left largely unfulfilled by Haider Ali and Tipu Sultan, because of constraints of time imposed by the British conquests, their plans for modernization provided true Britons with a sure guide to the making of profit, which by cruel coincidence worked to the greater glory of the cholera morbus.

Under the old generally cholera-free rural order that existed when Clive and Haidar Ali came on the scene, each settlement had been a geographically mobile community under a warrior who was headman, disputes adjudicator and distributor of use-rights in communal lands which he made no claim to owning. Indeed in most of India, village life had been based on the premise that a village consisted of a people and their customs rather than a fixed place and set of buildings.

Further complicating rural reality was the fact that around 1817 the subcontinent was still underpopulated relative to its potential resource base; much of it was covered by forests. Particularly in the central plateau of the Deccan, there were vast sparsely populated tracts where people moved around at will. Under this sort of land-use regime, fertile land would be cultivated until it seemed to tire, then the village would move on somewhere else, returning two or three generations later to recolonize the land. Equipped with this attitude towards place, if the rains failed, or if a disease threat appeared, the village would move to a more healthy site.[50] This flexibility doubtless largely explains why in pre-British days epidemic cholera and smallpox had not been continental-scale phenomena.

In addition to its semi-mobile agricultural populations, India contained a large number of wandering pastoralists, the tribal peoples. In the course of his life an individual tribal might have several professions, serving as mercenary soldier, cobbler, trader, healer, or in whatever other niche opportunity provided. Based during the hottest months in the hills of western India (the Ghats) or in the uplands and mountains of the north towards Afghanistan and the Himalayas, tribals moved to the lowlands during the cooler months, there to circulate goods of all sorts (some honestly come by, some stolen) among ordinary semi-monetized peoples. Tribals also cared for the pasturage and breeding of the horses and cattle which provided settled villagers throughout the subcontinent with the herds which were the principal form of wealth needed for their rites of passage.[51]

Into this complex of life-worlds in which settled, semi-settled and wandering tribal peoples all had their accustomed roles in a harsh natural environment with which they managed to cope, burst the English war machine and fiscal state. Building on precedents created by Haidar Ali and Tipu Sultan, it coerced people to settle permanently on fixed village sites so that they could be regularly taxed and regularly governed. As a direct result of British policies of compulsory settlement and monetarization, tens of thousands of people became demoralized, hunger-weakened wrecks whose inner organs seemed incapable of generating the acids and alkali needed in time of emergency to fight off the cholera vibrio.

What imperializing early and mid-nineteenth-century Britons failed to take into account when, for example, creating small tenancies held by the *ryotwari* system in South India, was that such policies quickly resulted in a massive increase in the amount of *sub-standard* land brought into cultivation. Rather than worrying about the consequences of this, government statistician W. W. Hunter and others of his sort thought that the increase in the area of cultivation—in the twenty-five years after 1853 the increase was 66 percent—spoke well for the British civilizing presence.[52] Reality was quite different. With *ryots*' greater dependence on marginal land they also became more reliant on usurers to tide them over when taxes fell due. When the rains either failed or came with so much force that they destroyed crops, arrangements with usurers led to default and confiscation, with predictable results: famine and—if the vibrio happened to be around—an epidemic of cholera.

In their own perceptions of the origins of cholera, Indian village people could be found (no one village being typical) who posited a connection between the coming of the British and the catastrophic killer disease. Writing of the region around Bombay, the retired civil servant, E. E. Enthoven, reported that:

> There is a popular tradition that in ancient times cholera was subjugated by King Vikrama, and was buried under ground. Once upon a time the British excavated the place of burial in the belief that treasure was concealed there, and thus cholera was released. After many soldiers had fallen

victim, the disease deity was at last propitiated by an oblation, and was handed over to the Bhangis [untouchables].[53]

Enthoven's words spark off four thoughts: first, the association in the popular mind between British greed for gold and the coming of cholera. Secondly, that soldiers were particularly prone. In the year of the Great Rebellion of 1857–58 (an event of cosmic significance certain to be remembered in oral tradition), in the provinces in revolt one in ten Sepoy or British soldiers died (100.6 per thousand). Of these deaths only 4.3 per thousand were chalked up to military action; nearly all the rest died of diseases, led by cholera.[54]

The third Enthoven spark concerns the oft-reported Indian village assumption that the disease was sent by a controlling force, a disease goddess, who was willing to enter into negotiations with humankind and, when satisfied with the propitiatory offerings received would withdraw the disease. True Britons scoffed at this, holding it to be another of the superstitions of the ignorant black population.[55] However, in light of modern understandings, what bigoted people might term "superstition" and progressive people recognize as a healthy form of tension release was not confined to India. In July 1866, during the worst of Europe's cholera epidemics, the populace of Brussels (now the capital of Europe) entered into negotiations with the Holy Virgin Mary indistinguishable from those undertaken with another goddess in village India.[56]

In India, Enthoven's observations of popular customs raise a fourth point: the transference of the disease "to the Bhangis," the lowest caste, the untouchables. It would seem that in Bombay such people were regarded as having a touch of magic about them that enabled them to deal with catastrophic diseases before which ordinary indigenous professional health workers were helpless.

Moving now to medical responses to cholera in India, it will be seen that almost from the beginning of continent-wide cholera epidemics in 1817, British health provisioners made a point of *not* communicating with their Indian counterparts. This was a new departure. Some decades earlier, in the 1660s and 1670s, the occasional European medical person who travelled in the subcontinent—doctors like François Bernier and surgeons like John Fryer—had accepted that Indian medical professionals were more or less on the same wavelength as themselves despite their unwillingness to practice bleeding, the patent western cure for fevers.

Bernier and Fryer had found that there were two principal *learned* medical systems on the subcontinent. The oldest, the *Ayurvéda*, was based on texts written in Sanskrit between 1 CE and 1000; practitioners were known as *vaids*. The second system, *Unani Tibb* (the medicine of Hellenistic Greece), came in slowly after the eighth century with Muslim traders and in a big way with the Turko-Arab conquests of the 1400s. It was cousin-germane to the humoral medicine used in West Europe until the birth of the clinic in the eighteenth century. *Unani Tibb* practitioners were known as *hakims*.

In undertaking to become a *vaid* in the Sanskrit tradition, apprentices generally lived in the household of their master, who was often either their father or their uncle. The live-in apprenticeship system was sometimes also used in the *Unani Tibb* system, though many *hakims* were associated with a great school, temple and library complex where they assisted in the training of apprentices. The *Unani Tibb* training program was undermined when the British, using bogus legal precedents, claimed that property titles were faulty and confiscated the endowed lands needed to keep Muslim institutions in being.[57]

However, the difficulties faced under Company rule by practitioners of learned medicine in the *Unani Tibb* and *Ayurvéda* traditions had only a *marginal* impact on the sort of medical provisioning available to ordinary village people. In pre-colonial days *vaids* and *hakims* had generally confined their practice to well-off clients in princely courts. It was only when this patronage began to dry up with the slaughter or compulsory retirement of dissident princes and their replacement with British collaborators (who used British doctors) that *vaids* and *hakims* widened their catchment base to include the new Indian middle class in cities such as Calcutta and Bombay that were fully in the British sphere. These developments still left the rural world—where 95 percent of all Indians lived—virtually untouched by any formal system of medicine.[58]

Straws thrown into the air early on showed which way the wind would blow for indigenous learned medicine. In 1814 the directors of the EIC suggested that the expatriate doctors consult Indian practitioners about the sorts of cures they used for the special diseases of the place. Doctors however were by that time already aware that Indians used calomel as a cure for fevers and felt that they had nothing else to learn. After 1814 they came to hold all Indian medical systems and practitioners in contempt.[59]

This attitude reflected the impact which the philosophic code of conduct devised for gentlemen, known as "Independency," was having on colonial minds. As reworked by Adam Smith in his *Theory of Moral Sentiments* (published in 1759, with many later editions) building on John Locke's *Thoughts on Education* and the Stoic writings of Marcus Aurelius and Epictetus, independency exalted mind over matter, and reason over passion. Its goal was "self-command" and a sense of "independency upon Fortune, and contempt of all outward accidents of pain, poverty, exile, and death." Quoting Locke and Epictetus, Smith moralized that "Death, as we say, is the King of Terrors" but the "man who has conquered his fear of death" demonstrates his complete control over his passions and thus is able "to breathe the free air of liberty and Independency."[60]

This moral uplift found expression in medical responses when cholera first broke out. In 1817 it was learned in Calcutta that cholera was nearby at Jessore. Asked to make recommendations, the Calcutta Medical Board reprimanded the English magistrate at Jessore who had forgotten to conquer his fear of death and instead closed down his court and sent people home. With their own stiff upper lips still intact, the Medical Board then claimed that the cholera was "the usual epidemic of this period of the year" and, with a bow to Church of England cleric Thomas Malthus, pointed out that "it is probable that the consequences . . . may in the present instance have been beneficial, correcting the influence of an *overcrowded population*." As we saw earlier, Indian numbers were actually already in decline.[61]

In 1827 when the second all-India epidemic was intensifying preparatory to its advance through Europe, R. H. Kennedy, an Anglo-Irishman writing from Bombay, opined that the epidemic failed to offer "a more distressing image of desolation to our view than what we are in the habit of beholding with philosophic calmness, and ranking among the ordinary casualties of Indian life."[62] Here then on the Malabar Coast was a medical person invoking Epictetus and his Roman Stoic phrase, "the lecture room of the philosopher is the hospital," mediated through Adam Smith's *Moral Sentiments*.[63] One wonders if Kennedy knew about the final agonies of the highest British official on the other side of the peninsula on the Coromandel Coast. Dying of cholera in 1827, the creator of the *ryotwari* system, Sir Thomas Munro, presumably passed through the standard stages: uncontrollable vomiting, passage of rice-stools, dehydration, screaming in pain, living death followed by spasms of rigor mortis.

Western medical doctors' closure of minds to *Ayurévda* and *Unani Tibb* medical systems after 1814 was followed by another setback for medicine in 1835. In that year, in a response to a request by Governor-General Lord William Bentinck, Thomas Babington Macaulay issued his definitive "Minute on Education." This held that any educational institution funded by tributary exactions from Indians (taxes) must use the English language as its sole medium for instruction. Indian revisionist historians have recently seized the initiative from romantics of the "timeless India" school who have always regarded the "Minute on Education" as insulting. Instead they have highlighted the contributions of Rammohun Roy (1772–1833) and other Bengali Brahmins. Running contrary to the stereotype timeless Indian, Rammohun fully accepted that Indians had fallen behind in conceptualizing and producing the "ingenious contrivances and useful discoveries which have made such giant strides in Europe in late years." To set things right he demanded (in 1823) that the English permit the recycling of funds to support *English-language* teaching institutions that would enable Indians to catch up with the West. As a result of the head of steam Rammohun Roy built up the Calcutta Medical College was established in 1851.[64]

That this promising beginning did not lead to much progress in medical education can be credited to pre-existing and new attitudes regarding the "nature of Indians." As interpreted by a modern historian (who himself posited a "colonial divide"), "these held that Indians were a single reified 'Other.' "[65]

This mindset was part of the British reaction to the Rebellion of 1857–58, when for a time it seemed that Britain might have to abandon the subcontinent. Yet at a deeper level, failure to make any significant headway in public health in India was linked to attitudinal and political developments back in England. It is to these we now turn.

Cholera in Britain

Writing up his impressions of cholera in Manchester during the first epidemic to hit Britain, medical doctor James Kay (later known as Kay-Shuttleworth) affirmed that:

> the invasion of pestilence . . . unmask[s] the deformity of evils which have preyed upon the energies of the community. He whose duty it is to follow in the steps of this messenger of death, must descend to the abodes of poverty . . . where pauperism and disease congregate around the source of social discontent and political disorder in the centre of our large towns, and behold with alarm, in the hot-bed of pestilence, ills that fester in secret, at the very heart of society.[66]

Freighted with paranoiac fears of social discontent and dissolution, Dr Kay-Shuttleworth's cholera statement is part of an epidemiological past which can only be understood within the context of the extraordinary circumstances in which Britain found itself in the early 1830s.

Beginning with the contextual strands that impacted most directly upon the decision-makers in the upper echelons of society, we should remind ourselves that in 1830–31 Great Britain's ruling elite had only recently reinvented itself. Emerging from the humiliation of defeat at the hands of American colonialists at Yorktown in 1781, the thousand or so English families in the London orbit who were in hegemonic control of the two islands decided to widen the basis of elite recruitment to include the landholding classes of Scotland, Ireland, Wales and northern England. Various carrots were offered. These included promises of preferment for younger sons for prestigious posts in India and in the royal navy. They also included government support for the phenomenon known as Agrarian Patriotism. This policy encouraged accelerated extinction of ordinary country dwellers' customary rights, the enclosure of common land, the demonization of the peasantry, and the flight of dispossessed country people into towns.[67] In some regions, the impact was particularly dramatic. North and west of Glasgow and Aberdeen, in an ethnic cleansing known as the Highland Clearances, modernizing landlords who took their clue from Edinburgh's Scottish Enlightenment massively increased their profits by bringing in sheep to replace Gaelic-speaking customary tenants who had been on the land since time immemorial.[68]

Located several rungs lower down on the ladder of social esteem than the great landed proprietors were broad conglomerates of people still known as the middling sort or the middle classes (plural). Within this spectrum were the atypical entrepreneurial manufacturers who no longer felt quite at ease in the company of high-grade artisans, even though most manufacturers still did. The middling sort also included lawyers and barristers, merchants and bankers with modest incomes, town clerks and other bureaucrats, engineers, architects, the town-based pseudo-gentry (widows and pensioned family members of genuine landed gentry), and the triad of medical professionals—apothecaries, surgeons and second-rate physicians. What all men within the broad middle range of society had in common was that they kept their womenfolk at home. Beyond the domestic sphere, their commonality of experience was that they had *not* attended a public school and did not have a relationship based on equality with any of the landed gentry and aristocrats (the true Britons) who ran England, commanded her armies and navies, and determined foreign policy. Lacking true Britons' *rentier* incomes and inherited broad acres, young males in the middle social grades had to scout about for ways to make a living which would be both respectable and remunerative.[69]

Emerging from the ranks of this ambitious middling sort was a group of ideologues or visionary theorists. Determined to make something of themselves in a splashy sort of way, many of them saw a future in adopting Jeremy Bentham's ideology of moral rectitude known as Utilitarianism. This had as its slogan the catchy, but utterly misleading words, "the greatest happiness for the greatest number." Rather in the manner of Rousseau's famous concept, the General Will, the Utilitarian credo took it for granted that its adherents alone knew the true path to the "progress" promised by the Enlightenment. To make their voices heard in the general babble of the times, they tended to speak and write in arrogant acerbic tones. Violently opinionated, they let the world know that they were spokesmen for a new social category, the Middle Class, and that this was the keystone in the arch on which the stability of the whole social fabric depended. So successful were they in making this claim that it is only in very recent times that historians (themselves usually middle class) have discovered that the actual keystone—as late as 1914—consisted of gentlemanly capitalists, a mix of modernized aristocrats, upper-crust bankers, merchants and money-changers.[70]

For our purposes, other than elderly Jeremy Bentham himself, especially important among the ideologues of the middling sort was Bentham's one-time secretary, Edwin Chadwick, his particular medical friend, Thomas Southwood Smith and Bentham's young protégé, James Mill, author of the infamous *History of India*. Among the next generation of Utilitarians—until he suffered a nervous breakdown from its effects—was John Stuart Mill, son and successor of James Mill at the India Office. Seen in retrospect as a leading founder of the English ideology of liberalism, in writing his touchstone book *On Liberty* (1859), J. S. Mill made it clear that the privilege of being a free individual did not apply to any of the denizens of India.[71]

All but concealed from modern historians' eyes by the ideologues' invectives against the landed classes was their adoption of one of the principal elements in the agrarian patriot code: Adam's Smith's revamped Stoic construct, Independency. Using this as their conceptual core, during the years of the French wars and Anglo-Scottish reaction from 1793 to the time of the first cholera epidemic (1831–32) and the Reform Bill of 1832, British theorists constructed their own not so distinctive moral code. This stressed rugged individualism and hard work, moral rectitude, "manliness," dedication to family life and family recreations, clean speech, and avoidance of outward shows of emotion, public drunkenness or other unseemly forms of behavior. England and Scotland being Protestant countries, it also paid lip-service to church attendance. Closely allied to this secular ideology were various forms of evangelical Christianity.[72]

Standing in stark contrast to what R. J. Morris refers to as the "confident arrogant lunge for world cultural hegemony" by English and Scottish ideologues were the groupings in the artisan ranges of society. It was for people of this sort (unaffected, natural and sincere) that Thomas Paine wrote his tracts on the rights of humankind. Consisting of nearly two-thirds of the adult population, this broad social spectrum was made up of men and women who used their hands and skills to produce goods ranging from processed foodstuffs to high-quality household furnishings for sale on world markets. Only a few years earlier, in the late seventeenth and early eighteenth centuries, people of this sort had created the revolution in consumer habits on which the modern world economy is now based. Not being clairvoyant, they had been unaware that the consumerism monster they helped create would destroy the life-worlds of their descendants.[73]

In the early nineteenth century, before this final denouement came to pass (helped along by cholera), English and Scottish artisans thought in terms of hierarchies based on skill, honor, integrity and age. Though by then the old-style status gradations—apprentice, journeyman, master—were no longer as firmly fixed as they were in the German lands at the time, British masters continued to regard any of their number who used his surplus wealth to hire the services of another master to help meet production deadlines as just another artisan like themselves rather than as a member of some other class (an artisan undergoing upward social mobility). Tenacious in their blindness to what was going on, artisans placed a high premium on personal independence and their ability to hire out their skills to whomever they chose, when they chose. They looked askance at any master who carelessly borrowed money to buy raw materials from a ruthless entrepreneur, defaulted on repayment, and so fell into the trap of keeping bread on the family table by working as a full-time wage slave under his creditor.

Independent working men also placed a high premium on mutualities established in the overlapping worlds of the workshop, the alehouse, beer hall or tavern, and in the rough and tumble of leisure-time sports and festivities in streets and lanes. They enjoyed violent wrestling matches, bull-baiting, setting dogs on bears, betting on fighting cocks, and the use of "rough music" to enforce neighborhood behavioral norms among men and women. When it came time to say goodbye to a dead workmate, family member or neighbor, they insisted on the proprieties of a proper funeral and burial in consecrated ground. Though seldom likely to attend church services, they expected that at the Last Day the dead would rise from their graves to rejoice in the company of risen family members and workmates.[74]

Seen from the perspective of 1809 (the year in which Thomas Paine was both alive and dead) it seemed to some that this artisan life pattern was secure and timeless; yet it was doomed. Ill-equipped at law to protect the ways they took leave of their dead, found their recreations, and worked, ordinary people were unable to counter the violent thrusts of the visionary theorists who sought to destroy their world. In retrospect it would seem that ideologues' acts of despoilment (so much in evidence during the cholera months in 1831–32) were a response to their own felt need to differentiate themselves—the moral few—from the amorphous lower class *many*, so to win the approbation of the actual rulers of Britain, the great landed proprietors.

Even before cholera hit in 1831, late-flowering French jacobinical radicalism of the sort that flowed into the radical republicanism of Thomas Paine provided ideologues with a sense of urgency in their dealing with the mob (their general term for ordinary people). In addition to this political threat, and equally worrying, was the huge surge in the British population: from a base of around 5 million in 1700, it had increased to nearly 10 million by 1800. Building up a head of steam after around 1780, by 1850 it doubled again. As early as 1798, Thomas Malthus, a fearful parson in the Church of England (d. 1834), warned that all these surplus humans had no right to exist. Malthus also held that Nature, in its wisdom, would cut their numbers through famine, war or plague. In the first edition of his *Essay on Population* in 1798, he was unaware that cholera might be *the* purging agency he required.[75]

Adding fuel to the Malthusian specter was the suspicion that among the laboring classes the average age at which a woman was first impregnated by a man was steadily dropping from the twenty-six or twenty-five that had obtained before the homeostatic controls known under rural communitarianism had collapsed (a victim of Agrarian Patriotism) to the present twenty or twenty-one. In the absence of contraceptives and an appropriate mindset, a lower age of marriage meant higher rates of birth and more mouths demanding to be fed. On the eve of cholera in 1831, it was all too apparent that just under half the members of the laboring classes were under the age of twenty and that nearly three out of four were under thirty (the age of full discretion). Adding further to what ideologues perceived as the threat of urban riot were the sizeable numbers of distressed Catholics who were coming from Ireland to find work in mainland towns.[76]

Confronted with social dissidence, a typical British middle-rank male response was to join one of the social-activist voluntary organizations recently founded to promote social and moral uplift. One such group was the Proclamation Society which, under the guidance of Hull-born William Wilberforce, instituted lawsuits against a man who published tracts written by Thomas Paine. When the printer was thrown into prison and his wife and children were evicted from their London flat, Wilberforce was heralded as a moral hero. Working from other London bases after 1802 were the Society for the Suppression of Vice and the umbrella organization for the dissemination of western values world-wide known as the Society for the Suppression of Slavery. In North Britain, among Scots setting moralization campaigns in motion was the Glasgow preacher Thomas Chalmers, to whom Dr James Phillips Kay (a graduate of Edinburgh University), dedicated his 1832 study of Manchester cholera. Another Scot was the peripatetic preacher of temperance, John Dunlop. Dunlop's special recipe for moralization was to persuade *working* people to give up alcohol entirely, though he would allow elites to drink fine wines.[77]

At a time when it was known that the cholera morbus had broken out of India and was making its way across the domains of the Romanovs and the Habsburgs (causing riots among peoples who saw it as a medico-aristocratic scheme to rid lands of surplus population), a further stimulus to social tension in England was provided by the parliamentary progress of a bill much favored by the Utilitarian clique. This was the Anatomy Bill, introduced in 1828. The bill can be seen as an Anglo-Scottish response to the famous French Enlightenment "birth of the clinic" which held that the way forward in medicine was through a more detailed understanding of human anatomy.

In Britain the first clinic to be established—in operation by the 1780s—was at Edinburgh. Early in the next century, medical entrepreneurs, seeing that they were onto a good thing, opened anatomy schools in scores of provincial towns. Following market demand, aspiring middle-class students who saw clinical medicine as a promising career option, clamored for entrance. This meant that there was a new and growing demand for dead human bodies.[78]

In order to provide anatomists with fresh dead, in the late 1820s ambitious school directors—including King George IV's own physician—took to hiring grave robbers. Sometimes, as in Edinburgh, unscrupulous minions such as Burke and Hare saved time by murdering their catch to bring in bodies that were still warm. Notwithstanding rumors of foul play, in 1828–29 Utilitarian ideologues openly asserted that mere ignorance and superstition prevented the laboring classes from willingly giving over their dead to their local middle-class anatomists.[79]

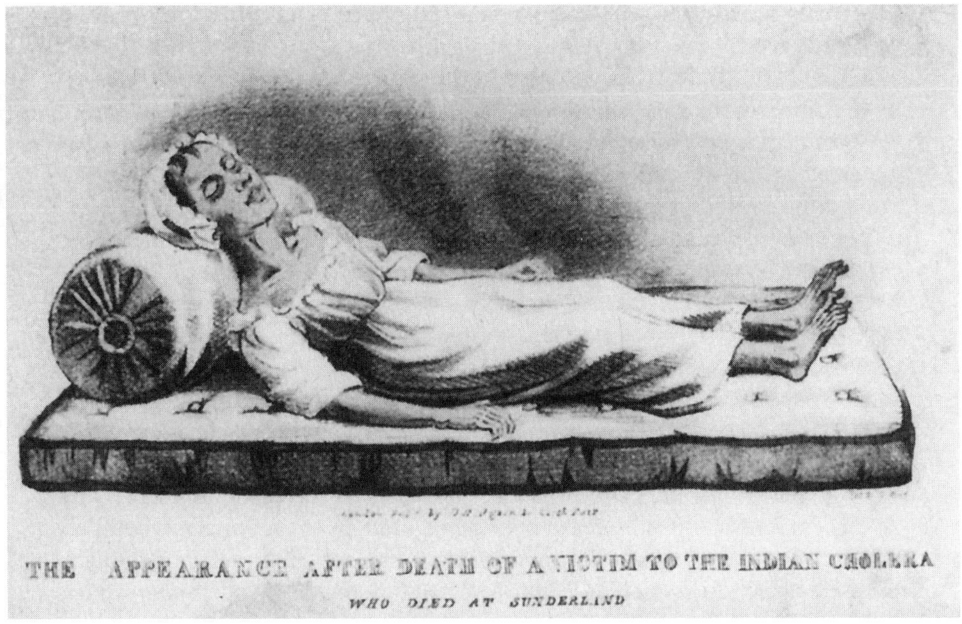

13. A dead victim of cholera at Sunderland. A colored lithograph, 1832, by I. W. G.

Confronted with intense hostility from laborers (left unenfranchised until fifty-six years later), in 1828 the Anatomy Bill was introduced into Parliament. When it received the Royal Assent in 1831, it ordained that poor people who died in workhouses who had none to claim their body would legally fall into the clutches of their local school. Delighted with this triumph of enlightened reason in which his protégé Thomas Babington Macauley (of later Minute on Indian Education fame) had played a major role, the eighty-year-old Jeremy Bentham gave orders that at his own death his dear friend, Dr Thomas Southwood Smith, should carve him up in the interest of science. So it was that at his demise in 1832, the great Utilitarian's mortal remains were mounted on a special "Auto-Ikon" and put on display in Bentham's foundation for higher education, University College, on Gower Street, London.[80]

With the triumph of the Anatomy Bill, ordinary people's terror of cholera (already present in German Baltic ports by the summer of 1831), was much heightened by fear that they would become part of an "anatomy soup." When in October 1831 cholera finally touched down in England at the port town of Sunderland in County Durham, it killed among others, old man Sproat aged sixty and William Sproat Jr, "a fine athletic young keelman who had attended on his parent." Eager to have a go at carving up cholera dead like young Sproat, medical doctors from Edinburgh and London descended on Sunderland.[81]

In the fearful weeks that followed, ordinary Britons (of the sort defined by Tom Paine) set their teeth in opposition to medical doctors and managers of for-profit anatomy schools. One of the most famous of the cholera riots occurred at the Swan Street Hospital in Manchester. On 24 March, John Hase, a laboring man, was told by hospital authorities that his three-year-old grandson, already bereft of both parents through cholera and suffering the disease himself, was on the road to recovery. Next day, when Hase went back to the hospital to take his grandson home, he was given the run-around and then told the boy was dead. Suspecting foul play, grandfather Hase rounded up his friends and, joined by a crowd of working women, invaded the hospital burial ground and dug up the boy's coffin. On opening the lid, they found that a brick had been substituted for the boy's head. Outraged, grandfather Hase and friends stormed into the hospital, and liberated other cholera patients who they believed were at risk of being murdered by medical doctors. Then, bearing the coffin aloft in triumphant procession, they marched into Manchester city center. In the end, they were put to flight by a troop of Hussars. *The Times* of London made much of the affair, describing Hase and his associates as a "*mob* numbering several thousand" and "ignorant rabble." Thus did the acerbic language made fashionable by James Mill serve as the tool of discourse—among the middling sort—in the troubled cholera months.[82]

In facing cholera in their own homelands, the British (and Continental) medical community were still at sixes and sevens. Though some of their number had been in India and witnessed cholera epidemics there, there was no agreement as to whether this particular fever-like disease was contagious (here defined as spread directly from person to person) or whether it was non-contagious and caused by identifiable predisposing causes. If the new cholera were indeed contagious, medical and administrative logic—working on the analogy of the way bubonic plague had been contained in the seventeenth century—would require quarantines and cordons sanitaires.[83] However as every Briton knew, since the era of the Continental Blockade imposed by Napoleon, Britain's prosperity had depended on its mercantile fleet and world-wide freedom of trade. Fortunately for Britain's continued commercial well-being, an alternative, non-contagious, explanation was at hand.

In 1817–19, just a decade before cholera struck England, the Galenic argument about predisposing causes and Non-Naturals had been dusted off for application to the "Irish disease" then sweeping through England's oldest colony. The illness was probably typhus, the disease of filth. At the time it was noticed that rich members of the Anglo-Irish Protestant Ascendancy had by and large escaped the epidemic unscathed, though tens of thousands of Irish Catholic poor had perished. By linking "superstitious" Catholicism, poverty and death through disease, then contrasting it with "enlightened" Protestantism, wealth and good health, the credibility of "predisposing causes" was greatly strengthened.[84] Yet as we will see, out in India, the explanatory notion of predisposing causes—with its stress on individual people—would, in the interest of political correctness, be overruled in favor of an explanation stressing the importance of "place."

With the arrival of cholera in Sunderland late in 1831 and later in nearby Newburn and Newcastle upon Tyne, conflicting perceptions, constructions and ideas about what the disease actually was were much in evidence. One drift of argument was found in reports filed by Dr David Craigie, who had come down specially from Edinburgh to investigate the cholera situation in the town of Newburn, Northumberland. According to Craigie, during the initial attack in which twenty-three people died (out of forty-six attacked) one of the victims had been the much respected and virtuous vicar of Newburn himself. Craigie had found that during a second epidemic attack when 356 people were laid low there had also been a good mix of social types. In his estimation, most Newburn folk were "good specimens of the human race, both for size, figure and strength." Their occupations included glass working, the coal trade and agriculture. Attesting that "I saw many stout young people of both sexes attacked by the disease, and not a few carried off," Craigie strenuously denied that cholera specially targeted "only the feeble, the broken down and the dissipated" or that its victims were characterized by any special "habit or pre-disposition" to disease.[85]

Yet in another statement contained in the same medical journal in which Craigie had published his report, a correspondent pointed out that local Durham, Northumberland and Newcastle "coal-owners, coal-merchants and other traders" had warned medical reporters that their claim that the cholera was a new disease, probably contagious, brought in by ship from India, was "*a rash, ignorant and erroneous judgement.*" Following this tongue-lashing by these influential local employers, a committee of eighteen medical doctors "are said to have delivered their unanimous opinion at a public meeting" that the disease was in fact *not* the Indian epidemic, but was instead some standard English fever which required no administrative response that would cut off trade and shipping. Appalled at this subservient grovelling to local capitalists, the medical reporter could only advise members of the profession elsewhere "whose feelings and private interests were not concerned in the matter" to take note of what had happened and to act accordingly.[86]

They did. Coached by medical doctors who in turn were coached by interregional traders and bankers, Government after November 1831 saw cholera as "non-contagious." It was a variant of an English fever which could be expected to target those who were predisposed to it by their immoral living, their poverty, their neglect of family values, their holding of opinions about political matters, and their heavy drinking.

It was against these predisposing causes no less than the disease itself that local boards of health directed their attention when carrying out preventive and clean-up campaigns among the working classes during the actual cholera months. Taking up the temperance campaign of John Dunlop and his like, men from the middle-class-in-the-making on local boards of health posted notices warning working people that cholera's first victims *were always* those who had drunk strong spirits.[87] Typically, at Oxford some days before cholera arrived, the board of health posted warnings to:

> All Drunkards, Revellers. . . . You are now told for the third time, that Death and Drunkenness go hand in hand. . . . Death smites with its surest and swiftest arrows the licentious and intemperate.[88]

Writing of east London, a highly influential medical man, Bentham's friend Dr Thomas Southwood Smith, claimed that fevers (for him cholera was simply a fever variant) were caused by immorality (sex and the bottle) and by victims' general lack of self-reliance and proper habits.

And so it went throughout the two kingdoms. Ideologues and incipient liberals, seizing the opportunity provided by cholera, strove purposefully to smash the moral world of the artisan classes. In the interests of middle-class-defined "respectability," sporting events were forever cancelled and working men's drinking establishments were vilified and closed down.[89]

In the introductory comments of this chapter, I stressed the importance of eschewing the Whig approach to medical history. Here, as a case in point, is the middle-class vendetta against lower-class drinking. In the modern medical understanding, it is thought that any form of *excessive* drinking or eating may led to a stomach upset which may temporarily prevent that organ from secreting the appropriate antidote to invading *Vibrio cholerae*. However, for the 1831–32 moral rectitude crew—who of course knew nothing about biological responses to biological threats—*any drinking* at all by rough working people was an act of immorality which necessarily predisposed them to sicken and die from cholera.

Allied to the ideologues' attacks on drinking were their assaults on laboring men's habits of mourning and paying tribute to the dead. In popular communitarian culture, seen as of central importance in the face of death were the final laying out, washing, keeping watch all night, attendance at the funeral, and walking in the procession to the graveyard in recognition of the common humanity of the dead and the living. Because of work schedules and the felt need to bring in next of kin from distant places, the whole affair might take more than a week. Yet driven on by the morally righteous few who were intent on smashing artisans' life-worlds (seen as relics from the dark ages) administrative regulations required that the corpses of the cholera dead be handed over for proper disposal. Writing of the horrible things he had witnessed in 1832, the parish clerk of St Stephen's, Coleman Street, London recalled corpses being laid in lime in coffins from which only a few minutes later horrible liquids slurped out as burial attendants—fortified by strong drink—carried the mess out to carts waiting in the street. From there it would be carted off for disposal in unhallowed ground in places unknown to the surviving family and their friends.[90]

Figures available to historians (the General Registry Office was not established until 1837) suggest that in 1831–32, 31,474 people died of cholera in England, Wales and Scotland. However, what we know of popular attitudes towards human bodies and towards officialdom suggests that many cholera dead were kept out of their clutches and disposed of in an honorable way. In Sheffield in 1835, months after ideologues had conveniently forgotten that cholera had ever passed through, laboring men ensured that their own cholera dead would not be lost to mind. Working through their own voluntary organizations they raised a special monument to 339 cholera victims, "our kindred, our neighbours . . . our friends" who had been callously buried in unhallowed ground "without the camp" in 1831–32.[91]

Casting its gloomy shadow over ordinary English people during the first cholera epidemic were the discussions among respectable sorts that led up to the Poor Law Amendment Act. Summing up ideologues' interpretation of the sort of provision which had obtained earlier, Jeremy Bentham had fatuously claimed that:

> In this country, under the existing poor laws, every man has a right to be maintained, in the character of a pauper, at the public charge: under which right he is in fact, with a very few exceptions, maintained in idleness.[92]

At issue was the fraught question of who should pay the costs of keeping unemployed people alive—property-holding rate-payers or the unemployed's own family members. The old solution based on modifications of the Elizabethan Poor Law of 1601 had directed that each parish be responsible for providing *outdoor* relief or sheltered housing for those in need. At a time when life expectancy at birth was seldom more than forty (dropping back to thirty-five after the mid-seventeenth century), the Elizabethan expectation that the elderly, the crippled, disabled, orphaned or otherwise incapacitated receive parish relief as of right seemed reasonable. However, coping abilities faltered under the twin pressures of massive population increase after 1780 and the fallout (hordes of dispossessed people) resulting from government-sponsored Agrarian Patriotism.[93]

In the event it was Jeremy Bentham's trusted secretary, Edwin Chadwick (a Mancunian lawyer who saw his career future in central government) who took up the task of creating a new system of poor relief which would at one and the same time maintain the fiction that England was a Christian country and cater to the ideological needs of the propertied classes. Though a preparatory hearing had been held before cholera broke out—causing much melancholic worry among susceptibles during the epidemic—it was not until the size of the English political nation had been marginally enlarged by giving the franchise to some of the better-off urban middling sort (by the Reform Bill of 1832) that full-scale parliamentary hearings got underway.

The end result, the Poor Law Amendment Act of 1834, created a nationwide system (a Scottish system would be created in 1845) based on groupings of parishes into Poor Law Unions. Management went to Poor Law Guardians elected by a weighted franchise of local rate-payers. Property holders who owed high rates might have up to six votes; marginal property holders would have only one. As things worked out, these Poor Law Guardians (the word coming from Plato's authoritarian guardian class) would take on all the new functions which central government chose to extend to the localities. But because they were elected on the understanding that their main function was to keep rates low, local guardians were loath to undertake any enterprise that required money. In August 1833, central government had already announced that any future occurrence of cholera "should be left to the prudence and good feelings of those communities where it may occasionally show itself."[94]

For its intended clientele, the new Poor Law mandated the building of union poorhouses in which conditions of life would be so barren that no able-bodied person would choose to request admission. Following the Chadwickian principle of "less eligibility," people who volunteered for incarceration were dressed in a standard basic uniform, fed minimal food, forbidden alcohol or tobacco, forbidden any reading matter but the Bible, and were harassed by religiously obsessed lay preachers. Even worse (at a time when the middle classes were putting a new high premium on family togetherness in well-appointed homes), inmates were segregated by sex in the interest of cutting down further population increase. In practice this meant that old people who had been married to each other all their adult lives were made to live apart and, depending on the whim of the poorhouse beadle, might never be permitted to see each other again.

The response of ordinary men and women was to dub the union poorhouses "bastilles" and to keep clear of them. Within a generation, the idea that it was degrading, dishonorable and depraved to allow oneself to be carted away to the poorhouse had become central to laboring people's system of values. The alternative—starvation or suicide at home—was seen as preferable. Writing of the situation in poorhouses during the cholera epidemic of 1848–49, William Farr (himself the son of a rural laboring family and after 1837 Registrar-General) held that cholera death rates there were usually two or three times what they were among the population as a whole. After laboring people's efforts at parliamentary reform (the Chartists' petition of 1838–39) were laughed out of Parliament, all hope that social justice for the poor might be restored was lost. Bitterly disappointed, thousands of English people including my Northumbrian kin began their mass migration to North America.[95]

Just prior to the Chartists' débâcle at Westminster, Poor Law chief Edwin

Chadwick's acerbic tongue finally proved too much for his aristocratic patrons. Yet rather than being sent off to obscurity, he was promised the top post in public health. Using his Poor Law position to ease himself into his new job, Chadwick oversaw the creation of a Royal Commission to study the health of English towns. Knowing before he opened proceedings that he wanted to prove that the Poor Law had effectively solved the problem of poverty by forcing the willfully idle to work for their bread, Chadwick used his well-honed manipulative skills in gathering witnesses whose testimony would prove his point. Evidence surviving from the hearings suggests that no witness actually dared to claim that poverty still existed or that tens of thousands of people in want of common necessities were falling dead from diseases associated with malnourishment. Chadwick could not conceal the reality of illness among the masses—coroners' reports were still being kept—but in order to prove that he was on top of this problem, he claimed that all diseases were caused by miasmas. With this, he was well on the way to giving the Sanitarian position the official sanction of government.[96]

In organizing his report on urban sanitary conditions (when published in 1842, it become something of a middle-class bestseller), Chadwick saw fit to take the advice of two Edinburgh-trained medical doctors. One was James Phillips Kay (Kay-Shuttleworth) whose paranoiac fears of people of the sort struck down by cholera in Manchester in 1832 ("the deformity of evils") I quoted at the head of this section. Chadwick's other medical confidant was Thomas Southwood Smith, the anatomizer of Bentham and the false-knowledge expert who insisted that all fevers including "cholera" were simply different manifestations of the same, miasma-caused, disease. Margaret Pelling holds that it was Southwood Smith who was chiefly responsible for forming a coherent bundle of the rag-bag of ideas which thereafter was known as the Sanitarian ideal.[97]

Soon after publication of the Health of Towns report (*Report on the Sanitary Condition of the Labouring Population of Great Britain*) in 1842, Chadwick jettisoned his alliance with the doctors and instead took up with a sanitary engineer who held a consultancy in Holborn and Finsbury. Thereafter engineer John Roe had unique access to Chadwick's ear about the best—and of course in Chadwick's view the *only possible*—way to proceed in improving the health of British towns.[98]

In the Roe–Chadwick scheme which emerged, the way forward in public health lay in the provision of a network of sewage disposal and water supply pipes laid beneath public streets. For this Chadwick had two stated rationales. The first was that since all diseases were ultimately caused by the miasmas arising from decaying animal and vegetable matter, by removing the cause of stench, *engineering* genius (rather than medical genius) would remove the principal cause of illness. Further, by removing the cause of disease (miasmas), engineering genius would remove one of the principal causes of poverty, and with it, family dissolution, alcoholic parents, and malnourished adolescent children given over to a life of crime under their local Fagin organizer. Chadwick's second rationale was that since his engineering panacea only involved digging ditches and laying pipes in public streets, there would be a minimum of conflict with the legal rights of slum landlords and the great aristocrats (like the Russells) who owned half of London's fashionable West End.[99]

In the long term, it can be assumed that Chadwickian schemes to pipe human sewage away from built-up areas and from sources of drinking water did have some impact, at least in the few towns in which piping systems were actually laid down. Yet because Chadwick at no time took any particular interest in cholera other than as fodder for his propaganda mill (after all he was *not* a medical doctor), only token credit can be given to him for any improvement that may have occurred in overall British health. For him—just as with the 1891 Disease Commission in India (Thomson, Rake, Buckmaster)—cholera was merely a social indicator, rather than a disease phenomenon which was scientifically interesting in its own right.

Other than his own abrasive personality, which in 1854 forced him out of office (this time for good, though he lived until 1890), Chadwick's problem was that neither he nor his aristocratic patrons nor his middle-class expert friends were much interested in creating the climate of opinion needed for the promotion of innovative medical thought or indeed of innovations in civil engineering (water and sewerage). Lacking shared paradigms of what post-moderns see as scientifically credible knowledge and practice, Britain's medical men and engineers flannelled about. Meanwhile cholera continued on its killing way.[100]

In London, John Snow of York, credited in retrospect with publishing useful studies on drinking water and fecal matter as causal agents of cholera in 1849 and 1854, did not bother to back up his hypothesis with microscopic analysis. At the time, however, microscopes *were* found at Göttingen University. Thus it remained for the man who had Göttingen-style expertise, Robert Koch of Prussia, to make the necessary lab-based scientific experiments needed to back up initial hunches.[101]

If Snow's unscientific approach can be regarded as Alice-in-Wonderland curious, so too can the actions of Joseph Chamberlain in Birmingham. Heralded as the pace-setting voice of the gospel of urban renewal, Chamberlain allowed the city council to prohibit the installation of water closets (our modern toilets). This decision was made on the pretext that since water closets required link-up with an under-street sewage system, they were infinitely more costly than the portable pan-toilets, then standard. The contents of these archaic vessels had to be put into bins to await periodic collection in honey-carts.[102]

In 1848–49 cholera returned to Britain. To confront it, at the center of government, was the General Board of Health effectively headed by its only paid executive member, acid-tongued Edwin Chadwick. Standing by to face the crisis in the localities were the locally elected Poor Law Guardians, loyal still to their commitment to keep rates low by not spending money. Confronted with this non-existent defense, cholera worked its way through England, hitting old people in union poorhouses particularly hard. According to official statistics, this epidemic left some 62,000 dead, nearly twice the toll of cholera in 1831–32.[103] Writing of its impact on the sensibilities of men of his own rank and class, a gentleman named Thomas Frost opined:

> But then we had been used to these evils since the days of the Plantagenets, and though they had become intensified with the increase of population and the growth of the large towns, had not Malthus taught us that epidemics of disease were one of the means used by divine providence to prevent the numbers of the human race exceeding the means of subsistence?[104]

Acerbic James Mill could not have put it better.

In 1853–54 cholera returned in force, heavily targeting Newcastle upon Tyne, not far from where its cholera predecessor had created chaos thirty-two years before. Standing in place to defend the lives of 90,000 Newcastle folk and tens of thousands of others in the surrounding counties were the local Poor Law Guardians, whose attitude remained unchanged. As cholera bore down on Newcastle in August 1853:

> The effect on the town was devastating. Business was reported to be "in compete stagnation". People from the surrounding countryside kept away from the town and the important markets were very thinly attended. Some of those who could afford to closed their houses and fled to other places to escape the cholera. The doctors worked night and day, often overcome not only by exhaustion but by nausea, especially at night after people had emptied their wastes into the street gullies . . . the people in the poorer districts were naturally terrified . . . the cemeteries could not cope with the number of dead [which in the end totalled 1,527].[105]

In 1866 cholera again returned, this time taking care to hit populations in most English counties. As in 1853–54, standing by to resist the disease was—effectively nothing. However, as a result of the emergency generated by the anticipated arrival of the scourge, Parliament finally got around to passing an Act *permitting* (not requiring) local authorities to purchase for-profit water companies and to establish medical officers of health. Yet after compulsory legislation was finally passed (the Public Health Act of 1872) and given a few more teeth by Benjamin Disraeli's Public Health Act of 1875, local councillors found they had reason to worry that their personal savings might be confiscated to satisfy awards granted by courts to plaintiffs whose property interests were at odds with councillors' sanitary policies.[106]

In this, the legal establishment, the third professional grouping involved in the struggle against cholera (medical men and engineers being the others), was making itself heard. Barristers and judges, all financially well off and living and working in areas where they could avoid any personal risk from the disease, took it for granted that it was up to the experts in medicine and civil engineering to solve the cholera problem. As they saw it, their own responsibility lay in protecting the Common Law rights of landed property. By their rigid defense of these twelfth-century principles, lawyers, barristers and judges made it extremely difficult for town councils to make substantive progress in providing ordinary townspeople with clean drinking water and functioning sewage disposal systems. Meanwhile out at Windsor in 1861, the German-born Prince Consort, Albert, was reputed to have died of a waterborne *disease of filth* (typhoid).[107]

In the end, it is a cause for wonderment that the English were not regularly decimated by epidemic cholera in the decades following what was in fact the last major visitation—that of 1866–67—which left 14,000 dead.[108] Aside from the contingencies of chance (cholera is a great gamester), what probably saved the English was the imposition of quite rigorous quarantine controls between India and points west.[109] After the international meeting of the cholera control commission in Istanbul in 1866 and the establishment of rigorous quarantine measures by Egyptians staffing the Suez Canal station after its opening in 1869, British ships were forced to keep at sea while any of their crew or passengers were dying of cholera. However, mean-spirited British ministers of state like Lord Granville made it clear that compliance with quarantine regulations was in gross violation of the principles of Free Trade as codified and laid down by parliamentary legislation in 1846.[110] Mindful of this defiant British disregard of what other nations regarded as the norms of civilized behavior, we return to British India in the wake of its Rebellion.

Cholera in India after 1857

Writing in the year that cholera first swept through England (1831–32), the Indian intellectual Jambhekar commented on the achievements of western science. As paraphrased by T. Raychaudhuri, Jambhekar held that:

> the inhabitants of Europe had achieved "pre-eminent superiority . . . over the rest of the world, in almost every department of science . . ." through the selfless dedication of intrepid individuals to the pursuit of knowledge for its own sake. Their disinterested labours added to the stock of human knowledge, and promoted "the good of man, by discoveries and inventions which enlarge his powers, or augment the means of his usefulness to his fellow creatures".[111]

Unfortunately, among most of the British people who had a hand in the governance of India before 1920, reality was somewhat different. At root, their failings were due to an over-rigid compartmentalization of categories of knowledge. After post-Rebellion reforms (1859) gave direct control over Indian affairs to the UK government, ending the amateurism of the EIC, salaried specialists coming out to perform one particular task invariably carried on with it, oblivious of what anybody else was doing. Because of this mindset, any holistic understanding of the problems of India (25 million cholera dead) was clearly impossible. Laying aside for the moment the role of gentlemanly capitalists (the true Britons back home), one can identify two profession groupings who more than any other contributed to the successes of the cholera vibrio in reaping its harvest of human lives. These were the engineers (both royal army and civil) and the medical professionals.[112]

Wherever cholera was endemic—as in the lower reaches of the Ganges—interaction between works undertaken by engineers and *Vibrio cholerae* occurred almost daily, leaving a few people dead. However, in any region being swept by one of India's great periodic famines, cholera mortality could be extremely high. David Arnold went part-way in explaining correlations when he pointed out that:

> One of the best documented illustrations of the relationship between cholera and famine comes from the Madras Presidency in the 1870s. From a low point of 840 reported deaths in 1873 . . . the provincial total rose sharply in 1875 to 94,546 with the start of a new epidemic cycle. In 1876 mortality reached 148,193. . . . The epidemic peaked in 1877 at 357,430 deaths (a rate of 12.24 per thousand of population) before falling back to 47,167 in 1878. . . . In 1877 the ten principal famine districts had a cholera mortality rate of 18 per thousand, while the five in which famine developed later averaged 11.1.[113]

But what Arnold did not go on to say was that in time of famine distress, the engineering establishment known as the Public Works Department (PWD) was usually given responsibility for overseeing relief. According to principles laid down by Government, starving men, women and children were expected to leave their villages and come into central camps to be assigned tasks involving strenuous physical labor. In practice this meant that during a famine crisis, tens of thousands of people might be gathered in a single locale. Ninety-nine times out of a hundred these work-camps lacked adequate supplies of safe drinking water; this situation was obviously tailor made for cholera. During the terrible famine of 1897, in the North West Provinces and Oudh a million and a half people were put to work on PWD relief projects. Three years on, writing of the famine disaster of 1900 when large gangs were employed on PWD projects, the Sanitary Commissioner for the Central Provinces stated a general truth: Cholera was "a disease which finds in famine its chief ally."[114]

In a PWD-managed famine camp which followed Chadwickian dictates of "less eligability," to qualify for food handouts every person, however malnourished, had to dig away in heavy soils for road works or for irrigation canals. If they refused, they were marked down as having failed the "work test" and were scratched from the rolls of those eligible for food. During the Madras famine in the mid-1870s, the local sanitary officer, Surgeon-Major Cornish, hinted that the quantity of food doled out to workers was inadequate for people "undergoing severe physical exertions." In response, the government's special famine investigator, Sir Richard Temple, gave Cornish credit for quoting "abstract scientific theories" about the amount of food required for normal Europeans, but pointed out that Indians had been making do on much less food "from time immemorial." Temple's penny-pinching policies won the day, and he was duly promoted, becoming the Lieutenant Governor of Bengal.[115] Yet in fairness to him it might be noted that investigation of the food requirements needed to keep people in good health was not of interest to any European scientists (in this case German) until the 1880s. In Britain, the first study of human nutritional requirements was published as recently as 1933.[116]

In 1935 when the Raj still had twelve years to run, a Crown-appointed committee on nutrition found:

> There is abundant evidence indeed that a very large proportion of the population is undernourished and this . . . not only affects the mental and physical energy of the individual but increases the morbidity and mortality of the multifarious infections to which he [*sic*] is subjected. Furthermore, the more the matter is investigated the more sufferers from disease due to specific food deficiencies do we recognize. On the other side we have the very low economic status of the population . . . a factor . . . of exceptional importance.[117]

Since the mid-1980s Oxfam and other disaster relief organizations have accepted that malnutrition (which contributes to a person's predisposition to cholera) and famine (leading to death from starvation) are *man-made* disasters rather than the result of natural phenomena.[118]

In 1881, one Alexander Fraser, a royal engineer about to retire from his post in the North Western Provinces and Oudh, drew up an assessment of PWD relief work in time of famine. Fraser suggested that it was folly, indeed criminal, to bring starving people to a huge central work site—where they were exposed to lethal disease—in the expectation that they would perform unaccustomed heavy manual labor. He recommended that it would be far better to provide relief for people in their home villages. Going further, he held that it was more humane and professionally sound to limit work requirements to male household heads and to allow specialized craftsmen to carry on with the sort of tasks to which they were accustomed—weavers weaving, carpenters carpentering, brick-makers making bricks—rather than forcing every man, woman and child to dig ditches or starve. As the retiring RE rather awkwardly put it, "the main point I think in all organization for famine relief is not to adapt measures which have a tendency to break up the homelife of the people, and if this be true, *our great system of great central workhouses, and great centers of works is to be depreciated.*"[119]

Responding to this scathing criticism of Chadwickian dogma, Major Colin Scott Moncrieff, a highly placed royal engineer who would shortly transfer to Egypt to inflict his irrigation mania upon peoples along the Nile, rudely said, "Rubbish! rubbish!" It would seem that Scott Moncrieff calculated that professional interests would be best served by using the opportunities presented by famine to build up the size and competencies of the PWD whatever the cost in lost subaltern lives.[120] In the same year, the true Briton responsible to Parliament for supervision of the finances of India, one Evelyn Baring (the later Lord Cromer, of Egypt), noted that "every benevolent attempt [we have] made to mitigate the effects of famine and defective sanitation serves but to enhance the evils resulting from [Malthusian] overpopulation."[121]

In a chapter entitled "'Meeting Her Obligations To Her English Creditors': India, 1858–1914," Cain and Hopkins found that debt repayment, interest, pensions and the like necessitated the transfer *from* Indian taxpayers *to* England of several million pounds sterling annually. Well aware of this, but perhaps worried lest he be implicated, in 1881 Sir Thomas Seccombe, a retired finance officer with fifty years' experience in India, told a committee of the House of Commons that "the very mistaken idea that a *tribute* of £15 or £16 million is paid annually by the people of India to this country . . . is, in my opinion, a mis-application of terms." One might however just as well call a spade a spade. Other spades also need to be clearly displayed. Trade deficits working through India were generally made good by balancing in profits from the huge quantities of Indian-grown *opium* which the British required that China buy. As estimated by Evelyn Baring, profits from opium accounted for one tenth of gross Indian revenues.[122]

Because they feared that default in India might cause a crisis in the British financial world, men at the helm after the Rebellion tended to be singularly nervous. Writing in 1869–72 Lord Mayo the Governor-General warned that:

> We hold India by a thread. At any moment a serious danger might arise. We owe now £180 millions, more than 85 per cent of which is held in England. Add £100 millions to this and an Indian disaster would entail consequences equal to the extinction of half of the National Debt. The loss of India or a portion of it would be nothing as compared to the ruin which would occur at home.[123]

Given that much of the £150 million "held in England" gave gentlemanly capitalists a solid return of 5–7 percent annually, one can readily see why India was regarded as the Jewel in the Crown. Much of this money in outstanding debts was in the form of loans for construction of infrastructure.

Among the more important infrastructural tasks giving employment to engineers in India was the laying down of railways, and with it, the wholesale destruction of forests. Starting from a base of only a few miles at the time of the Rebellion of 1857–58, by 1887–88 14,383 miles of track had been laid. By 1893–94, mileage had been increased to an impressive 18,500. But as David Hardiman has recently pointed out, in time of famine, access to a local railhead did not necessarily mean that Government would bring in food to feed the starving. On the contrary, citing its well-entrenched doctrine of free trade and non-interference, Government usually did nothing to prevent local entrepreneurs—who had bitten deeply into the European apple of possessive individualism—from using rail to transfer food reserves held in places stricken with dearth to another part of the country where they would fetch a higher price.[124]

Accompanying these murderous policies, government officials very often claimed that few, if any, Indians actually died of starvation. What they died from instead were the filth diseases like cholera that accompanied famine. Authority also repeatedly claimed that there was no "empirical evidence" that cholera causal agents (whatever they might be) travelled by rail. As they saw it, the "fact of the matter" was that in the age of steam, epidemics advanced no faster than they had in any previous era. In this fiction Anglo-Indian authority buttressed its position as late as 1892 with the writings of the south German cholera soil-poison expert, Max von Pettenkofer. However in that year the railway-driven events leading up to the great Hamburg cholera epidemic (thirteen dead per thousand) proved Pettenkofer to be disastrously wrong.[125]

In addition to the construction of Indian railways, royal and civilian engineers also oversaw the construction of massive networks of irrigation canals. Starting with some gigantic projects in the north and coastal east in the 1830s, the project of irrigating India surged forward after 1862 when Sir Richard Strachey was appointed head of the Public Works Department (created in 1854). Never one to hide his light under a bushel, Strachey was quite open in admitting that no canal would be built unless an early and satisfactory return for the money invested could be guaranteed. Returns would come in the direct form of interest payments on loans and on enhanced land revenue collections, and indirectly from returns on irrigated crops such as the cotton grown specially for export to the mills of Manchester.[126]

Writing in 1888, Sir Richard Strachey's brother John reported that some 10,000 square miles of India were being irrigated by 28,000 miles of canals. Seven years later, in the annual account of the "Material and Moral Progress of India" it was reported that there were now some 14,114 miles of major canals, supplemented with 26,119 miles of minor canals, all built under PWD supervision with money borrowed from gentlemanly capitalists back home. Writing of the hundreds of miles of canals in the Punjab in 1904, it was reported that all the major canals, with one exception, yielded 7.15 percent net return compared with outlay. Much of this had been achieved by totally disrupting the ecology of the region [127]

Boasting of his brother's works, Sir John Strachey held that: "no public works of nobler utility have ever been undertaken." True enough, India was well on the way to becoming the most heavily irrigated territory under imperial rule anywhere on the globe: by 1901, 20 percent of its cultivated land was watered by irrigation.[128] It was also the corner of the world where cholera took its highest toll. The connection needs to be more fully explored.

Before around 1899, any provincial sanitary office who suspected a connection between canal irrigation and the spread of cholera—following in the footsteps of John Snow of 1854 Broadstreet Pump fame—knew full well that anything they said publicly would rebound adversely on their careers. It escaped no one's attention that the great men at the top of the Army Sanitary Commission with the Government of India adamantly insisted that cholera was caused *solely by local* sanitary imperfections centered on bad air, bad water, bad conservancy and all the other "filthy habits" of the local people.

In 1877, the righteousness of this idea was confirmed by old Edwin Chadwick himself in his vitriolic opening address to the health section of the Social Science Congress. Thus fortified, authority repeated time and again that it was heretical ever to claim that the causal agent of cholera (whatever it might be) could actually be imported or, indeed, that the particular sort of cholera found in Europe was one and the same as the cholera found in India. In 1881, Dr J. M. Cuningham (Edinburgh), chief sanitary commissioner since 1868, laid it out clearly: "It may just as well be said here that any officer who feels he is under a conscientious necessity of framing his procedure on 'contagion' should avoid sanitary work." As understood at the time, "contagion" was of course the code word for policies of quarantine and land-based cordon sanitaire which would cut off Indian trade, obviating the true purposes (milch-cow economics) for which the British were in India.[129]

What then were the peculiarly "filthy habits" of the people of India and how did they relate to canals? In the nature of things, most people then, as now, tended to regard these aspects of life as strictly private affairs. Accordingly, we actually know very little about where people choose to defecate, how they disposed of their bodily wastes, how they cleaned their private parts, their teeth, their cooking and eating utensils and so on. Unable, as historians, to investigate through personal observation the habits of people now dead, one must fall back on analogies.[130]

Particularly useful is a study conducted in 1967 by Khwaja Arif Hasan in a north Indian village he called "Chinaura." Here the researcher discovered that Muslim men and Hindu men and women generally went out early in the morning to the fields near their houses to relieve themselves. Where a canal, pool or other water source was available, they tended to squat nearby, having first collected water to wash their parts in a small bowl they carried with them. Their tasks done and parts washed, they then threw the water out, sometimes into the canal or pool from which they then drew water for drinking, cleaning their teeth and washing. The bowl itself was cleaned with mud, so that it could later be used for other purposes, some of which involved water which might be brought to the mouth. As Robert Koch might have noted, these behaviors were tailor made for the spread of the *Vibrio cholerae*.[131]

Complementing Hasan's statement about the habits of village people is a report on Hindu *urban* habits written in 1880–81 by Sreenath Ghose, a Bengali doctor trained in western medical ideas at Calcutta. According to Dr Ghose, most families had indoor "privy wells" which they emptied into the gutter in the street during heavy rains. Ghose considered this practice to be contrary to "enlightened ideas of conservancy," but went on to explain that the children of Indian collaborators in city schools were being taught to recite Shakespeare and Milton and to quote Bentham and John Stuart Mill, yet were never taught elementary principles of personal hygiene. This situation would remain unchanged until the Montagu–Chelmsford Reforms of 1920 placed responsibility for local education firmly in Indian hands.[132]

Mention of education, or—in the case of how to cope with personal hygiene and canals—its absence, brings us to the topic of the quality of training offered to potential British engineers at the two special engineering schools set up after the Crown decided to irrigate India. One was Thomason College near Rorkee (in present-day Himachel Pradesh) established in 1856. The other was the Cooper Hill College in England, established in 1871 with a view to attracting public school boys into what the middle class regarded as the eminently respectable profession of engineering. Without commenting on the relevance of the courses on offer for those who intended to build canals in England or mainland Europe, one is struck by the lack of attention the Cooper Hill program paid to the special geological, geographical and meteorological conditions of India.[133]

What was particularly tragic, in view of the massive harm it inflicted on the peoples and terrain of India, was the failure to stress that every network of canals must be accompanied by a network of drainage ditches. Since not all the water introduced from a canal into a field would sink into the soil at once, nearby ditches were always needed to drain away surplus waters in order not to destroy the crops. Standing water would also leave residues of salt on the soil, in time converting productive fields into barren wastes. Literature reviews suggest that it was not until well after 1930 in India, and until after 1965 in British-irrigated Egypt (enlarging on the work of Scott Moncrieff), that engineers fully realized that for every unit of water brought in through irrigation, it was necessary to make provision for its removal through a system of ditches.[134]

Of direct relevance to cholera was the harsh reality that in the absence of a network of clearance ditches, canal waters swamped great patches of surrounding land. If these surplus waters were infected on one of their shores by the defecations of a cholera carrier, the actions of wind and waves soon spread the infection over a wide area. It must be noted as well that these waters also provided ideal breeding places for mosquitoes. In its various forms, malaria was in fact the principal killing disease of nineteenth- and twentieth-century India.[135]

Drainage ditches were, one assumes, a straightforward engineering problem, a part of specialized knowledge, which it just happened that profit-minded Britons ignored. Beyond this was the larger problem caused by the absence of the holistic approach. In this context what was critically lacking was engineering knowledge about the culturally determined ways local cultivators chose to grow, water, harvest, market or consume their crops. Even more tragic, in a land repeatedly racked by famines, was the absence of proper agricultural training colleges given over to the study of local crops, soils, water needs, food and dietary preferences. As a commentator pointed out in 1904, in the absence of locally based experimental studies, most of the information available to irrigation engineers was taken from journals published by the US Department of Agriculture in Washington, DC. With all due respect, one cannot believe that much of that information was of any relevance to the special climatic conditions (monsoons) of India.[136]

In 1902, while India was still firmly in the grasp of the Raj, its situation was summed up by John Hobson. Rather than speaking in triumphalist terms of "the despotism of custom" in the East as John Stuart Mill had done in 1859, Hobson contended that:

> The idea that we are civilizing India in the sense of assisting them to industrial, political, and moral progress along the lines either of our own or of their civilization is a complete delusion, based upon a false estimate of the influence of superficial changes wrought by government and the activity of a minute group of aliens. The delusion is only sustained by the sophistry of Imperialism, which weaves these fallacies to cover its nakedness and the advantages which certain interests suck out of empire.[137]

Sophistry, delusion, nakedness, advantages, certain interest groups: these are harsh words. Yet added to their number is *cholera*, the disease that imperialism kept in being for 130 years at the cost of some 25 million Indian dead.

Even as Hobson was writing, highly placed medical authorities adamantly denied that the devastations wrought by cholera could be halted by the application of the paradigm of disease causation introduced by Robert Koch as a result of his studies in Calcutta cholera waters. In 1899 (fifteen years after Koch) writing from the Presidency of Madras—where there had been 65,444 cholera deaths in the last twelve months—the sanitary officer bravely suggested that the cholera microbe might have been transmitted from village to village "by means of lengthy channels liable to contamination due to the insanitary habits of the people." Commenting on this, the Army Sanitary Commission sourly noted that the Madras report "would have had more weight . . . had it been supported by statistics [irrefutable 'facts'] showing that the opening [and closing] of these channels" corresponded with the arrival and departure of cholera. As everyone who cared about job security knew, cholera was generated by local sanitary deficiencies: it was not imported.[138]

These dismissive comments replicated those that had regularly come out of the office of the Government of India Sanitary Commissioner during the long reign (1868–84) of J. M. Cuningham. A Scot born in 1829 in the Cape of Good Hope (seedbed of somewhat strained racial relations) and educated at the University of Edinburgh, Cuningham was the sort of dinosaur that British government authorities liked to keep at the helm of Indian medical affairs.[139] Coming under his whip were two successive sanitary officers in the Punjab: A. C. C. DeRenzy—pushed out in 1876—and H. W. Bellew—pushed out in 1885. In a nutshell, both adopted the then revolutionary idea that it was possible to design preventive programs to improve the overall health of India. In their estimation, John Snow's theory about the way cholera covers a country was correct. This meant that rural needs could best be served if villagers were provided with safe sources of drinking water, village-based soak-away systems, and given elementary education in personal hygiene. In the predominantly Muslim Punjab, the latter could be provided by village *hakims*. Bellew also thought that village people's physical condition would be much improved if they were allowed to retain enough of what they grew in their fields to provide their families with a decent level of subsistence. Convinced, however, that Bellew's theories about cholera and economics were "unsound" Cuningham had government reply:

> it was beyond government's resources to increase "the comforts of so large a proportion of its population . . . it is certain that the attempt to do so would lead to a very large increase in the number [of people] to be dealt with" [and that] so long as poverty existed, its concomitants must be accepted as inevitable "however painful they may be to contemplate."[140]

After Bellew was passed over for promotion in 1885, he retired to England, leaving no one in India to take up the cudgels of preventive health care.

In 1889, an interesting article appeared in *Scientific Memoirs by Medical Officers of the Army of India*. Written by Dr D. D. Cunningham, the double "n" head of the research laboratory recently set up to advise the Sanitary Commission in Calcutta, it held that detailed, long-term, microscopic research had shown there were "many different species of common bacilli and that therefore Koch's theory of the existence of a single specific choleraic comma *must finally be abandoned.*" Cunningham was willing to admit that Koch's comma bacilli might, in some cases, be resultants of cholera, but denied that they were the actual causal agents. Instead, he and his superiors fell back on the weary old explanation. Cholera was caused by local sanitary imperfections; it was a disease contingent on place rather than on individuals.[141]

Writing their memo covering Cunningham's report in 1894 (ten years after Koch), the Army Commission warned that "to teach the people that safety is to be found in avoiding others" (i.e. the rice-water stools and vomit of cholera patients) is "calculated to do much harm because it diverts their attention from [standard sanitary improvement]." In this the army heads were confusing their own interests (or rather, that of gentlemanly capitalists at home) with two quite different types of action. Had they given the matter rational consideration, they would have realized that personal avoidance of the sick (an action of which R. Koch strongly approved) was not necessarily in the same category of action as quarantine and cordon sanitaire (techniques about which even Koch had some doubts). Further reflecting their reactionary mindset, the Army Commission went on to claim that in the "present undetermined state of the etiology of this mysterious disease," the sudden emergence of an epidemic of cholera followed by its sudden disappearance must be dependent "on some great natural laws" (perhaps Aristotelian), which were still unknown.[142]

A year or two earlier (in 1894), the Secretary to the Governor-General of India, C. J. Lyall, wrote a circular warning government officials not to spread rumors that cholera could be imported into one place from another. Sparking off the Governor-General's ire was an incident in which someone in a letter home had claimed that British troops had been the agents who had brought cholera into a certain cantonment and district. Following this allegation, questions had been asked in Parliament and highly critical articles published which, according to Lyall, "had no foundation whatsoever *in the facts of the case.*" Officials were now enjoined never to give "expression to opinions not warranted by the facts established by the evidence." They were also warned that "theoretical discussion should be avoided as far as possible." The Governor-General's advisory note ended with the stern admonition: "It is hardly necessary to add that general statements made by villagers and subordinate officials . . . should only be accepted after careful scrutiny."[143]

A few years later readers of the *Journal of Tropical Medicine* were regaled with an unsigned article claiming that

> When keen and scientific officers recorded facts tending to prove communicability they were accused of "theorising" and deliberately ordered to delete the facts from their official reports, so that a reputation for a

weakness for research was about the worst a man could earn who desired to succeed in the service.[144]

Writing soon after 1828, Governor-General William Bentinck confessed that:

> Europeans generally know little or nothing of the customs and manners of the Hindus. . . . We understand very imperfectly their language. . . . We do not, we cannot associate with the natives. We cannot see them in their houses and with their families. We are necessarily very much confined to our houses by the heat; all our wants and business which would create a greater intercourse with the natives is done for us, and we are in fact strangers to the land.[145]

Half a century later, the army medical commentator on the annual sanitary report coming in from the Presidency of Madras made much the same point. He pointed to

> a great want of accurate knowledge among European officials in India in regard to the social habits and mode of life of the Native poor. The food they eat, its amount and variety, the number of meals daily and, in fact, all matters relating to the domestic life of the people are hidden from the gaze of the European official who . . . may pass a lifetime in the country without attaining any accurate information on such subjects.[146]

One of the reasons for the popularity among middle-class English readers of Rudyard Kipling's *Kim*, published in 1901, was that it recounted the story of an English boy who seemed entirely able to pass as a native Indian, a boy who was *not* a stranger to the land. Yet coming out of Kipling's own lived experience (he was born in the subcontinent in 1865 and remained there until near puberty) was his mature assessment of Indians. Writing in 1899 he depicted them as: "fluttered folk and wild . . . new-caught sullen peoples, Half devil and half child."[147]

At the end of the nineteenth century it was grudgingly conceded that young Indians be allowed to train as hospital assistants in specially created subordinate medical colleges. In 1906, an article on "The Problem of Medical Aid to Semi-Civilized [*sic*] Countries" noted that 250 students at the new Punjab college had lodged a complaint against their all-Indian faculty. One grievance was that instructors were elderly men thirty years out of date who refused to teach in English. The 1906 commentator felt obliged to mention that

> the young educated Indian is, very naturally, apt to inveigh against his rulers as invaders and oppressors, but where his personal interests are

concerned he will generally be found to prefer English professors and judges to his own countrymen.[148]

In reality, as early as December 1823, Bengal reformer Rammohun Roy had pleaded for schooling in English on full parity with English standards. And as for books, according to the 1906 reporter: "those available are practically obsolete *rechauffés* of English text-books, designed to meet the requirements of European students of a past generation." It would seem that these texts made no mention of Robert Koch's breakthrough in the understanding of cholera made in the tanks of Calcutta in 1884. In the year in which this critique was published (1906), the all-India cholera death rate (three cholera dead per thousand) was the highest it would be at any time in the twentieth century.[149]

During World War I, Edwin Montagu, Secretary of State for India—a Jewish gentleman who, as a permanent outsider in English society, sympathized with other underdogs—pushed a bill through Parliament which became the Montagu–Chelmsford Reforms. According to its clauses, public health policy decisions—other than those which might include the remission of taxes in time of famine or personal disaster—devolved to Indian-elected local authorities. The reforms took effect in 1920, a few months after General Dyer slaughtered 379 peaceful Indian protesters at Amritsar, destroying what little was left of the mystique upon which rested British rule.[150]

By coincidence, in the two decades that followed the assumption of something resembling Indian control over public health the man-created phenomenon known as famine lost its hold. And though only a few Indian villages had as yet been provided with access to secure, safe supplies of water, tolls from cholera also began to drop. WHO figures show total deaths from cholera falling from 3.8 million in the decade 1910–19, to 1.7 million in the decade 1930–39, to 380,100 in the five-year period 1950–4.[151] However, in a book published in 1940 which was banned in India, the nationalist leader, R. Palme Dutt, was probably not far off mark when he claimed that

> provision for the most elementary needs of public hygiene, sanitation or health is so low, in respect of the working masses in the towns or in the villages, as to be practically non-existent.[152]

In the end it remained for American research teams after World War II to create the liquid glucose-electrolyte solution that replicated the vital fluids the body had lost: when taken orally, this can reduce cholera mortality to less than 1 percent. The catch is that people must come in for treatment. This is not always possible in remote areas not served by modern health provisioners equipped with modern facilities or with oral re-hydration kits.[153]

Cholera continues to be infinitely mobile and may be going beyond El Tor and *Vibrio cholera* 0139 in mutating into new forms not amenable to cure by western expertise. As of this writing cholera remains a lesson . . . in the need for humility.

6 Yellow Fever, Malaria and Development: Atlantic Africa and the New World, 1647 to 1928

> The Cerberus that guards the African Continent, its secrets, its mystery, and its treasure is disease . . . (which I would liken to an insect). But for these . . . many curious and dangerous diseases . . . Africa, instead of following up as a very bad fag-end in the race of civilisation, would probably have been well to the front. We all know what Egypt is, and has been. Why is . . . Africa a "very bad last"?
>
> Sir Patrick Manson, 1907[1]

Introduction

Yellow fever, "the hurricane of the human frame . . . dark and inscrutable in its cause," seems to have come to the New World aboard ships carrying slaves from Africa; its first documented appearance was in Barbados in 1647.[2] Long thought to be one of the awful fevers harbored by the foul airs and soils of a particular place, in early years it was commonly claimed that its preferred targets were "unseasoned" newcomers from northern Europe. With death rates ranging from 20 to 55 percent, local promoters interested in attracting settlers usually clamped down hard on medical doctors who alleged the disease was present.[3]

An account written by Dr George Pinckard of England newly arrived in the West Indies in 1806 tells of his own experience with yellow fever. Suddenly overtaken, he found:

> The light was intolerable and the pulsations of the head and eyes were most excruciating . . . conveying a sensation as if three or four hooks were fastened into the globe of each eyes and some person, standing behind me, was dragging them forcibly from their orbits back into the head . . . the calves of my legs [felt] as if dogs were gnawing down to the bones. . . . No place, no position afforded a moment's rest.[4]

Pinckard was fortunate to survive.

Falciparum malaria, the second disease discussed in this chapter, also appears to have been brought to the Americas by slave ships from Africa, though we don't know precisely when. As late as 1639, European travellers in the Amazon River Basin (now horribly plagued) made mention of many lethal things, but not of *falciparum* malaria. However, soon after 1650 it was recorded along the north-east and eastern coasts of Portuguese and Spanish territories. By the 1680s it was found far to the north among English settlers on the eastern side of the Appalachians.[5] Transmitted by a bite from a mosquito infected with *Plasmodium falciparum*, the incubation period within a human victim was from ten to fourteen days. Among adults, death rates could be as high as one in four.[6]

An underlying theme of this chapter is that the complex of processes known as Development—involving the movement of huge numbers of humans and ships—greatly assisted the causal agents of *falciparum* malaria and yellow fever in causing plagues of disease on both the African and the American sides of the Atlantic. As suggested in the "Introduction," Development was a multi-layered, pyramid-shaped affair in which the minuscule number of top-men organizers in Europe were several stages removed from what was going on in Africa, in the two Americas, and on the ocean-going vessels linking the four continents. With few exceptions, stay-at-home investors were not interested in Development's human costs.[7]

Until the abolition of slavery (in 1865 in the United States of America, in 1886 in Cuba, in 1888 in Brazil), Development processes brought to the fertile lands of the Americas slave laborers taken from Africa. Once there, they produced the sugar, tobacco, indigo, cotton and other agricultural products in high demand in Europe. In the Americas, the processes were lubricated by credit extended by agents representing the merchant bankers of London, Amsterdam and Lisbon.

Credit and credit relationships were also found along the central west African coasts (extending northward from Angola to Senegal) and their inland slave-raiding frontiers, albeit in rather unsophisticated forms. Here, enforcement on defaulters was done by pre-emptive confiscations or by smearing a debtor's reputation to cut off access to the loans he needed to keep his existing creditors at bay. A man thus made insolvent had the option of suicide or of going into the interior with a slave-raiding party to hunt down blacks for sale in collection centers on the coast. If the rascal survived these feats, he might use the proceeds to pay off enough of his debts to re-establish his credit and begin borrowing again. In the course of these activities undertaken by miscreants on behalf of thugs, the frontiers of slavery were pushed further and further inland, bringing with them the lethal disease environments of the coasts.[8]

Throughout the late eighteenth and nineteenth centuries the ultimate goal of Development remained the same—the remittance home to Europe of profits earned through the speculative lending of money. However, over the years some of the instruments for profit-making were either transformed or withered away. This brings us to *the* greatest of the discontinuities in south Atlantic history after 1492: the abolition of slavery. This was undertaken first by the revolutionary French in 1789 (repealed in 1806) then, with more lasting effect, by the English.

In England, abolition was carried out by people of the middling sort who were on the way to converting themselves into the new middle class.[9] Straining to break their ideological dependence on the old territorial aristocracy while at the same time putting deep water between themselves and the revolutionary "Liberty, Equality and Fraternity" bourgeoisie of France, English theorists for the still unformed middle class saw the abolition of slavery as a useful unifying cause. Working through the gentlemanly Grand Assize of England (Parliament), abolitionists succeeded in having the trade in slaves within the British Empire abolished in 1807. Limited of course to British domains, the abolition of slavery followed in 1833.

Yet in such matters, the balance between what committed abolitionists claimed was *morally* just and what development agents knew was *economically* sound was always set right by men of affairs working behind the scenes in the Admiralty, the Foreign Office and the City.[10] Thus when dealing with slave shipments coming in from Africa, British anti-slavery patrols were always given instructions calculated not to harm true Britons' global interests. Falling in with these was the British naval commander who haplessly reported in 1849: "During 26 years, 103,000 slaves had been emancipated [by anti-slavery patrols] while in the same period, 1,795,000 slaves were actually landed in the Americas." This was a slippage of 95 percent.[11] Still following the logic of top people, in the new territorial empire which in the 1890s Britain called into being in West Africa, ostensibly to end slavery, slavery was permitted to function until the 1930s.[12]

In the newly independent Spanish colonies in Meso- and South America, and in Portuguese Brazil, and in English North America, the move—starting in the 1830s—to wind down slave imports was offset by a great flood of immigrant white Europeans. The relationship between the new labor supply and the old seems to have differed in each culture zone, and south of the Rio Grande has been comparatively little studied. However for North America, masses of well documented studies show that whites felt that slaves and their freeman descendants should either return to their ancestral Africa or accept that they should take only menial jobs in America. This would free up better-paid positions for incoming Europeans or for Euro-Americans. Until 1868, federal law, and thereafter state-mandated Jim Crow laws, ensured that African-Americans would not think of themselves as fully emancipated US citizens entitled to vote or to hold public office.

Topping off populist arguments that blacks were inferior to whites was the intellectualist clutch of ideas known as scientific racism.[13] In the world of medicine, scientific racism merged with what I term Construct yellow fever and Construct malaria. Among other things these constructs held that black people were immune to yellow fever and nearly immune to malaria. Propagated by otherwise quite admirable medical doctors, the constructs were used to justify the continuing economic and social subordination of blacks to whites. They remained an undercurrent in *medical* consciousness well into the twentieth century. However, they suffered a major setback at Cairo in 1928, when at an international conference on tropical medicine, W. H. Hoffmann of the Instituto Finlay in Havana, Cuba, advised the world that for yellow fever "a racial immunity does not exist."[14]

In this chapter I will sketch out shifts in attitudes to yellow fever and malaria and suggest how they informed medical and community action. I will begin with Hoffmann's understanding of disease reality as it stood at the time of the Cairo conference and then touch on yellow fever and malaria hot-points, beginning with West Africa. I will then cross the ocean to the Americas to examine the situation in the Caribbean (Barbados and Haiti), in the United States, Brazil and Cuba. Leaving US-occupied Havana, I will again cross the Atlantic to finish up in West Africa during the era of the "legitimate trade" in primary products ostensibly grown by non-slaves.

The Diseases

When the Cairo conference on tropical medicine convened in 1928 it had been known for several years that both yellow fever and *falciparum* malaria (in fact all the malaria types) were caused by specific living disease organisms. As early as 1880, as part of the Pasteur Institute crash program to advance settler penetration into Muslim North Africa, Alphonse Laveran discovered the causal agent, the *plasmodia*, of malaria. Amongst the enlightened, this medical knowledge replaced the old idea that malaria (from the Italian word *mal'aria*, bad air) was caused by the vaporous fumes arising from the swamps and stagnant waters of a particular malodorous place and that, being indigenous and place specific, it could not be imported.[15] In the case of yellow fever, a causal viral organism was suspected, but not actually isolated until 1928 (by Adrien Stokes and others in West Africa).[16]

By then, it had been known for around thirty years that malaria *plasmodia* and the yellow fever virus were both transferred to humans by the bites of specific sorts of mosquito. In the case of yellow fever, it was thought that the species *Aedes aegypti* served as the *only* mosquito vector. This was overly optimistic. Present-day knowledge recognizes some thirteen species of mosquito capable of carrying the yellow fever virus and does not rule out the possibility that it might also be harbored by certain tropical ticks.[17]

Experts at the 1928 Cairo conference were aware that the presence of a flourishing population of *Aedes aegypti* mosquito in a given territory did not necessarily mean that yellow fever was also there. A case in point was Asia: it had plenty of *Aedes aegypti* but no yellow fever. Life-enhancing though this situation was for the hundreds of millions of Chinese who stayed at home, the absence of the disease impacted rather badly on the thousands brought over to Brazil in the mid-nineteenth century as contract laborers. Having had no opportunity to gain immunity through previous exposure as children, once in Brazil Chinese laborers tended to be carried off by yellow fever before they had time to meet girls and add to the local gene pool. Yet for developers, the cost-benefits had been obvious. Though the Chinese were generally diligent workers, because of high levels of yellow fever mortality, few of them survived to the end of their contract term when, by law, they could demand passage money to their homes on the far side of the Pacific.[18]

In the case of the malarias and the Americas, it is now known that mosquito types capable of serving as intermediate hosts for one or other malaria form were present in large enough concentrations to have hosted the disease before Columbus arrived in his viral-freighted ships in 1492. Seemingly absent however were malaria *plasmodia*. This meant that malaria, like yellow fever, was unknown in the Americas before the coming of the Europeans.[19]

In his report to the 1928 Cairo conference Hoffmann of Havana held that yellow fever had not succeeded in establishing a reservoir in the vast interior spaces of South America. This, together with his presumption that the early twentieth-century United-States-supervised eradication campaigns in Cuba had cleared the island of household-hovering *Aedes aegypti* mosquitoes, led Hoffmann to conclude that the only remaining yellow fever territorial base was West Africa. Unfortunately, on both counts he was wrong. In 1935 distressed investigators found that certain species of monkey living in the Amazon Basin could serve as hosts for the yellow fever virus just as well as human beings, and were doing so in great numbers.[20]

This discovery gave rise to the distinction between what was called "urban" yellow fever (human to human via mosquito), and "sylvan" yellow fever (transmitted from monkeys via mosquitoes to humans). Recently, this terminology has been replaced by terms descriptive of *three* transmission cycles: interhuman (via mosquito), sylvatic (monkey to human via mosquito) and intermediate (a mix of human and monkey transmissions). In West Africa, it was this intermediate type that caused fifteen yellow fever epidemics among rural Africans between 1958 and 1982. Since then more horrendous epidemics have occurred, most notably the outbreak in and around Oshogbo, Nigeria, in 1987 in which 120,000 people developed the disease and 24,000 died.[21]

Though Hoffmann's 1928 terms of reference were overly optimistic, he was correct in asserting that in West Africa infants and young children often underwent an attack of yellow fever so mild that their parents and attendants were unaware that the child was sick. This mild case gave victims lifelong or long-term immunity. Hoffmann termed this sort of illness *endemic* yellow fever and contrasted it with an *epidemic* situation when hundreds of non-immune adults took sick and died.[22]

Up to a point, Hoffmann was also correct in assuming that the presence of *endemic* yellow fever formed a link in the chain of transmission. During the first three or four days that infants and young children were suffering their mild bout, their blood was infective. If this blood was tapped by a non-infected mosquito of the relevant species, which after several days' rest bit a non-immune person (during the interval the virus reproduced within the mosquito), the disease virus might cause a case of yellow fever that served as yet another link in a chain of transmission. The blood of people who had developed immunity to yellow fever was not infective.[23]

With knowledge superior to that of 1928, we now know that what I have just sketched out is not yellow fever's only way of perpetuating itself. In wet savannah zones in West Africa and continuing eastward to southern Sudan, Ethiopia and Kenya where the mosquito population is now exceptionally dense, the yellow fever virus is capable of *vertical* transmission. This means that it works through a female's eggs to infect the next generation of mosquitoes. Unfortunately, it also means that biting female mosquitoes (numbering billions) rather than humans or monkeys are the actual reservoirs of the virus. This new knowledge gives added poignancy to the awareness that continuing deforestation, in response to the demands of Development, creates new water-catching crevices which can serve as breeding places for mosquitoes. In these circumstances yellow fever's threat to humankind is self-sustaining and will continue *ad infinitum*.[24]

Two other points can be made about yellow fever, one as disease, and one as Construct. It is now known that the most distinctive feature of the illness, black vomit, is displayed by only a relatively small percentage of victims. From this it follows that many cases of what experts in a properly equipped laboratory could recognize as yellow fever but which occur in remote rural areas serviced by untrained health workers are erroneously taken to be viral hepatitis or malaria. In a worst-case scenario, such as that in Ethiopia in 1960–62, before qualified authorities were aware of what was going on, a horrendous yellow fever epidemic was well underway. Out of an at-risk Ethiopian population of a million, 100,000 fell sick and 30,000 died. Nearly all these deaths could have been prevented had the vaccine developed in the late 1930s been rushed in at the onset of the outbreak.[25]

The second point involves yellow fever as Construct. Because yellow fever was so often confused with other diseases and because of what Dr Rubert Boyce (in 1911) termed "notification fear," official counts of the yellow fever dead tended to under-report the actual number of people killed. Current World Health Organization guidelines suggest that official morbidity and mortality rates in West Africa represent somewhere between a tenth and a thousandth of actual numbers. This has had serious consequences. Thus, during the Nixon years when the US was bombing North Vietnam at the cost of billions, in order to save a few millions on a massively under-reported yellow fever presence in South America the US calculated that its anti-mosquito campaign was expendable and withdrew funding. Given a reprieve, those mosquito yellow fever hosts which had evolved an immunity to the chemicals used in earlier eradication campaigns came to supersede rival mosquitoes of the sort that chemicals could actually kill.[26]

Also important after the early 1800s in keeping yellow fever in being was the special kind of under-reportage associated with Construct yellow fever. Since white medical doctors, slave plantation owners, free-labor employers and white persons in general were convinced that blacks were immune to yellow fever, it follows that they deliberately kept themselves in ignorance of any sickness of that sort suffered by African-Americans or Africans.[27]

We turn now to our other major mosquito-borne killer, *falciparum* malaria, brought from West Africa to the New World. On either side of the ocean this malaria type weakened the unprotected victims it did not kill (enlarging the poison-filtering organs of the body; the liver and spleen), giving these unfortunates the appearance of being listless and lazy. In her assessment of the disease in North American pre-Civil War coastal lands, J. Dubisch suggested that:

> The most serious problem posed to health by malaria is the general debility it produces, often making its victims susceptible to other more serious diseases. This means that even when reliable *mortality* statistics are available, they can serve, at best, only to provide a rough indication of actual *morbidity* patterns for malaria.[28]

Like its European-based cousin, *vivax* malaria which also entered the Americas in the seventeenth century, *falciparum* malaria is known to cause especially high mortality among infants and young children under the age of five, whose brief passage through life was often never recorded.[29]

In the matter of temporal perspectives, Mark Ridley assures us that malaria's role as the most successful killer of masses of humankind is relatively recent. As he goes on to say:

> To introduce malaria to a human society, the trick is to cut down the forest and have the humans living at a reasonably high density. The mosquitoes—which had previously been absent, or rare, or were flying around in the forest canopy—can then make a living at ground level, particularly if there is standing water.[30]

In the timing of its first New World appearances malaria seemed to work along the moving frontier on a delayed time fuse. Ten or twenty years after settlers had cleared a forest and built their barns and houses, epidemic malaria struck. Typically, a visitor coming into settler Maryland in the 1690s observed "the washed countenances of the people standing at their doors . . . like so many standing ghosts . . . every house was an infirmary."[31] The same thing happened as the frontier crossed the Appalachians into Ohio

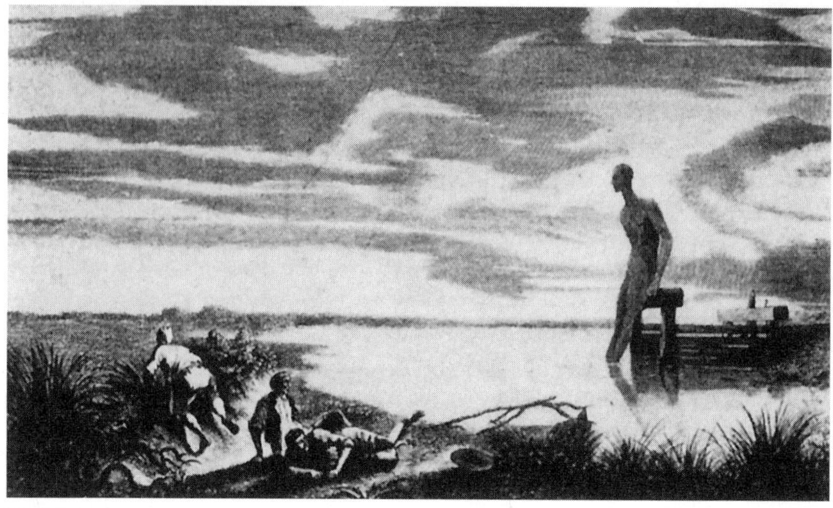

14. An allegory of malaria: "The Ghost of the Swamp." An engraving after M. Sands (1823–89).

and Indiana in the late eighteenth century.[32] It *may* have happened earlier in West Africa.

Some time ago it was discovered that in the Nigerian regions and westward to the Gambia and Senegal, agricultural tools made of stone were replaced by tools with cutting edges of iron around 1000 BCE. On the basis of this supposed "fact," a hypothesis was spun to account for what was posited to have been ever-present malaria. This theory held that using the newly invented tools after 1000 BCE West Africans had gone ahead to clear extensive tracts of virgin forests. It went on to suggest that by alternately clearing land and then letting it return to bush to regain its fertility and replacing it with another newly cleared strip, iron-tooled cultivators created the near-constant supply of unevenly broken soil needed to provide the myriad holes that became the pools required for the optimal breeding of *Anopheles gambiae* mosquitoes. In recent times, *Anopheles gambiae* is one of the principal intermediate hosts of *falciparum* malaria; it flourishes in greatest numbers during the wet season.

Complementing this wet-season pest in fine-spun theory was the behavior of *Anopheles funestus*. This host mosquito did best during the dry season when it laid its eggs in water-catching discards, such as potsherds, found near human habitations. Taken together, the pools formed in newly cleared land (for *A. gambiae*) and those provided by man-made containers (for *A. funestus*) would have provided enough breeding places during the last 3,000 years for large numbers of one or the other of the two mosquito hosts to be almost constantly within range of man.[33]

Behind this hypothesis lies the unexamined assumption that after 1000

BCE West Africa had always been what it is now—the seedbed of epidemic malaria. However, what we have already seen of European ideas about the timelessness of the disease environment of India (in the case of cholera and smallpox), bids us be cautious when attributing timelessness to African disease environments. Granted that both *A. gambiae* and *A. funestus* mosquitoes are known to have existed in West Africa in the recent past, it does not necessarily follow that human use of iron tools 3,000 years ago brought together all the requirements for widespread year-around malaria.

Whatever forest-clearing techniques may actually have been used in the distant past, the fact is that in the course of my own extensive travels in Nigeria in the 1970s and 1980s I found that cultivators cleared bush and trees, not by using iron tools, but *by setting them on fire.* This labor- and energy-saving technique neither disturbs the ground-cover and soil nor does anything to provide special breeding sites for *A. gambiae.*[34] This bit of empirical research suggests that the old hypothesis about Africa having been afflicted by malaria time out of mind may have to be rethought.

Beginning in the mid-1940s, various researchers who claimed their work was validated by the criteria of objective science rather than by the mindset of Social Darwinism suggested that peoples in West Africa whose ancestors had lived in heavily infected malaria regions since time immemorial inherited genetic responses to the disease. These responses prevented permanent liver damage or death. Beavering away in this research, biochemists have shown that in West and west central Africa local variants of malaria thought to have occurred in the last 1,500 years contributed to the development of four different locally centered types of human biological feature. These are known as sickle cell traits. One of the four is centered in Senegal, another in Benin, another in the Cameroons and the last, the Bantu, in west central Africa. It would seem that these discrete traits are genetically transferred from one generation to the next. However, it is important to bear in mind that this process is not unique to Africans. It also occurs among Italians (descendants of world-conquering Romans and their Germanic successors) who live in what in the nineteenth century was the malaria zone south of Rome.[35]

As Anderson and May point out when referring to sickle cells, it is not altogether clear that the trait actually provides protection against local forms of malaria.[36] Moreover, if the trait was an adaptive technique used by natural selection to preserve locally present representatives of *Homo sapiens* from death, it certainly left something to be desired. Since any child who inherits sickle cell genes from both parents will die before reaching reproductive age (of sickle cell anaemia), it is difficult to see how the trait contributes to species perpetuation.

Among some Africans born of lineages long resident near the coast (before European penetration this would have been only a small percentage), there was another localistic characteristic: the genetically transferred Duffy negative factor in the blood. According to biologist Frank Livingstone, writing in

1990, the Duffy negative factor made its bearers immune to the *vivax* form of malaria.[37] But as Anderson and May point out, only regional pockets of Africa are currently subject to *vivax* forms; elsewhere it may have died off. Another curious thing is that recent research in Ethiopia showed that two different, but ethnically similar groups living adjacent to each other had very different levels of susceptibility to *vivax* malaria.

With respect to Africa's own deadly *falciparum* malaria and its mosquito hosts, recent research found that the bodily systems of ethnically identical populations living in the same locale reacted very differently to the disease. Some people bitten by an infected mosquito shake it off without becoming infective themselves, while others do not.[38] Obviously in these instances it was the particularities of the group and of its individual members rather than ethnicity *per se* which made the difference. Recognizing, as suggested here, that the path labelled "genetic inheritance of resistance to malaria" has failed to explain why more than a million African children died of malaria each year during the 1980s and 1990s, many scientists have been turning their attention to the less contentious mysteries of *acquired* immunity.

In West Africa, this line of inquiry begins with the understanding that in pre-colonial, colonial and post-colonial situations the most healthy place for any African to live was the disease environment in which she/he had been born. As in any human population, during the first few months of life an infant shared some of the disease immunities which the mother had built up in her own blood. Then, as this non-genetic, inborn resistance wore off and breast-feeding was replaced by pap, it was up to the child to acquire its own immunities. In the case of *falciparum* malaria, a child would begin to build this up by surviving an initial case. However, in the course of this endeavor, millions of infants have died.

Though generalizations are becoming increasingly hazardous as mosquito and *plasmodium* populations mutate and become more subtle in their differences and in the plenitude of their types (each requiring its own immunity), it has been found that, once established, immunity to *falciparum* malaria lasts only six months to a year. This means that any immune person who was away from home longer than that and then returned would have to start building up immunity from a much-depleted base.[39] It follows that the compulsory long-term movement of tens of thousands of enslaved Africans from the places of their birth after *c.* 1690–1750 may have resulted in a near-catastrophic increase in malaria morbidity and mortality. The implications of this will be discussed below.

The malaria Construct which came into being in the medical worlds of Liverpool and West Africa in the 1890s held that the children of Africa were the principal bearers of malaria. This was based on a double misunderstanding. The first was failure to recognize that mosquitoes are color blind when it comes to identifying which hosts to bite and may react to two people with identical skin pigmentation in very different ways. Allied to this, was

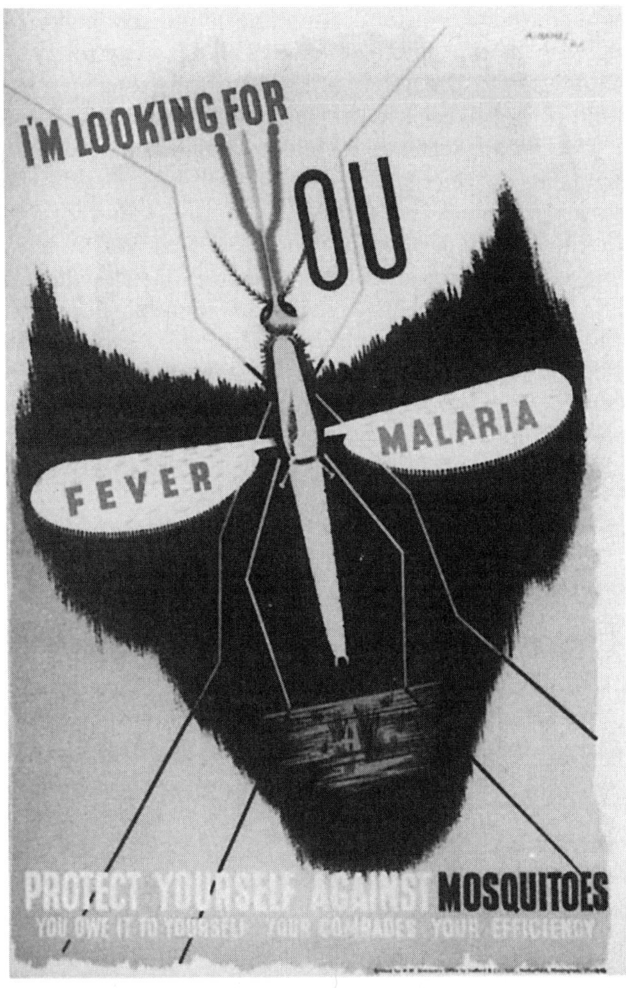

15. A twentieth-century poster warns of the dangers of malaria.

the fact that, whatever their skin pigmentation, any human adult who had acquired effective immunity to a particular malarial form which enabled him or her to shake it off without any visible ill effects, was very often infective. This meant that if a now-infected human happened to be bitten by an *un*infected mosquito, the mosquito would in turn become infective and be capable of infecting other people. To counter earlier prejudiced reading, the point which needs to be stressed here is that since *any* human host would do (Caucasian, Asian, African) the *plasmodium* did not exclusively, or even primarily, depend on black children to continue its chain of species renewal.

The second colonialist misunderstanding hinged on faulty assumptions about personal behavior. Bitten, infected children (regardless of ethnicity) who had not yet had time to build up their personal immunity would be listless and obviously sick, whereas long-experienced well-bitten adults, personally immune but infective to others, would be able to carry on with work as usual. Given the context of a colonized West Africa in which most married couples with children sent them back to England for schooling, the majority of the young persons present were Africans. In the colonialist mindset, this led to the conviction that black children—whether listless or not—were the principal bearers of malaria. From this, Social Darwin logic held that both personally, and as members of a despised ethnic group, African children were responsible for the continuing lethal presence of malaria.[40] On this white-held conviction was built a dangerously misguided understanding of malaria.

Slavery and the Fevers in Atlantic Africa to c. *1840*

Arabic and European language records pre-dating the 1840s provide only snippets of information about the disease environments of West Africa. However, in 1820 an English official named Joseph Dupuis wrote about the situation on the Gold Coast (modern Ghana). Reflecting on his recent visit inland to Kumasi in Ashantiland, and obviously thinking in then fashionable terms about the fevers (place-specific and miasma born), Dupuis held that:

> As regards climate or atmosphere, the Gold Coast and places adjacent to the settlements [on the coast] are more or less known to be unhealthy. But I will hazard an opinion that the countries inland are infinitely more salubrious, the aire more pure, and the soil less humid and vaporous than at any station on the coast.[41]

Writing about Kumasi three years earlier, H. Tedlie, the first western medical doctor to visit the Ashante, asserted that:

> The diseases most common in the Ashantee country are the Lues [syphilis], Yaws, Itch, Ulcers, Scald-heads, and griping pains in the bowels. Other diseases are occasionally met with, I should suppose in the same proportion that they occur in [other] countries.[42]

It will be noted that Tedlie and Dupuis said nothing about yellow fever, *falciparum* malaria or any other epidemic disease. If the fevers had been present, theirs would have been curious oversights indeed. For the sake of argument, let us posit a fever-free environment.

Environments of this sort were often associated with a lived-world in which community members were geographically stable. This situation comes close to those found in West African regions still unblitzed by the commercial trade in slaves. Here in time of peace, the generality of the population seldom travelled far from the cluster of villages or the large urban settlements in which they had been born. Within this *pays* and those immediately adjacent, they found their spouses, did their farming and marketing, buried their dead and did whatever else normal people do. Biologically, this relatively restricted region served as a unified disease environment.

This is not to say that West African societies didn't engage in a considerable amount of trade with distant places; it is well known that they did. Yet as Ralph Austen has shown, in the conduct of this trade, it was the *goods* that travelled great distances, rather than the traders. For reasons that doubtless had to do with rivalries between neighboring groups which elders saw fit to keep quiescent through no-trespass policies, the movement of trade goods was carried on through a system of relays. Here products would be carried across the territory of one ethnic group by members of that group, then at a frontier they would be handed over to traders from the neighboring ethnic group, and so sent forward.[43]

Another important factor that tended to keep the disease environments along the coast separated from disease environments further inland was that the trade which West Africans regarded as really interesting took place across their own great inland sea of sand, the Sahara Desert. Since the eighth century of the present era camel caravans had been regularly crossing this sea. Some provided linkage with regions in the west (Senegal and Gambia), others with regions in the east (Sudan and Ethiopia), and others with the port cities of the Berber coast (Morocco, Tunis) and Egypt. Some of this last-mentioned caravan linkage involved the movement of Muslim pilgrims to Cairo's Al-Azhar University; many then crossed the Red Sea and went on to the holy sites in Mecca and Medina in present-day Saudi Arabia. In addition to pilgrims, other elements in this south to north linkage were high-value goods.[44]

In the early fifteenth century—and having long-term consequences from which Africa continues to bleed today—one of the high-value goods carried northward was the *gold* from Mali which excited the cupidity of Portuguese merchants trading in Berber ports. Thinking that the cost of the gold might be much reduced if they could seize it directly at the places where it was mined rather than having access only through a long chain of pagan and Muslim intermediaries, the Portuguese took action. Beginning in the 1440s they devised navigational skills and invented ships that could sail south along the West African coasts and then—this was the really crucial point—*return* home by sailing a roundabout way north. Before this nautical trick was sorted out, sailings south from Portugal had been one-way voyages to oblivion.

As we saw in the earlier chapter on smallpox, by the middle years of the sixteenth century Portuguese navigators backed by Development agents in

Lisbon had rounded the Cape of Good Hope and established trading emporia at Goa in India and Macao in China. In the construction of their global trading network, two other sites were of great significance: Luanda in Angola and, just across the South Atlantic, landing places in Brazil. Through the accidents of papal politics, both were in Portuguese rather than in Spanish hands. Through a parallel set of accidents—the Spanish discovery and enforcement of claims to the rest of the New World—it was the Spanish who urgently needed vast numbers of laborers to work their American mines of gold and silver. This deficiency the Portuguese undertook to make good using their fortified base in Luanda and others along the "slave coasts" stretching from Senegal to the Nigeria regions.[45]

This is not the appropriate place to rehearse pro-and-con arguments about the role that coastal chieftains played in the enslavement of other Africans who happened to live inland. One or two points however need to be mentioned. First, such was their own progress in the manufacture of cloth, iron goods, palm wines and the like that African chieftains really did not need to accept the fine Indian-made goods the Portuguese brought in from Goa and demanded that they accept on credit. Yet, after initial hesitations, many African chiefs fell in with the Portuguese ploy. Why they did is one of history's unanswered questions.[46]

A second point is that once *credit* relationships between Portuguese/Portuguese agents and African chiefs/warrior adventurers had been established—this sort of thing has been most intensively studied in the case of Luanda—the brutal logic of debt reclamation, risk-taking and the exploitation of inland African victims by debt-racked coastal Africans was carried along on its own momentum. And as their teachers, the chieftains of Angola and the regions further north had Portuguese Old Christians and Portuguese New Christians who were at ideological loggerheads in their natal land. Drawing on deep historical roots well watered during the era of the emperors Vespasian and Titus (69–81 CE), it would seem that the Portuguese excelled their ancient mentors in their delight in gratuitous cruelty. Like the ancient Romans—whose classics ruling elites memorized in their youth—the Portuguese had recourse to spectacularly faulty policies of state. But rather than emulating the ploy of *bringing in* German barbarians to serve as soldiers (the Germans had ultimately taken over the Roman Empire West), in the Portuguese case it was a matter of forcing people out. Following the lead of Isabella and Ferdinand in the neighboring Spanish kingdoms, in 1497 the Portuguese Crown decreed such rigorous controls over the descendants of Jacob and Isaac that most decided to leave the country. Many took up residence in what after various vicissitudes became the independent United Provinces. Here Dutchmen old and new took to exploiting the Portuguese world trading network—for the greater glory of Development.[47]

Within Africa, long before the slave-raiding Portuguese came, there had existed institutionalized forms of slavery. However, these contrasted markedly with the plantation slavery that was even then being devised in Portuguese provisioning stations at São Tomé and Principe and which, from there, would be transferred to Brazil and to the Caribbean. European-managed slavery operated on the principle (except in the few years just before the United States Civil War) that black African lives were expendable. Within old Africa itself, other principles obtained. These held that humans were humans and that being in rather short supply they should be cherished. The first system—the European—was tailor made for the widespread dispersal of epidemic holocausts of yellow fever and malaria. The second (the African) was, as far as can be determined, disease neutral.

Before the rise of commercial slavery for the Atlantic trade (in being by 1500, but not extensive until the 1690s–1750s), indigenous African slavery usually involved young men who had been taken captive in war or who were domestic troublemakers unwilling to accept the behavioral norms set by their elders. Once elders had decided to rid the village of an unwelcome youth or a maid, common practice was to send them to a distant place many days' journey away so that they could never return to meditate before the graves of their ancestors. Permanently separated from kin, the slave living in an alien land became the dependant of a household head. Yet in the course of his life a male slave might rise to a position of authority and come to hold slaves of his own. In the case of a maid, it was not unlikely that she would marry her owner, perhaps as a second or third wife, and, if fertile and pleasing in her master's sight, rise to a position of authority in the household, honored in her middle and old age. It was likely that the children of this mother would be regarded as ordinary village members and share in the privileges and duties inherent in this status.[48] As is too well known, in the Americas after 1500, nothing like this ever happened, even at the landed estate at Monticello owned by the Virginian who in a ringing declaration in 1776 affirmed that "all men are created equal."

During the era of European-sponsored slave raiding, an African was heard to say that any person, white or black, who aided the white man in his trade in slaves had "gone dead in the heart."[49] No other judgment seems possible. One can simply report that between the beginning of the trade in the late fifteenth century, its massive take-off after 1690–1750, and its effective suppression in the mid-nineteenth century, some 12–20 million Africans were shipped in bondage across the Atlantic. To this human loss must be added the several million people—perhaps 40 percent of the total captured—who died of disease, starvation or torture on the trail between the place they were abducted and the coast where they were loaded onto white men's ships for the Middle Passage. Added to this were the perhaps 4 million souls who were forced to walk across the Sahara for sale in the slave pens of Cairo, Damascus and Istanbul. For West Africa and west central Africa, the total number of people lost comes to somewhere between 24 and 37 million.[50]

In the realm of ideas which would impact upon perceptions of blacks and black men's diseases just before and after Europe's territorial invasions of West Africa in the 1890s, one must report a mirror image. Some Africans believed that white men were cannibals and that enslavement was intended to bring fresh meat to the Americas. This fantasy was drawn on by H. G. Wells when writing his prototype science fiction novel in 1895. In that year and in those that followed, young people in church halls in England and Scotland were mesmerized by lurid tales of missionaries being cooked in iron pots by the Devil's black African minions. Adding to the horror was medical men's assurance that African worshippers of Satan had been granted special immunity to yellow fever and *falciparum* malaria, diseases which "time out of mind" had made the coasts of West Africa "the white man's grave."[51]

Slavery, Yellow Fever and Malaria in the New World

Barbados

In its first New World visitation, epidemic yellow fever from coastal Africa struck Barbados in 1647. What followed then is significant for a number of reasons. First, and most obviously, was the special relationship established between this pioneer English example of New World Development and the disease environment which the settlers created (the ruthless clearance of virgin forests to free up land for the cultivation of sugar cane). As manifest here, Development brought together arable land and imported labor to produce the sugar marketed in England. This product did much to set in motion—through multiplier effects in allied industries—the larger consumer revolution on which the modern world is based.

For medical historians, also of special interest is the disease determinism which an historian has associated with Barbados. This claims that the island's plantations necessarily had to be worked by black African slaves because they were more or less immune to the yellow fever that killed off most Barbadian whites. In the recent past, this determinism has hampered objective study of the interrelationship of yellow fever and human populations in the Caribbean, in the American South, and in Africa.[52]

Located north of the mouths of the Orinoco, with a population in 1646 of 40,000 on a land area only 500 kilometers square, Barbados was the most densely settled chunk of territory in the overseas British Empire. Accordingly, it was a prime candidate for epidemic disaster.[53] In the course of the yellow fever visitation of 1647 (which lingered on until 1650), 6,000 Barbadians were carried off, roughly 15 percent of the population. Writing in 1673, the chronicler Richard Ligon, himself struck during the first epidemic, testified that newcomers lived in dread of the "Country Disease" and that frequent deaths caused much wearing of "Black Ribbon for mourning."[54]

In 1691 yellow fever hit again, and hovered around for several years. According to John Oldmixon in his history of Barbados, it swept away great numbers of "Masters, Servants *and Slaves*."[55] Alarmed by the continuing plague, many whites upped stakes and fled. Some, who had yet to make the great fortunes America was supposed to offer, moved to the virgin lands of South Carolina. By the end of the visitation, losses occasioned by flight and fever had cut back island numbers by a quarter, leaving a shrunken population of 25,000 white workers and proprietors, and 60,000 black slaves.[56]

Quite unlike the situation in other tropical islands—which typically after a disease disaster would enter a long period of decline—in Barbados it was during the era punctuated at either end by epidemics that the colony became the epicenter of a paradigm-setting revolution in consumer tastes. The product involved—cane sugar—was neither an essential foodstuff nor a particularly healthy one. Until it had become commonly available—thanks to Barbados—ordinary Europeans had sweetened their foods with honey.[57]

That the sugar revolution was initially based on that island was something of a fluke. Apparently void of any indiginous peoples, Barbados was first settled by the English in 1627. Within a short time these pioneers were able to avail themselves of the skills and credit connections of the Dutch. The latter people (both proper Netherlandish and Sephardic) had earlier conquered land in north-east Brazil and begun to grow sugar cane soon after 1637, only to be thrown out by the Portuguese eight years later. Murky deals between Dutch and English followed, leading in Barbados to the planting of stalks of cane and the building of some sugar-grinding mills.[58]

Then, working through Parliament, a mercantilist program was put in place which compelled colonial producers to market their goods in England. Sugar was included in the enumerated articles in 1663. Added to these happenings (fortuitous for planters and dentists) was the European "reformation in manners." This was a civilizing process that encouraged artisans and others in middling social strata to drink two products only recently imported in quantity from Asia: tea and coffee. Fashion dictated that to form a proper drink, a teaspoon or so of sugar be added. These new drinks contrasted with the fine spirits to which the aristocracy were said to be addicted as well as with the adulterated gin reputedly drunk by the gallon by the dissolute poor.

As early as 1655 London merchants imported 5,236 metric tons of Barbadian sugar. On arrival this was worth £180,000, an increase of 27 percent on its value on departure from Bridgetown. Thereafter, there was nowhere to go but up. Austen and Smith quote figures showing the rapid increase in British sugar consumption, from 4.6 pounds per capita in 1698–1700 (when Britain's population stood at 6.1 million), to 11.1 pounds in

1726–30, to 16.2 in 1766–70 (when Britain's population was 29.6 million). Added to this enormous increase in the amount of sugar absorbed in Britain (some 2.4 million metric tons), was the Barbadian sugar re-exported in English bottoms from English ports to France. There the product sparked off a similar revolution in consumer tastes and, following mercantilistic principles, led to French Development ventures in St Domingue.[59]

Far more than any other crop, cane sugar was capital intensive. Planted and harvested on a year-round schedule, after the stalks had been cut, they had to be brought immediately to a wind-driven or water-driven mill. There they were cooked down, cooled, recooked and processed until the sugar was ready to be poured out into special containers, preparatory for shipment to England. Because of the rapid decline in the sugar content of cane after it was cut, it was essential that each sizeable plantation have at least one mill constructed along the most modern lines. In case of breakdown, an alternative mill had to be nearby, lest the entire crop be lost. Considering that in England there was no machinery appreciably more complicated than a sugar-refining mill and that Barbados was on the periphery of the known world, it is something of a marvel that capital for this novel, risky enterprise could be found. Yet of course its provision was grist to the mill of London-based extenders of credit. For them, the basic rule was "the higher the risk, the higher the interest charged."[60]

Though funding processes during the early years of Enterprise Barbados remain obscure, it is known that after the 1690s second- and third-generation planters succumbed to the temptations offered by the gewgaws of Britain. These included the fine wallpapers, furniture and dresses, and the fine carriages drawn by fine horses which planters imported in great quantities *on credit*. Presumably the roots of their willingness to take financial risks to enhance their perceived status extended back to the time of the Civil War and the Restoration. During those years, for Dick Whittington types walking the streets of London or Bristol, Barbados was said to be the place to make one's fortune; anyone who failed there was obviously of no use to himself or anyone else. Lest these points be lost, Barbadian promotional specialists haunted English alehouses and bookstalls hawking word of the island's wondrous bounty.[61]

We now turn directly to the vexed question of the sort of labor that would be used in Barbados, and whether the situation that ultimately prevailed (blacks predominating) was in any way determined by the killing preferences of the yellow fever virus. Evidence strongly suggests that in the 1640s and 1650s resident plantation owners much preferred to use the same sort of non-family labor they had known at home in Britain: white indentured servants. Typical was the request which planter William Hay sent back to a friend in Scotland in September 1645:

> want of servants is my greatest bane and will hinder my designe. . . . In January next god willing I shall begin to make sugar. So pray if you come

neare to any port where shipping comes hither indenture procure and send me [servants] . . . lett them be of any sort men women or boys . . . what I shall not make use off and are not serviceable for mee I can exchange with others especially any sort of tradesmen.[62]

As this shows, most apprentices were indigent young English and Scottish persons who had lacked the passage money needed to cross the Atlantic on their own. Encouraged by promotional literature about Barbados the island paradise, they contracted to sell their services for a term of three to seven years to a ship's captain, who in turn sold them to the highest bidder in Barbados. In this manner, tens of thousands of Anglo-Saxon-Celtic semi-servile laborers sailed westward intending to make their fortunes.

Once in Barbados, indentured laborers might find themselves working in a mixed gang. Side by sweaty side, unfree whites and unfree blacks worked from before dawn to past dusk, turning over the land for planting. As they walked along in wet soil, their footfalls created potential mosquito breeding pools. Because Barbados was only a snippet of land (barely twice the size of the modern District of Columbia), both ethnic sorts often worked not far from broken shards near a jetty where sickly sailors and slaves fresh from Africa might unload the foodstuffs and commodities needed for plantation life. Their daytime work in the fields done, contract whites and slave blacks might then spend much of the night in the plantation mill. There, where overseers' whips enforced time-obedience, freshly harvested sugar was cleaned, ground and crystallized in huge vats cooked over wood-fires, eventually to be drained into containers and made ready for shipment to England.[63]

Day and night, night and day, African and Anglo-Saxon-Celtic gang-mates underwent the same harsh discipline and shared the same low-grade food, shoddy clothing and broken-down housing. For some, circumstances were even worse. In the 1650s, a literate pair of Englishmen reported that after having been convicted of royalist sympathies in republican England, they had been shipped to Barbados and put on sale to the highest bidder. They had then fallen into the hands of the:

"most inhuman and barbarous persons," who worked them hard, fed them meagerly, and in general reduced them to the "most deplorable, and (as to Englishmen) . . . unparalleled condition" in which they were "bought and sold . . . from one planter to another, or attached as horses and beasts for the debts of their masters, . . . whipped at the whipping-posts (as rogues) for their masters' pleasure," forced to sleep "in sties worse than hogs in England and [in] many other ways made miserable, beyond expression or Christian imagination."[64]

Yet so long as they were in a state to work, the productivities of white indentured laborer and black slave were considered to be equal. Cost accountants calculated that either ethnic type should be able to process cane equivalent to their purchase price in twenty to twenty-four months. After that, any finished sugar they contributed was pure profit for the owner's home-based English creditor.

Why then did the percentage of white laborers in Barbados decline so dramatically relative to the number of blacks after *c.* 1690? The answer rests almost entirely on changing economic and social conditions in Europe. For any on-the-make young person in England, Scotland or the Continent considering whether to undergo the risks of Barbados, the deciding factor was what geographers term the "perceptual environment."[65]

Contrasting what he heard of the life-shortening risks in going to any large European city where fortunes were reputedly made—London, Amsterdam, Cologne—and the situation said to exist in Barbados and other New World colonies south of the Chesapeake Bay, there was nothing particularly unusual about Barbados. In comparison with the grim reality of urban life in Europe—where at nineteen a new arrival could at best expect to live only another ten or fifteen years—Barbados offered the off-chance that a bondsman, once liberated and paid off, might marry the widow of a rich planter and be able to set up as a person of substance. In most men's perceptual environment, opportunities such as this would be more common in Barbados than in London.

What finally tilted the balance away from white indentured labor towards black African slave labor in Barbados in the late 1660s, and in Maryland and Virginia thirty years later, was *not* fear of yellow fever (as disease determinists claim), but instead the gradual drying up of the supply of under-employed and unemployed young adults in England. A motherland which in 1600 was thought to be swarming with too many people (all 3 million of them), by the 1680s was coming to be perceived as a country suffering from labor scarcity.[66]

The key transforming factor in the perceptions of English people about what their own land had to offer was the dramatic growth in the production of a great range of hand-crafted manufactured goods for sale on distant markets (proto-industry).[67] Now that they had a way to pass their time doing something which would bring them a small disposable surplus that they could use to become consumers—in addition to meeting mere subsistence needs—young people elected to stay at home rather than going out as indentured servants to the Caribbean. Those few who *were* brought out in the late 1690s—like those whose agonies visiting French missionary Father Labat witnessed—had very often been kidnapped or "barbadoed." But once there, the "barbadoed" sort, having nothing to lose, gloried in the drinking, gambling, fist-fighting, sodomizing and other forms of violence for which the island was famous.[68]

Other than the rise of proto-industry in England and parts of mainland Europe, a further reason why the prospects of working as an indentured laborer in Barbados attracted fewer and fewer takers after 1670 was the general stagnation of Europe's population growth. Here again, what *really* mattered were developments in the cosmopolitan core rather than the presence of the frightful country disease, yellow fever, in the Caribbean periphery. Had Europe been experiencing vibrant demographic growth on the order of that which it would undergo between 1840 and 1914—when at-home populations doubled and 50 million Europeans emigrated, mostly to the Americas—there simply would have been no need to flood the Caribbean islands (and the American South) with slave labor abducted from Africa.

In the Netherlands, this stagnation in population size was also in evidence after the 1670s. Here any young man who wanted to go to the ends of the world to make his fortune would obviously join the services of the Dutch East India Company in spice-rich Indonesia. And in the German lands, after the Thirty Years War ended in 1648 with pre-war numbers cut by a fifth, the next two generations of young people had more than enough to do filling up the employment gaps caused by the long war. When in the 1690s and 1700s the Germans began to recover their numbers—causing much anxiety among village elders of the J. F. Osterwald sort (see p. 140)—adventuresome young souls generally elected to go out to the best poor man's country, Quaker-run Pennsylvania.[69] Few could be found who were willing to go to the god-forsaken island of Barbados where white indentured laborers were "whipped at the whipping posts (as rogues) for their masters' pleasure."[70]

Though conditions in Barbados were harsh for white bondsmen, they were undoubtedly even worse for "salt-water" slaves brought in by Portuguese and Dutch traders. Around 1700, Father Labat reported that:

> [owners and overseers appeared] "to care less for the life of a negro than that of a horse," . . . and [worked] slaves "beyond measure . . . [beating] them mercilessly for the least fault. [Escaped slaves were] burnt alive or exposed in iron cages in which they [were] attached to the branch of a tree or . . . left to die of hunger and thirst."[71]

Though the statistics of slave imports into Barbados before Father Labat's time are shaky, information is a bit more firm after 1708. To the Barbadian slave population, which in that year numbered 52,000, were added in the next quarter-century 80,000 new imports brought in from Africa. By 1735 the surviving slave population numbered 68,000—which works out at a gross loss of 64,000 black African lives in the intervening years. Added to uncounted thousands of deaths from yellow fever, were added deaths from strokes, hernias, torture and other causes.[72]

According to an early eighteenth-century visitor, plantation owners commonly allowed young slave males to take all the black women they wanted for their pleasure "and to leave them as they please, provided that they produce[d] a large number of children . . . work[ed] well and" did "not become ill."[73] Archaeologists digging in Barbadian graveyards dating from the days of slavery have found the bones of many infants who, after weaning, died of malnutrition. Doubtless the situation there was much as it was in the sugar plantations of Jamaica, where a white overseer put it on record that he kept pregnant women at work in the fields until the day they gave birth and called them back only three or four weeks later. Under such a regime a high infant mortality rate could be expected. This meant that in order to keep up the number of slaves needed for efficient sugar production, a constant flow from Africa had to be maintained.[74]

A hundred years after Fr. Labat's tour in 1700, another professional man visited Barbados. This was the military physician George Pinckard whose run-in with yellow fever we mentioned earlier (p. 213). Proud of his education in the Greek and Roman literary classics that provided a medical doctor with his intellectual stock in trade, Pinckard found most white Barbadian health provisioners woefully ignorant, "and the very *negroe doctors* of the estates do justly vie with them in medical knowledge."[75] When treating yellow fever, African healers used hot baths and herbs which soothed the system. Such practices contrasted sharply with those frequently used by whites. Their standard practice was:

> Treatment: The inflammatory character of the disease should be kept in view from a very early stage of the disease. Begin the treatment with bloodletting from the arm. Saline cathartics. Second day, bleed again. Apply leaches to the abdomen, 2 dozen, warm poultices, gentle evacuants. Third day, apply leaches . . . Third night, a large blister. . . .[76]

Yet in treating his own case, Dr Pinckard preferred alternative techniques and had his shipmates dose him with bucket after bucket of ice-cold water.[77]

Later in the century, another medical visitor confirmed Pinckard's discovery that Barbadian slaves had no confidence in white plantation doctors and whenever possible concealed their illnesses from them. One suspects that black persons' secrecy goes a long way in explaining the peculiar ideas that nineteenth-century white health provisioners (and late twentieth-century southern historians) had about the diseases suffered, or not suffered, by persons of color. Had they chosen to investigate black people's burial preferences—near their habitation rather than in some special pit for yellow fever victims dug far from any built-up place—they would have realized that Africans who had not gained immunity through a childhood case of "endemic" yellow fever (using Hoffmann's term) died of yellow fever quite as frequently as did non-immune whites.[78]

For people earnestly concerned about Development, whether they be English, Dutch, Sephardic, French or Spanish-Creole, progress required that the Caribbean and Continental basin lands best fitted for cane sugar be brought into production. Following this logic, production methods pioneered on tiny Barbados moved on, in the British sphere to the much larger island of Jamaica and, in the French, to Saint Domingue. Then, after an ideological hiccup or two (occasioned by the French Revolution and its wars), Brazil and Cuba came forward to become major producers. It is to these societies we now turn, beginning with the most maligned of them all, St Domingue, after 1804 known by its Native American name, Haiti.

Haiti

We visited this once happy island earlier just before it was brought under the burning rule of Christopher Columbus. As we saw, through the linked agencies of disease (smallpox) and Spanish genocide, Hispaniola's indigenous Taino people had rapidly become extinct. To replace them as panners of non-existent gold, the Spanish had the Portuguese bring in slaves from Africa. Then with the conquest of Mexico and Peru and the discovery there of bounteous mines of silver and gold, the Spanish lost interest and allowed Hispaniola's salt-water Africans, creoles and half-castes to go their own way as subsistence cultivators.

Two and a half centuries later, the vicissitudes of history enabled entrepreneurs from France (ruled by a Bourbon cousin of the Spanish king) to establish plantations on the western third of the island. This collection of plantations, upland wastes and urban places (Port au Prince and Cap François) came to be known as St Domingue. Development progress was astonishingly rapid and by 1775 St Domingue had been transformed into the most lucrative colony in the world. Approximately the same size as Maryland, it produced more than half of the world's sugar. Together with its exports of cotton, indigo and coffee, sugar gave St Domingue a gross colonial product greater than that of the thirteen English mainland colonies combined.[79]

Following the pattern established after 1690 in Barbados (the result of Europe's flourishing proto-industry and static population size), on St Domingue nearly all the cane sugar field work, processing and final preparation was carried out by African slaves. In the year revolution broke out in France, the colony contained some 480,000 slaves; of these a sizeable proportion were recent imports. In the last normal year of the old regime (1791), 25,000 "salt-water" slaves were brought in to supplement decaying numbers.

Distressed, disorganized and unruly, St Domingue's slaves were subjected to what by now had become standard forms of discipline. As reported by one of them:

> Have they not hung up men with heads downwards, drowned them in sacks, crucified them on planks, buried them alive, crushed them in mortars? Have they not forced them to eat shit? And having flayed them with the lash . . . have they not lashed them to stakes in the swamp to be devoured by mosquitoes?[80]

In addition to its other hazards, mosquito-borne yellow fever and several types of malaria were endemic in St Domingue. No figures or guesstimates of the numbers of blacks who died from these killers have survived. However, for the sort of people record-keepers thought important—white troops—there is considerable information. One snippet tells of the fate of 100 men stationed in the town of Port au Prince. After having become acclimatized to the town's particular disease environment, in 1777 the hapless 100 were transferred to a post fifty miles away. Within six weeks, twenty-five of them were dead and only nineteen remained healthy. Two years later, of the original 100, only seventeen survived.[81]

Tied by bonds of credit and kinship to metropolitan France, after 1791 St Domingue's white elite were caught up in the maelstrom of its revolution. Contributing to their difficulties were local social fissures. Pitted against the great white planters (who expected on retirement to live comfortably in Bordeaux or La Rochelle) were groupings of small white planters and of landless artisans. In addition, there were freed black and half-caste planters who themselves owned slaves. It was from this grouping that Haiti's revolutionary leadership would emerge, men like Toussaint Louverture and Jean-Jacques Dessalines.

Early in the complex of events that led in 1804 to the liberation of the slaves and establishment of Haiti as a black-ruled independent republic, the great white planters took flight. Beginning in 1793, some returned to France and others took ship to Philadelphia, the then chief city of the United States. There they and their mosquito companions caused a famous epidemic of yellow fever. Since most of these high-ranking refugees had acquired immunity to the disease as children (following Hoffmann's endemic yellow fever scheme), nearly all the 5,000 yellow fever Philadelphian dead were either citizens of the new United States or imported slaves.[82]

In Haiti itself after 1791, ordered disorder left effective leadership in the hands of a coalition of mulatto and black militia captains who had long since been seduced by the glamor of European consumer goods. No longer in sympathy with locally born black subsistence farmers and salt-water immigrants who simply wanted to be left alone, revolutionary captains like Toussaint thought it essential that European and North American consumer goods keep flowing in. Aware that this would make them dependent on resident white agents, at the same time the black leadership saw that the backbone of their revolutionary movement lay with the 90 percent of the population who were enslaved or in some lesser form of bondage.[83]

Emerging from revolutionary councils was a two-pronged program to maintain links with the sources of the gewgaws of the West while providing the mass of the population with a modicum of social amelioration. Probably not aware that they were following a model provided by Eastern Europe and Russia during the era of the Second Serfdom (after 1500), Haiti's revolutionaries proposed that outright slavery be replaced by a serf-like status which gave workers some control over their daily lives. The problem with this program, as far as Europeans in control of powerful armies and navies were concerned (no one asked the serfs their opinion), was that it was being carried out by "persons of color."

Seen from the perspectives of London and Paris, it seemed that the only way to prevent further slave rebellions on sugar-rich Caribbean islands (the domino theory) was to invade St Domingue. Using the pretext that war had broken out between England and France, Prime Minister William Pitt, the most effective of Europe's *ancien régime* leaders, sent troops to conquer the rebellious French colony. Between 1793 and 1798 some 20,000 British men-at-arms were landed at St Domingue's ports. This was followed by a French invasion that brought in another 35,000 warriors.[84]

Seldom in recent history had so many unseasoned Europeans "of the most dense or rigid fiber" come to a Caribbean island infested with yellow fever and malaria. Confronted with this concentration of potential victims in port city garrisons, both fevers had a field day. Some English troops who survived both yellow fever and the "heroic bleedings" performed by British doctors were later sent to their graves by *falciparum* malaria. Overall, of the 20,000 Britons who had confronted the bullets of risen Africa and "the yellow pest that stalks gigantic through the Western Isles," 12,700 died, and 1,500 required invaliding home, leaving only about 6,000 physically unscathed. Among the French, death by bullets and fevers sent 29,000 troops to the oblivion of death. Only 6,000 lived to return to French-ruled Europe.[85]

But for the French, the Haitian experience provided training for later campaigns in Algeria. Particularly useful were the ways used to deal with local populations. For this, action plans were drawn up by Napoleon's brother-in-law, General LeClerc. In the last letter he sent from Haiti before he was extinguished by yellow fever, LeClerc envisioned that:

> You will have to exterminate all the blacks in the mountains, women as well as men, except for children under twelve. Wipe out half the population of the lowlands and do not leave in the colony a single black who has worn an epaulet [in the rebel army].[86]

In the event, French troops carrying out punitive actions killed some 150,000 people and destroyed vast quantities of foodstuffs and farming equipment. Of the 342,000 adult Haitians still alive when the French withdrew, only 170,000 retained enough strength to hoe the fields and plant the crops needed for subsistence.[87]

In world-historical perspective, the fallout from the failure of Europe's schemes to subdue the independent black republic was multi-faceted. Of particular significance was the psychological blockage which prevented Europeans and Euro-Americans from accepting that a republic established by risen African slaves deserved recognition as a proper sovereign state. Exemplifying this attitude, US Army Major W. C. Gorgas provided a 1903

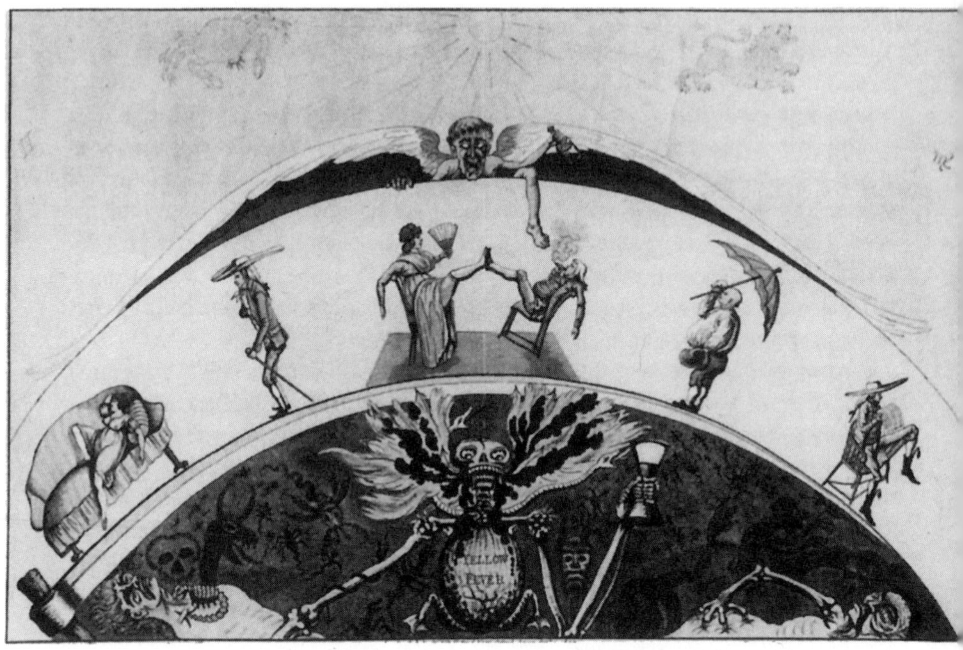

16. Caribbean island: the hells of yellow fever. A colored aquatint, *c.* 1800, by A. J.

international congress on tropical medicine with a history of the French expedition to Haiti. Gorgas held that: "out of 25,000 men, nearly 22,000 died of yellow fever in one season, leaving the remainder entirely at the mercy of the enemy, who scarcely had to fire a shot."[88]

Gorgas wanted the world to believe that blacks had never been able to defeat a white army on their own, whereas in fact a sizeable percentage of the French and English dead were victims of Haitian bullets. It will be noted that Gorgas's invented history was timed to provide a counter-example to offset memory of Italy's recent military defeat at the hands of the Ethiopians, at Adowa in 1896.[89]

In 1804, immediately after Haitians' hard-won victory which had left so many of their number dead, European and American imperial powers imposed a diplomatic and economic boycott. Amongst the English, manly teeth were set on edge by any hint that a black-directed republic should be recognized as a diplomatic equal. For their part the French insisted that the Haitian government pay full compensation to the great planters whose plantations had been confiscated.[90]

Yet there was more to the Haitian problem than differences in skin pigmentation. What influenced British attitudes as much as anything were the behavioral preferences of ordinary Haitians. Rather than accepting the need for economic domination by the world's greatest extender of credit so that they could purchase European goods, most Haitians preferred to remain subsistence cultivators. Working on the African model, Haitian women established a cycle of four-day markets which was perfectly adequate to meet the requirements of exchange for items such as salt, local foodstuffs and African-style clothes.[91] Content with what they had, Haitians felt there was no need for foreign trade.

But by rejecting the West's gift of Development, ordinary Haitians placed themselves in a position unacceptable to a Europe that was heir to the Enlightenment and convinced it alone possessed a universally valid moral code. Unfortunately (for those who like happy endings), not everyone in Haiti supported the rejection of consumerism. Particularly crucial was the attitude of heads of state. After 1804, most of them fell for the lure of imported goods. Increasingly tied by indebtedness to the West, and contemptuous of ordinary subsistence cultivators and their religious beliefs, presidents for life marched smartly down the road to disaster. As the nineteenth century wore on, the Haitian republic became a client state, first of the merchants of Hamburg (the "most English" of the German commercial cities) and then (as is still the case) of the independent United States.[92] This leads us to disease-related events and meanings in that continental giant.

The United States

After 1804, as before, black African slavery (the "Peculiar Institution") continued to flourish in the southern states of America. Yet its presence led to less difficulty with the former mother country than might have been expected. Though in principle the institution was regarded as infamous by the English moral reformers who brought an end to the slave trade in 1807 and in 1833 achieved Empire-wide abolition, as things worked out practice, London's gentlemanly capitalists and diplomats never seriously considered boycotting American goods or cutting off diplomatic relations. The contrast between British attitudes towards the USA—source of most of the cotton that fuelled the mills of Manchester and Oldham—and British attitudes towards Haiti—the one New World republic which *had* overturned slavery—is instructive. But rather than belaboring "perfidious Albion," let us turn to another concern. This is the role that America's Peculiar Institution and its post-Civil War control measures (Jim Crow Laws, the Ku-Klux-Klan, Supreme Court decisions) had in the making of Construct yellow fever. As will become apparent, this Construct became part of an endemic state of mind that shaped white and black relations in America and, to some extent, in the rest of the Anglophone world.

The United States acquired the vast Louisiana Territory by purchase from France in 1803 (with the help of Baring's Bank), thus funding the French military campaign against Haiti. Then during the Anglo-American war of 1812–15 the US usurped West Florida from Spain. Emptied of their Creek, Cherokee, Chickasaw, Choctaw and Natchez inhabitants by Andrew

Jackson in his capacities as military man and US president, those parts of the new territories facing the Gulf of Mexico to the south and the Mississippi River to the west became the regional setting for the new culture in which slave-grown cotton became king.

To keep things in perspective, it must be realized that in core–periphery relations, the newly developed South was a peripheral region for the provision of raw materials for conversion into finished goods in the north of England. England, lying at the operative center of core-zone Europe, provided most of the investment capital, short-term credit and transatlantic shipping facilities the South required for the expansion of its frontiers of cultivation.[93]

However, assessment of core–periphery relationships looked rather different when viewed from the front porch of a prosperous Mississippi or Louisiana slave owner's newly built Greek Revival plantation house. Masters of all they surveyed—with plantations running to thousands of acres—the Lower South's ruling families regarded themselves as the highest form of created beings. Many were descendants of planters who had come to South Carolina from Barbados during its 1690s troubles with yellow fever, and then, as new lands had opened up, moved into the virgin soils of the Lower South.

In the 1820s and 1830s, first-generation planters were not noticeably defensive about their way of life. They could afford to be complacent. The bottom line of their account books usually showed that black African slavery was more cost effective than the free white labor that northerners used on their owner-occupied farms in the North West Territory (i.e. Indiana, Illinois and Ohio). Then too, their finely tuned use of time-obedience while working their slaves put them in the forefront of advanced labor–management relations.[94]

However after the early 1840s, Southerners' nonchalance gave way to more aggressive attitudes. Looking at their region's position in the USA as a whole they found that northern politicians were regularly winning control of the US presidency and Senate; pessimists feared that this situation might become permanent. Threatening southern interests even more were reports that many northern politicians were listening to New England abolitionists who wanted to destroy slavery root and branch. And looking ahead to the future was the unsettled question of which regional grouping—slave holders in the South or northerners—would win dominant control of the vast new territories that American Manifest Destiny had yet to conquer, the whole of Mexico, South America, Cuba and Canada.[95]

Confronted with bothersome abolitionists (the editor of the Boston-based *Liberator* even claimed that black people deserved full equality with whites!) substantial southern planters and their professional clients went on the defensive. Terming themselves *Southrons* to make it clear they were entirely different from northern types, they held that theirs was a uniquely well favored civilization with roots going back to ancient slave-holding Athens and Sparta.[96] Conveniently at hand to help build this invented identity were locally educated medical doctors, experts on yellow fever.

As it happened, after around 1850 yellow fever epidemics became increasingly common in the South, striking at large cities—New Orleans, Memphis, Charleston—as well as at the several hundred small regional centers which provided planters with basic services. In an era in which yellow fever had all but disappeared from the northern states, these frequent epidemics of what modern southern historians term "the scourge of the South" were giving the region a bad name.

For medically qualified Southerners anxious to prove that black slaves were part of a distinctive servile "race" which was biologically different from the white master "race," yellow fever was a godsend.[97] Commonly thought to be imported by ship from Cuba to mainland America, it was perceived that each epidemic first broke out along the harbor fronts of Charleston or New Orleans and then moved up the Atlantic coast or the Mississippi Valley as the case might be.[98] However, in the light of current knowledge that yellow fever in endemic form can remain nearly invisible in any populated place where winter temperatures are above freezing, it is arguable that in some corners in the South yellow fever was actually endemic for years on end.

Included among these posited milieux were the closely packed slave quarters on large plantations. Heated by warm human bodies and by the hickory-wood fires that gave African-American settlements their distinctive smell, slaves' houses were capable of providing the minimal temperature needed to keep *Aedes aegypti* mosquitoes alive. Also kept warm and in a state fit to hatch later on were mosquito eggs (some perhaps vertically infected with the yellow fever virus). Hickory-wood fires also provided comforting warmth for the children who liked to play about indoors where they could be bitten by resident (daytime-biting) mosquitoes, made to feel slightly unwell, and so be (unwittingly) immunized against further attacks by yellow fever.[99]

Another point to be constantly borne in mind is that while in bondage African-Americans distrusted white plantation medical doctors and their curious ideas about bleeding and purging away fevers. Because of this antipathy, whenever possible slaves tended their own fever sick, using home remedies, such as bathing and administering soothing drinks. And just as black Americans liked to make their own clothes and dress in their own distinctive way, so too, they liked to tend their own dead and bury them in places known to them alone. Given that even today only a small percentage of people ill with yellow fever are diagnosed correctly (WHO figures suggest one in a thousand), it seems reasonable to suppose that many nineteenth-century blacks who died of this disease were not reported to authority. Indeed, until well after the Civil War, no state in the Lower South saw fit to register the vital statistics of *any* ethnic group.[100]

Among Southern practitioners of the special medicine of the South whose ideology was honed to the needs of plantation owners—"states' rights medicine"—it was self-evident that blacks suffered far less from yellow fever than did whites. Within the discourse I call Construct yellow fever, some medical ideologues went further and claimed that blacks were entirely immune. One of the first Southern doctors to commit these ideas to print was Dr J. C. Nott of Mobile, Alabama. Nott was a frequent contributor to the *Popular Magazine of Anthropology* and was generally taken to be an honest and respectable man.[101] Known in the 1840s for his sensible advice to people struck with yellow fever—he recommended plenty of liquids and rest rather than heroic bleedings—Nott declared: "I hazard nothing in the assertion, that one-fourth negro blood is a more perfect protection against yellow fever, than is vaccine against smallpox."[102] Another major contributor to the discourse was Samuel A. Cartwright, MD. As this locally famous New Orleans doctor put it:

> Although they [Negroes] are so liable to congestive and bilious fevers [malaria] . . . they are not liable to the dreaded *el vomito*, or yellow fever. At least they have it so lightly, that I have never seen a negro die with black vomit, although I have witnessed a number of yellow fever epidemics.[103]

Cartwright echoed southern planter opinion in claiming that: "Nature scorns to see the aristocracy of the white skin . . . reduced to drudgery work." According to him, recently arrived European immigrants who engaged in "laborious employments" under a "southern sun" and then fell to yellow fever died because they had violated "Nature's law."[104]

Printed notice of people who had violated another of nature's laws was found in the New Orleans newspaper *The Bee* early in May 1853. Among reports of the previous week's proceedings in the law courts, readers were told of:

> Routine matters . . . for example, cabaret-owner R. Jones was fined ten dollars for selling liquor to slaves. In another case, a fine was imposed on David King, free man of color, for permitting an illegal assembly of slaves in his cabaret; the *two* slaves who constituted the illegal assembly were given *twenty-five lashes apiece*.[105]

After the Confederate States of America in rebellion against the Federal Union were defeated by northern troops in 1865, their 4 million slaves were liberated and converted into impoverished rural share-croppers and urban slum-dwellers. Nourished now by home-grown racism as well as that imported from England, Cartwrightian biological determinism continued strong. Amongst its other redoubts was the oath of the Ku-Klux-Klan, the enforcing arm of post-war southern white supremacists. The KKK statement held that:

> History and physiology teach us that we belong to a race which nature has endowed with an evident superiority over all other races. [We have] over inferior races a dominion from which no human laws can permanently derogate.[106]

It was in this spirit that Henry Rose Carter, MD (1852–1925) wrote up the "scientific" perceptions of yellow fever that were published after his death, in 1931. Born of slave-holding parents nine years before the Civil War (and thus of an age to be heavily traumatized by the war itself), Carter was brought up on Clifton Plantation in Caroline County, in the much-fought-over state of Virginia. Viewing the disease through these perceptual lenses, in his published statement on yellow fever Carter concluded that "the negro . . . has a true racial resistance which is not dependent upon prior infection or exposure."[107] However, Cartwrightian–Carter biological determinism was not accepted everywhere.

Writing in 1901, Mary Kingsley, a noted north of England literary personage and inveterate traveller in West Africa, reported that in Freetown, Sierra Leone it was common knowledge that blacks repatriated to Africa whose ancestors and parents had lived for two or three generations in America, Canada or England had lost all immunity to yellow fever and malaria. According to her, among returnees, fever death rates had been nearly as high as among white susceptibles fresh from Europe.[108] But what was common knowledge in Mary Kingsley's rather select circle in England was apparently unknown in the American South.

In the Southern medical literature published after 1865, recently examined by Margaret Humphreys, virtually nothing was said about yellow fever among American-born blacks.[109] What however *did* interest "Southerners" was the negative impact that yellow fever had on immigration from Europe. It was also having a negative impact on the flow of finance capital from the new source that had recently come into its own: Wall Street, New York City. In responding to these difficulties, Southern chambers of commerce had three choices: (1) deny that any threat from yellow fever existed; (2) acknowledge the threat by imposing quarantine on ships coming from infected ports; or (3) meet a yellow fever epidemic crisis when it occurred by taking the usual defensive steps against the miasma which everyone knew was its cause by burning barrels of tar in the streets and firing off cannon.[110]

Typical of the first approach was an editorial in the New Orleans *Daily Picayune* early in May 1853, which boasted that: "Nature has placed no limits on [our city's] greatness, she must become . . . perhaps one day the greatest commercial emporium on the face of the earth."[111] That autumn, after the first frosts had settled, New Orleans newspapers were again given over to boosterism. From reading the local press no uninformed reader would realize that, the previous May, panic caused by reports that yellow fever had killed a few citizens had sent 50,000 New Orleans whites scurrying off for their lives. Between the great May exodus and the coming of the frosts, yellow fever had killed 9,000 people, one in ten of the population remaining in town.[112]

While Yellow Jack ruled New Orleans in 1853, Royale Street and the fashionable new American Quarter were deserted except for night-time robbers. Besides thieves, there were other problems. New Orleans was built below sea level and lacked a proper burial ground where bodies could be left undisturbed. This meant that during an epidemic when there was heavy pressure on services, one-year-dead bodies had to be moved out of their graves to some other site before the current yellow fever dead could be dropped in. Since no one at that time knew whether yellow fever was non-contagious (as Dr Rush of Philadelphia had insisted in 1793) or whether it could jump from yellow fever dead to graveyard worker, burial crews were chronically under-staffed.

As reported by Humphreys, in August, when 200 people were dying a day, "the coffins were deposited on the ground by the cartmen who then left." Worse horrors followed when "after two days in the hot Louisiana sun, the swollen corpses burst their coffins."[113] During the crisis, some 9,000 yellow fever dead had to be somehow dealt with. Further up the Mississippi in towns where there was enough dry land to bury the dead permanently, yellow fever killed another 11,000 people. This gave a grand total of 20,000 *known* victims in 1853.[114]

During the years of civil war (1861–65), 258,000 Confederate soldiers died of wounds or disease, out of a total southern white population of 8 million; at the time the region's blacks numbered 4 million. Had the whites killed while in the prime of life survived to breed at anything like the rate known among the 2,000 Dutch Boers in South Africa, who between 1713 and 1865 increased their numbers to 250,000 (doubling every twenty years to form the core of Afrikanerdom), by 1905 the Whitening of the Old South would have been well underway.

Whitening would also have been well advanced if a higher proportion of the 35 million European immigrants who came to the United States between 1840 and 1914 had chosen to live in the South. In explaining why most of them elected instead to put down roots in the North, the Middle West or in California, some credit should be given to the yellow fever epidemics of 1878, 1879, 1897 and 1905.

In 1878 yellow fever raced up the Mississippi from New Orleans to Memphis and beyond, spreading through 200 towns in eight states and claiming a total of 20,000 lives. In Memphis, at the first rumor of its approach, citizens of substance fled into the depths of Shelby County or upstream to Illinois, leaving only the rump of municipal government behind. Left to their own devices, council members tried to maintain essential services—feeding traumatized orphans found wandering naked along the river and burying the yellow fever dead—but in the process went broke. After autumn frosts put an end to the slaughter—5,150 Memphians were *known* to have died of yellow fever—survivors met and petitioned that the bankrupt city find a new way to govern itself; the State obliged by cancelling the city charter. While this was going on, it was seriously suggested that the site of Memphis be abandoned, levelled to the ground, and salted. Several opponents of this idea promptly sold their town properties at knock-down prices and moved on, just in time to escape the yellow fever epidemic of 1879.[115]

According to one report, in the course of this second epidemic, 2,000 Memphians took sick and 583 died. Humphreys however points out that such was the confusion of the times that no proper registers of the dead were kept. In any case, the reappearance of yellow fever (presumably kept alive locally over the winter) was the death knell of the city's reputation. What on the eve of the epidemic of the previous year had been a booming metropolis of 40,000—in commercial terms the capital of Mississippi—was, after the combined disasters of 1878 and 1879, a wizened community of 33,000 that had suffered a net population loss of 17 percent. During the next several decades, Memphis, rather than attracting great numbers of immigrant fair-haired Aryan Germans or Irish, drew to itself only failed black share-croppers and rural Arkansas and Tennessee poor whites. In statistical terms, the proportion of immigrants in the city fell from 17 percent in 1870, to 3 percent in 1900. By then, the black population of Memphis, which in 1870 had been outnumbered by whites on a ratio of five to three, had become equal to the white.[116] Almost until the outbreak of World War II, the reputation of Memphis as a slough of disease remained unshaken.

In 1897, four years after the cotton boll-weevil had begun to nibble its way through its staple crop, the Lower South was hit by another visitation of yellow fever. Other than the boll-weevil, part of the context of this new disaster was the South's reputation for public lynchings of blacks and its new Jim Crow laws. In northern financial centers these caused much clacking of tongues. Added to this was the new twist in the popular interpretation of Construct yellow fever: this held that yellow fever *was spread by* blacks and by all non-local people. Known to be countenanced by local law enforcement and health officials, the wave of southern violence occasioned by the Construct was probably more instrumental in blocking the flow of immigrants and finance capital than was the disease itself.

Alerted in 1897 by their local and KKK networks that yellow fever was being spread by refugees fleeing from New Orleans and river towns upstream, rural whites in the region bounded by the Kansas state line, the Ohio River and the Gulf of Mexico defended their local *pays* against all comers. At roadside crossings, township boundaries and wooded stretches, masked vigilantes popped out of bushes wielding shotguns, forcing strangers who were lucky enough to be travelling in a white skin into jerry-built quarantine camps. There is no report about what happened to black travellers.[117]

For a region critically short of capital and with a reputation already badly marred by violence, even more harmful was the damage done to capital stock at night. Working under flaming torches, local Southron protectors dynamited bridges and tore up railway tracks, fired the piles then twisted and deformed the rails so that they could not be relaid. At a time when even southern newspaper editors confessed that "the entire country south of the Ohio River . . . is dominated by madmen," railheads north of the Mason-Dixon line worked overtime diverting traffic from a South given over to mass destruction.[118] None of this escaped the notice of Wall Street capitalists, or of immigrants on Ellis Island, or of thoughtful men in the South itself. Speaking before a medical conference in Mississippi, a local physician warned that yellow fever

> keeps capital away, drives commerce from our door and keeps immigration at a minimum—thereby leaving millions of acres of fertile land lying idle, which if cultivated would make of this one of the most prosperous portions of the Union.[119]

In the violence-ridden year of 1897 no incidents involving blacks were recorded, which, given what we know of conspiracies of silence about night-time lynchings, is not to say they didn't take place. Then in 1905, during the yellow fever epidemic that broke over the Mississippi Valley, the customary veil of silence lifted, slightly. By that time KKK and other white supremacists had been apprised that yellow fever could be spread from person to person. A likely source of this notion was a report published in 1898 to the effect that members of a "negro railway gang quartered in a set of shanty cars side-tracked alongside the Taylor [Mississippi] depot" were from Jackson (Mississippi) where an epidemic was raging. The report alleged that these Jackson "niggers" had spread yellow fever to the Taylor people who had come to the town railway station.[120]

Among others broadcasting the notion that yellow fever was contagious was the State of Mississippi health coordinator, C. B. Young.[121] According to this person:

> It is a notorious fact that in the country towns of the South, negroes habitually move about from place to place in spite of quarantine restrictions, and it being a popular belief that they did not have the fever, any slight sickness passed unnoticed . . . many of the outbreaks of fever in times gone by . . . really owed their origin to fever imported by negroes.[122]

Another professional health officer, Dr C. M. Brady of Louisiana, sketched out a slightly more complex linkage. Brady held that recent immigrants from Italy mingled at night with blacks on terms of perfect equality and that in the course of this interchange, the blacks spread their yellow fever to the immigrants. As every Calvinist and Baptist knew, the European-Latinos were Catholics and devious no-accounts who moved about "stealthily by night."[123] At Tallulah, Louisiana, five Italian immigrants caught mixing with blacks were successfully lynched by the KKK. Because these victims happened to be whites, their deaths were reported in the newspapers. No notice was generally taken of KKK-lynched African-Americans.[124]

In all this, it is obvious that yellow fever (as disease and as Construct) contributed to the slowness of the South's post-Civil-War recovery. Seen by Wall Street, the City of London and Brussels financiers as particularly unpromising material for Development were the region's ordinary white populace. Functionally illiterate, physically debilitated by malaria, hookworm, etc., and in their back-country way too arrogant ever to submit to the discipline of the factory floor, they seemed doomed to perpetual marginality.[125]

But as in most things American,"perpetual" was of finite duration. In this case what helped to reverse it was the disappearance of the Southern Scourge after 1905.[126] It is still uncertain whether the yellow fever virus decided to vacate of its own volition or whether it left because it was denied a refresher base in Cuba. In any case, though yellow fever disappeared from the American South, one distressing fact remains: the *white racism* it helped to inspire lived on.

Brazil

Four thousand kilometers to the south-east, in Brazil, a linkage between Construct and disease yellow fever and Development also comes into view. But before we sort through this maze, let us first establish where Brazil stood in relation to the financiers who effectively controlled it after the Napoleonic Wars: London's gentlemanly capitalists.[127]

Constituting more than 45 percent of the land mass of South America, the Brazilian region was brought into contact with the West by the Portuguese discoverer Alvarez Cabral in 1501. By 1800, when its (known) population stood at under 3 million, Euro-Brazilian settlement was concentrated in the coastal cities of Bahia, Recife, Salvador, São Paulo and in Rio de Janeiro, the capital. These enclaves aside, the white presence was also found on groupings of sugar plantations in the old north-east province of Pernambuco. Another, more recently established block of plantations was found in the central coastal provinces of Minas Gerais and São Paulo. These grew cane sugar and coffee for the export trade.[128]

Ruled since 1500 by the Portuguese Crown (worn by the king of Spain from 1580 to 1640), after the French invaded the fatherland in 1808, Brazil became the residence of the Portuguese king, John VI. Easing his move across the Atlantic were the gray éminences behind the throne, the gentlemanly capitalists of London. For the rest of the century Brazil was in financial terms a British satellite.[129]

Until 1888 most of the field labor in Brazil was provided by black African slaves. Mortality rates being what they were (unknown in detail but generally high), fresh slave imports from Angola, Hausaland and elsewhere kept up numbers. During robust growth decades like the 1840s, some 19,000 Africans were brought in each year.[130] This situation seems not to have presented any insurmountable problems to the British. As we know, they had banned the trade in their own empire as early as 1807 and at the Congress of Vienna (1815) had persuaded other European powers to do the same.

In this context, British people can be taken to be of several sorts. One grouping, John Stuart Mill's middle class*es* on the way to becoming the middle class, tended to occupy themselves with political and social affairs at home. By tacit agreement, their Members of Parliament (beneficiaries of 1832 reforms) generally left matters touching the outside world to the great aristocracy and their gentlemanly cousins in the City. The duplicity to which this led was nicely caught by the old Duke of Wellington, the Prime Minister. Minuting the Foreign Minister in 1828, Wellington advised that:

> We shall never succeed in abolishing the foreign slave trade. But we must take care to avoid to take any step which may induce the people of England [i.e. the middle classes] to believe that we do not do everything in our power to discourage and to put it down as soon as possible.[131]

For their part, elite Brazilians (being clever people aware of which side their bread was buttered) always took care that dividends and debt repayments were delivered to the British on time. The British reciprocated these favors. In 1873 when bank failures in Vienna caused tremors throughout the capitalist world, Lord Rothschild (since 1855 in charge of the special relationship between the City and Brazil), put Brazilian bonds on sale in European markets on very favorable terms, thus preserving Brazil's liquidity.[132]

Britain's financial leaders recognized the need to allow its Portuguese-Creole milch cow freedom in the conduct of its own domestic affairs. Thus in 1822 they made no fuss when the Emperor of Brazil severed ties with his father (the King of Portugal) and declared Brazil an independent kingdom. By that time the wealth and population (4 million) of Brazil had come to exceed that of the fatherland (3.5 million). Calculating British financiers also weathered the Brazilian storm of 1888 when conservative military and financial interests overthrew the monarchy and established a republic. In the reactionary Old Republic era that followed, British financiers reaped some of their highest returns. Contributing hugely to this success was yellow fever, both as disease and as Construct.

Historians in an older historiographic tradition accept the official Brazilian claim that in the 150 years after the great yellow fever epidemic of 1685–96 Brazil remained free of the scourge until 1849.[133] One much-quoted source substantiating this is a letter written by an English physician who was sailing off the coasts in 1830. He maintained that:

> The inhabitants of the shores of this vast continent [of South America] whether permanent or occasional, enjoy a high and a singularly uniform degree of health. . . . Epidemic diseases are scarcely known; with wide-spread and destructive force they are totally unknown. The [yellow] fever which frequently makes such havoc in the West Indies never makes its appearance here.[134]

Some support for the doctor's Panglossian view of Brazil as health resort had been provided by the example of the Portuguese monarch, John VI. In 1808, he had sailed in from Lisbon accompanied by 8,000 judges, ecclesiastics and other staff who were not immune to yellow fever. After settling in Rio, the dignitaries do not seen to have encountered any killing fevers. However, it was unlikely that men of their rank would have ever come within mosquito flying range of any impoverished Brazilian child (with her/his virtually symptomless disease) who might have been in a chain of (Hoffmann-style) *endemic* yellow fever stretching into the Amazon forests wherein monkeys played.[135]

This brings us to the formulation of nineteenth-century Brazil's population policy. According to the census taken in 1872, 38.1 percent of the population were people of European descent; 38.3 percent were of mixed race (mulatto); 19.7 percent had African ancestry; and 3.9 percent were Amerindians. Realistically accepting that North American and English ideas about the biological inferiority of blacks could not be applied to Brazil—its massive 58 percent black or mulatto population contrasted with only 14 percent black in the USA—around 1850 Brazilian planners devised the policy of "Whitening."[136]

This held that people of mixed blood, even if only one quarter white, carried within them the vital seeds of progress which *all* Europeans were thought to possess.[137] As a corollary, it was held that pure blacks, being lackadaisical in all things, including sex, found it difficult to replace their numbers. From this it followed that to reduce the number of morally impotent genes in the population, the government must discourage further African immigration. Decrees to this effect were duly issued; in time, Asian immigrants were also banned. Complementing this was Government's all-out effort to attract European immigrants. For this a variety of devices were used, including subsidized fares and the provision of special hillside camps to help new arrivals acclimatize to the disease environment.

Among the results of Whitening was the long-delayed abolition of black African slavery (finally achieved in 1888). Aside from ineffectual abolitionists' campaigns that had been going on for fifty years, the compelling argument that finally led to action was that free white European immigrants were reluctant to take up jobs if they were placed in direct competition with black African slaves. And so abolition came to pass. Released from bondage in 1888, some freed slaves returned to Africa. Others flocked to the bright lights of Rio de Janeiro.[138]

Complicating Whitening was the re-emergence of yellow fever. In its first wave, in December 1849, the epidemic ripped through Rio de Janeiro, Salvador and other urban centers. Though the government took care not to release any official figures, medically informed outsiders thought that the fever killed 14,000 people in Rio alone. In view of the fact that everyone of consequence claimed that yellow fever had been utterly unknown in Brazil since the 1690s, it seems odd that the epidemic especially targeted recently arrived foreigners. Native-born whites, mixed and blacks were only lightly touched. In light of later knowledge, it can be suggested that yellow fever had been there all along in its endemic form.[139]

News of Brazil's epidemics (there was a second one in 1853 and many others followed) caused considerable alarm among southern Europeans who were contemplating emigrating.[140] By 1856, near-stoppage of immigration, added to flight, had reduced Rio's population by more than half. However, coming to the rescue of dedicated Whiteners were southern Europeans' own "perceptual environments." Many people living in Lombardy or Venetia under an alien Austrian regime or in the authoritarian Bourbon-ruled Kingdom of the Two Sicilies, felt that, on balance, they were willing to accept the risk of yellow fever in distant Brazil. The alternative was the even greater risk of death in their home region by firing squad, hanging or casual soldierly violence. Perceptual environment choices having been made, tens of thousands of immigrants crossed the South Atlantic. Many first settled in Rio de Janeiro. By 1890, 29 percent of its population were immigrant newcomers. It was from this number that Rio's yellow fever culled most of its 60,000 dead.[141]

These losses notwithstanding, other romance-language immigrants crowded in, giving the Brazilian government cause to think that its policy of Whitening was moving successfully towards its goal. In 1890, a census (not of course a neutral source of information) claimed that Brazilian whites had greatly increased in number and now formed 44 percent of the population (up from 38 percent in 1872). Complementing this nicely was the falling percentage of people of full African descent, at 14.6 percent, down from 19.7 percent in 1872. Even more satisfying, the numbers of mixed parentage had dropped from 38.3 percent to 32.4 percent. Perhaps reflecting deeper penetration of Developers into the Amazon Basin (or perhaps merely a change in statistical bias), the percentage of Amerindians had increased to 9 percent of the population; in 1872, they had been recorded at only 3.9 percent. What was curious about this, given what we know about whole Amazonian tribes being made extinct by smallpox around this very time, was that the total number of Indians, added to the total number of whites, worked out at an acceptable 53 percent of the population, putting mulattoes and blacks in the minority. Statistically, which is to say perceptually, Whitening was well on track.[142]

Though it obviously did not derail Whitening (as determinists, working on the Barbados model, would have us believe it should), yellow fever as disease and as Construct did have long-term effects on the making of Brazil. Of particular importance was the impact it had on high-level decisions about which sorts of Development should be undertaken and which sorts would be relegated to the sidelines. Carried away by the example displayed by Baron Haussmann's new-made city during the 1867 Paris Exposition Universelle, in the 1880s Brazilian policy-makers made use of the continuing threat of yellow fever to provide a rationale for the costly rebuilding of their own capital city.

Fortunately for Old Republic Brazil's relations with its financial backers in the City of London, at that time medical doctors continued to hold that yellow fever was caused by a miasma arising from unsanitary grounds and waters. Those most apparent in Rio arose from the harbor where, in the absence of a sewage system, much of the city's human fecal matter was dumped.[143] On hand to help authority tidy things up—following the miasma paradigm—was an English-owned engineering firm, the City Improvements Company.

Many of the Rio engineering marvels the City Improvements Company subsequently built were constructed according to specifications appropriate to European climatic conditions but utterly unsuitable for a city on the Tropic of Capricorn. London financial backers, perhaps realizing that something like this might happen, had been careful to stipulate—in writing—that Brazilian authorities were to be financially liable for any rebuildings, reworkings or repairs needed after construction was complete. For English investors, all this was grease to their elbows.[144]

In this and in other ways, the Haussmannization of Rio vastly deepened the burden of debt the Old Republic owed gentlemanly capitalists in London. Explaining what happened next, Cain and Hopkins report that:

> The funding Loan of 1898 was very similar to the loan devised for Argentina in 1891, and was also arranged by Lord Rothschild. The Brazilian government was advanced £10 million over three years to cover its debt service. . . . Lord Rothschild . . . took care to point out that . . . repudiation, would involve not only "the complete loss of the country's credit" but might also "greatly affect Brazil's sovereignty, provoking complaints that could arrive at the extreme of foreign intervention. Brazil's President . . . duly administered the medicine: harsh deflationary policies were applied."[145]

Yet for most of Rio's population, the fine Beaux Arts buildings, wide boulevards and expensively constructed engineering works of the showcase center were irrelevancies that they hardly ever saw. Municipal authority, working on the understanding that yellow fever was caused by "insanitary conditions" and that displays of poverty were incompatible with European civilized values, banned ordinary poor Brazilians from living or showing themselves where they might be seen by wealthy Brazilians or foreign visitors. This condemned unemployed blacks, mulattos and new immigrants to living far out from the center. There in their wilderness of slums, they lacked ready, or indeed any, access to potable water, sewage and waste disposal, clinics, hospitals, schools and modern-sector employment.[146]

Partially counterbalancing the marginalization of 90 percent of the people was the Brazilian government's apparent success in bringing yellow fever under control in Rio and major provincial towns. Working under the new 1900 US Army-tested theory—that mosquitoes rather than foul air spread yellow fever—was the Brazilian bacteriologist Oswaldo Cruz. After 1903 he devised a control program which as early as 1907 gave the appearance of having conquered urban yellow fever.[147] Yet during Cruz's own time as public health czar, the yellow fever virus may already have taken root in mosquitoes in Amazonian Basin forests amongst which monkeys played. First suspected in 1910, its presence was confirmed in 1935.

Cuba

If Brazil seemed to be a country without a future in the half-century after 1849 when its cities were repeatedly struck by yellow fever, the same could *not* be said of Cuba. Only a little smaller than the state of Louisiana, the Caribbean island was governed by a Spanish and creole (Cuban-born) planter class renowned for their entrepreneurial flexibility and what can euphemistically be termed their "empirical approach" to the welfare of workers. Under such men, after the collapse of the Jamaican sugar industry in 1838 (when the post-slave apprenticeship system was wound up), Cuba rushed forward to become the world's single largest supplier.

Since it was so immensely profitable, sugar cultivation encouraged plantation owners to take high risks. Ignoring the prohibitions on the importation of African slaves which Britain had forced on the island's Madrid-based overlords in 1817 and again in 1835, planters connived with privateers—from Bristol (Rhode Island) and Portugal—to bring in fresh consignments. If queried by British agents about slave sales at Havana auctions, faked papers would show that the African was locally born and a legitimate pawn in the internal trade: this trade remained legal until 1886.[148]

On the Cuban sugar plantations themselves, owners—seemingly aware of the dangers of entrapment by foreign loans—plowed a generous proportion of their slave-generated profits back into their enterprises. Using state-of-the-art steam-driven refining mills and the latest in time-discipline techniques, between the early 1800s and 1860 sugar output per slave tripled. Locally generated profits were also used to supplement money borrowed abroad to lay down a railway network which by the end of the century was second only in length to that on the North American mainland. New railways connected port facilities with inland parts used now for the cultivation of sugar, coffee and cattle but which in former times had been the haunts of escaped slaves and bandits.[149]

Dominating this well-balanced economy was the capital city of Havana. With its ethnically diverse population from Africa and southern Europe, its muddle of eighteenth- and nineteenth-century architectural styles, its public squares, its mix of shops, concert halls, galleries, mansions, brothels and slums and, above all, its grand Malecon seafront promenade, Havana, in its New World cosmopolitanism was second only to New York.[150]

Until the late 1890s Cuba's governing creoles took very little interest in the yellow fever which after 1761 was presumably sometimes endemic, and sometimes renewed by infected mosquitoes and eggs brought in on slave ships from Africa. Most creoles themselves had been painlessly immunized by a mild case as infants. Those who did happen to be concerned about public health knew that one of their own experts was conducting research. In 1881 Carlos Finlay (born in 1833, the son of Scottish immigrant medical doctor Edward Finlay and his French wife) published a paper in which he suggested that mosquitoes were the bearers of a yellow fever poison. However because Finlay was not of a mind to use human guinea pig volunteers (as the conquerors of Cuba did later), his hypothesis remained unproven until 1901.[151]

After the 1850s Cuba, in perceptual environments, was seen as a prosperous white man's land where risk-takers were well rewarded, and where yellow fever was not very important. Neither was the island seen as being overwhelmed by blacks, since it was obvious that abducted slaves came in, worked for two or three years and then died without contributing much to the local gene pool. Given all these favorable perceptual conditions, Cuba attracted tens of thousands of caucasian men and women from Spain, Portugal and the Canary Islands.[152]

Despite its rocky politics after 1868—when an attempt by small planters to throw off Madrid's imperial claims led to a major war—in 1898 a nearly independent Cuba was rich in sugar and in talented people. However, anyone who thought that the island's future was assured failed to take account of the leaders of the "billion-dollar-country" 250 kilometers to the north—the USA.[153]

After their conquest and annexation of the northern third of Mexico in the mid-1840s, Americans had grandly assumed that it was their "manifest destiny" to absorb Spanish Cuba as well. To their mind, this task became all the more urgent after 1878 when yellow fever struck New Orleans, Memphis and towns upstream: every Southron knew that the disease had been shipped in direct from Cuba. After the epidemic passed, the US sent a study commission to Cuba. Among its members was the Hispanic-American pathologist, Juan Guiteras.

Later (in 1902) Guiteras was one of the first in tropical medicine to denounce the old idea that native populations in the tropical world had some sort of a natural or racial immunity to yellow fever. Finding the old notion "quite erroneous," Guiteras posited instead that many people in the tropics had a symptomless yellow fever in childhood that left them with lifelong immunity.[154] Quick to jump to the defense of Carlos Finlay when the latter's work was rubbished by the School of Tropical Medicine in London, in America Guiteras had to contend with the yellow fever Construct put forward as a "scientific truth" by the product of antebellum Virginia we met before, Henry Rose Carter.

Carter by now had become a medical officer in the US military. In 1879 he had carried out yellow fever research in Ku-Klux-Klan epicenters in rural Mississippi and so sharpened his own perceptual environment. In 1897 he was on the US Army Yellow Fever Commission appointed to study the disease situation in Cuba.[155] Given that 1897 was the year in which a horrendous epidemic of yellow fever swept the South, perceptual conditions did not much favor anyone who did not believe that brute force was a better way to settle disputes than rounds of reasoned discussion and compromise.

On the pretext that America had to do battle against the twin evils of yellow fever and of old world Spanish imperialism, in 1898 the US invaded Cuba. During their triumphant little war, they also conquered the Philippines and Puerto Rico, two other Spanish colonies which, oddly enough, were also producing sugar.[156] Yet for Henry Rose Carter, the war in Cuba was about something far grander than sugar: it was about civilization itself. According to this patriot:

> When the American Army established itself, intelligent officers of experience took up the "white man's burden" with an individual sense of obligation and a devotion worthy of the American citizen soldier.[157]

A generation after Cuba had become an American satellite, the US Commission on Cuban Affairs provided it with an appropriate history. This held that:

> Yellow fever was once the curse of Cuba. It destroyed commerce, killed thousands of young virile white immigrants in a single year and checked the development of the natural resources of the island for three centuries.[158]

What the report neglected to say was that in the year of the invasion, USA per capita consumption of sugar stood at a whopping 60 pounds a person, four times what it had been in 1835 when the US population was only a tenth the size. The 1935 report also failed to point out that American entrepreneurs going to the island after the 1870s had often found themselves regarded by the better sort of Cubans as crude savages. By taking over in 1898, America avenged this social put-down while at the same time ensuring that profits from sugar ended up in proper American hands.

Between their first landing in 1898 and 1901, the US military under Major William Crawford Gorgas, acting on the advice of the medical mission headed by Walter Reed, removed the threat posed by yellow fever. Early in his visit, Reed allowed sixty-some-year-old Carlos Finlay to come to see him and let Finlay remind him that in his paper published in 1881, he had suggested that mosquitoes carried yellow fever. Reed said yes, yes, I know all about it, apparently intending even while Finlay was in the room to claim personal credit. Reed was aware that "hypothesis" would have to be converted into a discovered "fact" arrived at through rigorous testing and that he alone had the capacity to do just this. In the weeks that followed, Reed used live human volunteers and hence proved that he had made a valid discovery.[159]

Applying the scientific knowledge thus obtained, the US military systematically poured oil into the water-storage pots belonging to each Havana household, thus, they claimed, killing all the mosquitoes that hosted yellow fever. Cuban locals, out-gunned by the occupying army, retaliated by making a great show of being amused. This response greatly annoyed the Americans who reported that:

> The people of Havana, being mostly immune, took small interest in yellow fever eradication. . . . There was much ridicule of our methods at that time, but fortunately this spirit of raillery and its pernicious influence in encouraging active and passive opposition to sanitary methods is now decreasing.[160]

Part of the constitutional arrangement put in place when the Americans were preparing to withdraw from the conquered island was the instrument known as the Platt Amendment. Accepted by Cubans under duress, the Platt Amendment permitted US military intervention whenever the disease or political situation seemed to warrant. Following the outbreak of epidemic yellow fever in New Orleans in 1905, Americans troops again swarmed in.[161]

In 1903, Theodore Roosevelt, hero of the battle of San Juan Hill (July 1898) which had turned the tide in the Cuban war, and by then President of the United States, gave behind-the-scenes encouragement to revolutionaries (headed by a doctor of tropical medicine) working away in northern Colombia in the Isthmus of Panama. After the Isthmus fell to the US and its rebel friends, Roosevelt sent in Major W. C. Gorgas to clear it of yellow fever and malaria, just as he had earlier done in Havana. When he had effortlessly achieved his goal (which had earlier defeated famous engineers from France and cost the lives of 50,000 Latino workers) the Americans were able to complete the canal linking the Atlantic Ocean and the Pacific.

In 1906, for his efforts in "promoting world peace" Stockholm awarded Roosevelt the Nobel Prize. Given the spirit of the times, this commendation should perhaps be rephrased to read, "for his efforts in making the tropical world safe for standard Europeans."[162] This thought leads us back across the Atlantic to West Africa. There we will assess the epidemiological consequences of the *fin-de-siècle* decision by the United Kingdom to bring that vast region fully within the pale of resident-white Development.

West Africa and Tropical Medicine, 1895–1928

Legitimization of the "Development of West Africa Project" depended to a large extent on breakthroughs in the field of tropical medicine. In the case of malaria, the requisite breakthrough occurred in 1897 when a hot-tempered English medical officer serving in India, one Ronald Ross, took credit for the intuitive insights of his Indian field assistant, Muhammad Bux. Emerging from this exercise was identification of the *Anopheles* mosquito as the carrier host of *falciparum* malaria. Working on the problem of yellow fever in Havana three years later, Reed, Gorgas and their live-experiment volunteers conclusively proved that the carrier here was the *Aedes aegypti* mosquito. This new knowledge opened possible courses of action which, if rigorously pursued, seemed likely to make both diseases locally extinct. One strategy was to kill all host mosquitoes. The other was to render all potential human hosts non-susceptible to the virus.[163]

Given sub-Saharan Africa's vast size and the heavy seasonal rains that created countless breeding places for mosquitoes, in 1898 it occurred to Robert Koch while briefly in East Africa that it would be easier to break the chain of transmission at its human link. Because malaria seemed to be the greater killer, his scheme was directed towards it rather than yellow fever. As Koch knew, well-heeled European travellers had long recognized that a judicious application of quinine was an effective prophylactic. Accordingly, while winding up his African tour Koch recommended that every inhabitant be encouraged to take quinine regularly. What he had seen of Africans led him to believe that ordinary people were "obedient and intelligent" and that they would be glad of European assistance in eradicating a frightful scourge.[164]

In this Koch was the pure scientist humanitarian, well meaning, but naive. In the age of Social Darwinism, more in tune with the way top people in Europe actually thought was Ronald Ross's throwaway comment to Patrick Manson. Writing from Sierra Leone in May 1899, Ross held that "the native . . . is really nearer a monkey than a man."[165] Ross later expressed himself at greater length:

> Malarial fever . . . haunts more especially the fertile, well-watered, and luxuriant tracts. . . . There it strikes down not only the indigenous barbaric population, but, with still greater certainty, the pioneers of civilisation—the planter, the trader, the missionary and the soldier. It is therefore the *principal and gigantic ally of Barbarism* . . . it has withheld an entire continent from humanity—the immense and fertile tracts of Africa.[166]

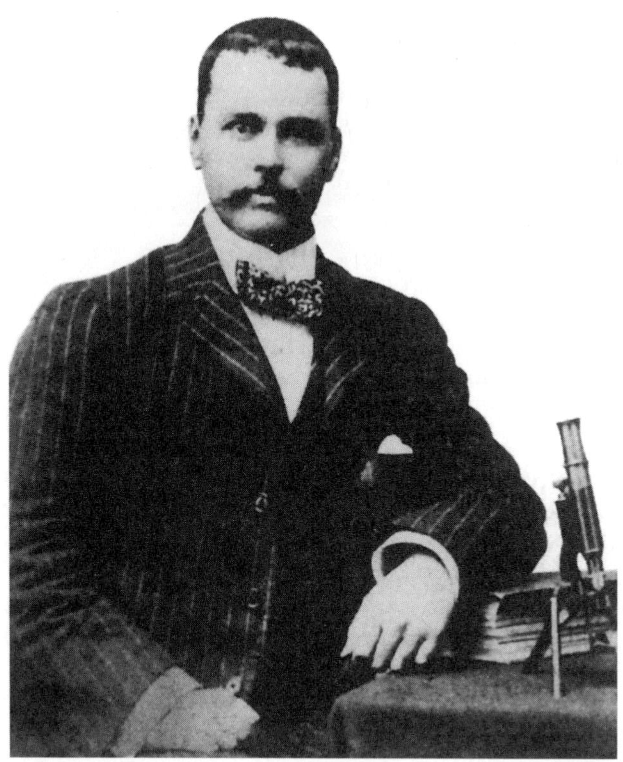

17. Sir Ronald Ross photographed with his diagnostic microscope in Darjeeling, May 1898.

Other medically informed authors were no less outspoken. Writing in the *Journal of Tropical Medicine* under the editorship of James Cantlie (of leprosy fame) a correspondent discussed the recent death of Dr Stewart in Sierra Leone. Noting that white men in the immediate vicinity of Cape Coast Castle were unlikely to attract cannibals' attention, he stated that "few who know the country would care to deny that [just a bit inland] cannibalistic tastes are still prevalent." Warming to his theme, Cantlie's contributor warned that:

> So inbred indeed, is this savagery, that even after generations of nominal Christianity [amongst black slaves] in the West Indies, the rising in Jamaica [in 1865] . . . was marked by such incidents as the scooping out of the brains of their European victims. . . . Surely such an incident shows *inter alia* that . . . it is essential that the negro should be ruled benevolently but despotically by the European. . . . [It] is quite possible that the very

> men who "chopped" poor Dr. Stewart may give trouble to his immediate successors in . . . an obstructive village sanitary committee.[167]

Writing in the *Journal of the African Society* in 1911, Rubert Boyce, founder of the Yellow Fever Bureau of the Liverpool School of Tropical Medicine, had this to say about Africans:

> From the earliest times [West Africa] was fixed upon as the spot where lowly organized human beings were developed, to become the slaves of the white man in every part of the world. . . . [The European traders who came in] found themselves face to face with . . . a veritable pack of children . . . a simple minded race. . . . In Africa there is little religious tradition, little art and little business capacity, as we understand it in Europe.[168]

Among the medico-political happenings which had helped ripen Social Darwinism in the UK was France's near conquest of the disease environment of Algeria. In 1830, 75,000 malaria-susceptible French troops and auxiliaries had marched in, usurped control of a wide strip of coastal land from resident Berbers and begun work on malaria control. The troops initially suffered heavily—a French general claimed in 1840 that the only part of occupied Algeria that was growing was the cemeteries—but in time malaria was brought under control. Long before Laveran located the *plasmodia* causal agent (1880), antique miasmic theory was used to justify large-scale swamp drainage near centers of population. After soldiers came down with malaria, they were treated with quinine; French doctors apparently ignored its prophylactic properties. By 1860, rigorous application of these *ancien régime* medical techniques had succeeded in bringing malaria mortality down from sixty-three white dead per thousand (in 1840–49) to less than one per thousand.

Heartened by this success, more and more *colons* from metropolitan France flooded in. By 1900, the usurpers, now numbering half a million, had confiscated great blocks of land from the 5 million Berbers and developed a hugely profitable export trade in citrus fruits, wines, cork and minerals. Accompanying this modernization, French developers pushed Muslim populations further and further south towards the edges of the Sahara, effectively marginalizing them in their own land.[169]

The collapse of Algeria's disease shield against invading white settlers did not pass unnoticed on the other coasts of the Sahara. Alarm bells seem first to have rung among the creoles of Freetown, Sierra Leone. Themselves descendants of repatriated slaves or half-castes and thus lacking kinship ties with people inland, Freetown creoles in overseas trade shared access to warehousing and distributing facilities with English traders; most of the latter were too uncouth to be accepted as business partners back home. Commenting after 1890 on the break-up of Algeria's "climatic estate", in the pages of the *Sierra Leone Weekly News* and the *Sierra Leone Times*, editors and correspondents with composite Portuguese-African names like Abdul Mortales showed their distaste for, and fear of, white settlers.[170]

Elsewhere in West Africa, thoughtful Africans could not forget that in the 200 years before the Trade wound down their ancestors had been unable to prevent millions of their fellows from being enslaved and carried off to die in the white man's New World.[171] Aware that they themselves lacked the military capacity to confine whites to enclaves along the coast or to ships at sea, western-educated West Africans tried to head off invasion by appealing to the sentiments of long-dead white abolitionists. Typical in its soft-spoken approach was an article in the *Lagos Times* in July 1882 advising readers that:

> We [Africans] respect and reverence the country of Wilberforce and Buxton and of most of our Missionaries, but we are not Englishmen. We are Africans and have no wish to be other than African.[172]

In 1867, in Abeokuta, a Yoruba community north of the British protectorate of Lagos, traditional religionists and former Christians had already attempted to head off the seizure of their ancestral lands by forcing the missionaries to move on; many of these proselytizers had come from Jamaica following the great revolt of 1865.[173] After showing these people the door, Abeokuta scholars then reduced the Yoruba language to European orthography and set up a vernacular press highly critical of European expansion. By such activities Abeokuta elders and scholars demonstrated that they, and by inference West Africa as a whole, were capable of moving smartly towards modernity on their own, and that they did not require physical occupation by a European power.

Yet in the event, the option of modernization without colonization was a non-starter. This can be attributed to a number of factors in UK decision-makers' psyche. Lying in the background was their nagging fear that their north country industries (such as cotton) were becoming obsolete in the race for markets. Even imperfect knowledge showed that the Americans (with their mills in New England and their cotton fields in the Old South), and the Germans (specialists in chemicals, electrical engineering and metallurgy) were pulling ahead. Also sharpening Britons' perceptions of decline was the slow-down occasioned by the collapse of Austrian finance banks in 1873. Twenty years into the Depression, it began to dawn on people of substance that to survive in an uncertain world, the UK must immediately secure whatever markets and raw materials it could. Waiting ready to gobble up whatever African territories remained unclaimed were the French. Though around 1890 French sub-Saharan colonies were relatively small, it was obvious they could rapidly expand, using African auxiliary soldiers recruited in the colonies the French already owned.

Yet viewing the continent as a whole circa 1895, London's gentlemanly capitalists remained of two minds about West Africa. They could not deny that since 1882 (when it was conquered) Egypt had paid them handsome returns; through this conquest they acquired indirect control over the huge unbounded land to the south known as Sudan. They were also receiving fine returns from South Africa, especially since 1867 and the discovery of diamond mines at Kimberley. In addition London financial interests were able to rake in nice profits from Angola, further north, thanks to their dominant influence in Lisbon.[174] Yet for statesmen far more concerned with dividend returns on investment than with profits from mercantile trade, several negative factors weighed against intervention in West Africa.

Of these, the most important was that since the mid-1880s West Africa's "legitimate trade" had been perceptibly dropping off. This trade was in raw materials—cotton, palm oil, ground nut oil and the like—used in north country industries.[175] However, influential northern industrialists like Alfred Jones were convinced that once proper plantations were established and managed by resident Europeans, West African cotton had the *potential* to become far more abundant than it was at present. Jones's great dream was to free Britain from its heavy dependence on American supplies (which of course had been cut off entirely during the Civil War of 1861–65), and to replace these with Nigerian cotton.[176]

Also promising better returns than those currently enjoyed were the gold mines in what is now Ghana. With the recognition that the edifice of British finance rested squarely on gold, as early as 1877 mechanization had been introduced into the mines and great numbers of African workers brought in. Given that the French were close by, to some it seemed vital to establish a massive British presence just to the east, in the Nigerian regions.[177]

So it was that pessimism about the present joined with optimism about the future encouraged (middling-status) chambers of commerce in Liverpool, Manchester, Birmingham and other northern and midland towns to put pressure on (high-status) men in government to assume direct control of the huge, still unclaimed territories of West Africa. To deal with the region's long-established reputation as the "white man's grave" and the old bogey of malaria, a well-connected northern woman—Mary Kingsley—travelled there herself. In her popular books *West African Studies* and *West African Travels*, directed towards ordinary, enfranchised, middle-class readers, Kingsley held that "malaria [was] not a thing to discourage England from holding West Africa, [though] it is a thing which calls for greater forethought in the administration of it than she need give to a healthier region."[178]

The key figure pulling together the threads of colonial expansion was Joseph Chamberlain, one-time reforming mayor of Birmingham. Chamberlain kissed hands as Colonial Secretary in 1895. Intending to cultivate what he prematurely and presumptuously called Britain's "under-developed estates," Chamberlain put the burden of actual conquest on the shoulders of unscrupulous warrior-traders such as George Goldie, agent of the Royal

Niger Company.[179] Anticipating a spot of trouble, Chamberlain had warned: "you can not destroy the practices of barbarism, of slavery, of superstition which for centuries have desolated the interior of Africa without the use of force. . . . you cannot have omelettes without breaking eggs."[180]

Setting the tone for much that followed was the expedition Goldie led out of Lokoja just after New Year's Day 1897. Taking the Colonial Secretary at his word, Goldie and his African auxiliary troops blasted their way through the territory of the northern Yoruba peoples with repeater rifles, cannon and maxim guns and swept to easy victory over the northern emirates of Ilorin and its Nupe neighbor at Bida. To the south-east, maxim guns ensured British conquest of Benin city, burnt to the ground after its fifteenth-century bronzes were stolen by British hands. Further north, in Hausaland in 1903, the English eccentric, Frederick Lugard, defeated the armies of the largest and most efficient Muslim state south of the Sahara, Sokoto. Lugard followed this up by stalking down and murdering the Sokoto Sultan. Regarded by its victims as standard behavior to be expected of Europeans (collectively known as Franks), this outrage forced 25,000 of the Sultan's followers to retreat to the Blue Nile lands of Sudan recently watered by the blood of the Mahdi's followers (defeated by General Kitchener in 1898). To the north of Lugard's new domains—termed the Protectorate of Northern Nigeria—the French in turn brought under their "hot burning rule" all that was left of non-European-controlled West Africa.[181] The only exception was Liberia. Founded as a refuge for returned slaves before the American Civil War, it was a satellite of America.

Once in occupation of the bulk of West Africa, it remained for the new British masters to deal with the disease environment of "the white man's grave" so that they could begin to export primary materials at a profit to manufacturing bases back home. To this end, Colonial Secretary Chamberlain worked through wealthy intermediaries such as cotton and shipping magnate Sir Alfred Jones to encourage the foundation of Britain's first school of tropical medicine (at Liverpool in 1899). A short time later Chamberlain was able to have his favorite medical person, Sir Patrick Manson, appointed head of the new London School of Tropical Medicine.[182]

The first of the new breed of tropical medical experts actually to visit West Africa was Ronald Ross. In 1899 he spent three fateful weeks in Sierra Leone and then returned to Liverpool. From there, together with Manson in London, he helped persuade the Colonial Office to send out a better-funded expedition. Resulting from this was the Royal Society West African expedition headed by Liverpool experts J. W. Stephens and S. R. Christophers; they were in West Africa on and off between 1900 and 1903. Another Liverpool expedition sent out specifically to study malaria in Nigeria was headed by three Canadian degree holders: H. Annett, J. Dutton and J. Elliott.[183]

Emerging from the reports these people made, and endorsed by Chamberlain's Colonial Office as the standard course to be followed wherever whites were found, was the policy of residential segregation. Adopting bogus science—which overlooked the fact that *anyone* of any age or skin pigmentation may be malarial infective—the founders of this policy agreed that:

> The anopheles which infect Europeans do not derive their infection from other Europeans, but from natives, i.e., from the native children who almost without exception suffer from continuous malaria.[184]

To escape from the presence of African children—and their swarming mosquito companions—the whites held it essential that all European residences be built a half-mile or so away from the nearest African habitation; this, it was posited, would be well beyond the flight range of a malarial mosquito. And to justify the use of tropical medicine as "an instrument of empire" largely to attend to the health needs of whites, these experts purposely refuted Robert Koch.

Just after Koch had found the inhabitants of East Africa generally "obedient and intelligent" and willing to take malarial prophylactics to deprive the virus of its human hosts (1901), Liverpool experts Annett, Dutton and Elliott scathingly claimed that:

> The native of Old Calabar—the seat of government in southern Nigeria—is stupid, unintelligent, and indifferent. . . . The natives of other parts of the delta and of the Niger banks are mostly uncivilized, and often run away at the sight of a European: while there are towns in the interior only occasionally visited by "white men," or which are absolutely unopened. It is true that the native chiefs are often intelligent and educated men, but these are exceedingly few . . . it can be safely stated that throughout the whole of Nigeria, we never met with a community which could in any way be classed as "obedient and intelligent."[185]

Segregation was accepted by the leading lights of the Liverpool and the London schools as (in Manson's words) "the first law of hygiene," yet the extent to which it was enforced depended on the personal prejudices of the local colonial administrator. In Lagos, governor William MacGregor (1899–1904), a medical man, regarded segregation as socially divisive and in total contradiction to the official reason for the British presence in West Africa, namely as humanitarian mentors for their African brothers. MacGregor's own approach was preventive. He stressed the importance of screening windows and doors (even though this blocked the free flow of fresh air) and undertook the drainage of the great Kimberley swamp lying near Lagos. Statistics from 1906 claim that thanks to MacGregor's work, malarial deaths among "those who are bearing 'the white man's burden'" in that coastal town dropped from forty per thousand in 1897 to virtually nil nine years later.[186]

Unlike the situation in Lagos, in the Northern Protectorate while Lord

Lugard was around (he was high commissioner 1900–6 and governor of united Nigeria, 1912–19), residential segregation was rigorously applied.[187] In addition to insisting on the half-mile barrier between white and black housing, Lugard was particularly keen to enforce the Christophers-Stephens admonition that white men should never sleep anywhere near Africans. For this there were two reasons: one was the "scientific" assumption that malarial mosquitoes bit only at night. The other was the *sub rosa* assumption that venereal syphilis was prevalent in the Muslim North and that the sexual activities through which it was transmitted similarly took place only at night. Lugard mentioned the VD problem as early as 1900, though the full extent of the hysteria was not spelled out until 1910. In that year, an official northern medical report advised that:

> Mosquito-borne, fly-borne and tick-borne diseases, water-borne diseases and leprosy need to have constant war waged against them; as is the case throughout West Africa. But, in the Mahommedan part of Northern Nigeria—by far the most important area of the country—I can say, without the slightest fear of contradiction, that venereal diseases work more havoc than do all the diseases, mentioned above, put together.[188]

Here where censorious European eyes saw syphilis (most of which was probably non-sexually transmitted yaws) lurking on the genitals of nearly the whole of the indigenous population, the Royal Society/Colonial Office directive requiring residential segregation (ostensibly to control malaria) was obviously welcome.[189]

Speaking in the name of Sir Rubert Boyce, founder of the Liverpool Yellow Fever Bureau, a medical man claimed in 1911 that "sanitary reforms may cause *momentary inconvenience*, but will soon greatly facilitate the progress of the colonies." The first phrase was the understatement of the century.[190] It overlooked the fact that segregation as "sanitary reform" reaped a whirlwind of resentment among African ministers of religion, African wholesale merchants and English-educated African medical doctors (prohibited from further employment in the West African Medical Service in 1909); its only positive success was to bring short-term gain to a small number of British firms. Thus in Sierra Leone, the 1903 decision to build a "hill town" for Europeans led to the importation from England of twenty-three pre-fabricated bungalows designed to be erected on stilts which rose from cement bases covering the surrounding (miasma-prone) soil. All the cement, building frames and other materials were specially imported.[191]

In 1911 Liverpool expert Sir Rubert Boyce undertook a three-month tour of the Gold Coast, southern Nigeria and Sierra Leone at the request of the Colonial Office. It is not quite certain why he was sent, given that he was an authority on a disease which UK businessmen preferred not to know existed.[192] While there, the coin dropped and Boyce suddenly confronted the *moral* illness he termed "notification fear."

At a time when West African gold mines were just beginning to produce significant yields, authorities were afraid to admit to a yellow fever presence that would force operations to close down. It was learned that when an unwary medical doctor named Baker had reported in 1901 that seven out of eight of his suspect patients had died of yellow fever, his superiors peremptorily warned him that: "if you have any more cases of *bilious remittent* to report, please do so."[193] In 1901, the year of Baker's humiliation, gold production had been worth £22,000. In 1903, when despite on-site yellow fever—the mines were kept in operation, production was worth £254,000. In 1907 production was valued at more than £1 million. Yields like this obviously justified the yellow fever deaths of hundreds of black miners and white denials that anything was amiss.[194]

This was the situation that Sir Rubert confronted in West Africa. On his return to London, he dropped a bombshell by telling an audience that included Sir Patrick Manson (founder of the London School) about "notification fear" and the way in which modern young doctors who recognized cases of yellow fever were put down by higher authority.[195] Responding to this, Manson turned nasty. With measured sarcasm he pointed out that:

> Sometimes medical men brought forward an erroneous though plausible idea which misled the official on the spot into acts for which he would be held responsible, and which might cost the country much before the error was detected. . . . he would like to see a little caution observed before adopting and acting on purely hypothetical views. . . .[196]

Perhaps it was on orders from London and its Tropical Medicine School that Gold Coast mining authorities suddenly enforced the housing segregation order earlier issued by the Colonial Office. At short notice, large numbers of African families were turned out in the rain and their houses demolished. Two years later, in 1913, Governor Hugh Clifford expressed his "concern" over the Colony's "overpublicised" and, so he claimed, unjustified reputation as an unhealthy place.[197]

One of Rubert Boyce's most pregnant insights (not necessarily accurate in detail) was that the spread of yellow fever by mosquito carrier/hosts was intimately connected with Development. As he rather awkwardly put it:

> It is not a swamp, gutter or puddle breeder (as a rule); it is essentially the mosquito which breeds in *all receptacles* which happen to contain clean water in no matter what quantity. . . . Hence it comes to be the mosquito of all discarded tins, bottles, &c., &c. Hence it is most abundant where there are traders, and is least abundant in the interior, where there is less trade. . . . Increased trade and commercial activity provide an increase of odd water-containers of all kinds, and therefore, an increase of the Stegomyia, and therefore a greater liability to yellow fever.[198]

Writing about malaria, a League of Nations commission noted in 1927 that: "Nothing is more favourable to a high incidence and severity of malaria than frequent movements of a population hither and thither."[199] Expressing a similar sentiment in Northern Nigeria thirteen years earlier, British medical authorities recognized that: "The ending of slave-raiding and internecine wars [courtesy of the Pax Britannica] has rendered intercommunication safe and has encouraged the spread of communicable disease."[200]

A pioneering insight into what the colonial intrusion meant was provided by a French government agent named Emile Baillaud.[201] Writing in 1905, Baillaud was already aware that European conquests and the panic-stricken flight of refugees had brought thousands of Africans into alien environments. He also seems to have understood some of the disease implications of new, on-site Development.

Of these, the most important was monetarization. This forced local people to use a metal currency transferable into European coin rather than the cowrie shells or other negotiables they had traded with in the past. Compulsory use of convertible currency was of course part of a colonialists' ploy to force local people to pay taxes. In order to earn the cash needed to pay off whatever they were assessed, they had to submit to the discipline of wage labor on newly established plantations given over to crops—such as cotton or groundnuts—grown for sale overseas.

Put into effect, monetarization worked a social revolution which transformed West Africa even more thoroughly than Atlantic slave-raiding had done: unlike the occasional raid, it affected everyone every year. Knowing that they would be severely beaten, even killed, by African collaborators if they did not pay taxes on demand, tens of thousands of Africans left their natal villages in the interior to search for work in regions where white-managed enterprise provided wage labor employment. In poor soil inland French colonial regions such as Bukina Faso and Mali, young people—driven by the need for solid coin—travelled hundreds of kilometers to work in Senegal or the Gambia.

After 1919, finding that inland villagers responding to the threat of tax collectors did not move quickly enough, French civilizers resorted to corvée labor. Complementing this, the population-scarce motherland (smarting from near defeat by Germany in the recent war) required all African males of nineteen or twenty years of age to serve in the military. This demand engendered much population movement as soon-to-be drafted young men in French-ruled lands fled in their thousands to British colonies on the coasts.[202]

Writing of "progressive" developments which caused mass movement of population in 1905, Baillaud reported that:

> At this moment in West Africa, the necessary hands . . . are easy to be had; and also at the coast the towns overflow with men going about looking for work. The captives having listened to our advice, and finding the way to

> freedom without dying from hunger, have come in numbers towards our enterprises, wherever it was possible to find work with the Europeans. They not only leave their masters, but also their countries.[203]

In retrospect, the consequences of medically unsupervised mass migration are clear. With immune systems unprepared for the local varieties of malaria they encountered (each variant type requiring its own immunity built up over time), voluntary and involuntary migrants died in their tens of thousands. No less tragic, the networks of mortality extended far inland from the coasts. Infected with a disease transmitted by a mosquito carrier just before they left coastal plantations at the end of the season and began their trek home into the interior, returning workers carried disease parasites in their blood. Wherever they stopped, they offered tempting targets to mosquitoes in search of blood meals. The same situation obtained when they finally arrived in their home village. Thus in places hundreds of kilometers inland, in which no woman or child could possibly have built up immunities to coastal malaria forms, victims were killed by a disease which to them was entirely new.[204]

Supportive of the thesis that traditional health provisioners were unable to cope with strange, unaccustomed malaria forms brought up from the south was the situation in the Northern Protectorate of Nigeria. Here in 1904, of the 13,356 "natives" admitted to colonial health clinics, 925 came in for treatment for malaria. In the next year when development processes in the South were far more extensive and labor-draining of the North, the European officer gave up even reporting the number of malaria cases attending.[205] Given that in Europe at the time, normal population increase over a twenty-five-year period might be well in excess of 5–6 percent, the situation in the Northern Protectorate was rather alarming. As a recording officer confessed: "I suppose there is a consensus of opinion that the population in 1926 did not differ essentially [in size] from that in 1900."[206]

Also working to convert what had been a localistic health problem into territorial-wide crises, was the bringing together on a single work-site or plantation of large numbers of African semi-wage, semi-slave laborers from diverse disease backgrounds. Throughout the southern and middle belts of what is now Nigeria, colonial authority permitted entrepreneurs like Sir Alfred Jones to set up large plantations for the production of cotton, cocoa, groundnuts and other goods marketable in Europe. But as the French agent Baillaud had already pointed out, people who were forced to work full time on an export crop had no daytime hours left to grow foodstuffs for their own subsistence needs. Supplying these needs—in ways which Europeans regarded as free enterprise and normal—were food crop producers drawn from a broad hinterland. Working their way back and forth through two or three disease environments (rather than through an old-style relay system in which goods, not people, travelled), these suppliers' movements contributed to the further spread of illness.

Linking export-oriented plantations hacked out of forests with port facilities on the coast were the railways which men like Chamberlain, Lugard and Clifford saw as harbingers of real Progress. Typically in 1906–7, the building of lines of track between Lagos and Ilorin 400 kilometers to the north brought together several hundred susceptibles in a moving front of epidemic disease.[207] This sort of malarial crisis would not be a once-only affair; because of the nature of the terrain, a permanent new disease environment would be established.

As Baillaud pointed out, the soils of West Africa were entirely unlike those of most of Europe, eastern North America, the flood-plain of Egypt or South-East Asia. Rather than consisting of a deep layer of topsoil, they were made up instead of a thin cover of humus over rock-hard laterite. In giant forest clearings created for plantation groundnuts or cotton, this thin soil lay exposed and open in a way it had never done under the mix-cropping regimes normally used by Africans.

Similarly, cutting down hundreds of trees for railway ties for every mile of trackage laid, left poorly rooted trees nearby open to buffeting by winds which soon toppled them over. These collapses greatly increased the area of thin soil exposed. Blasted during the dry season by the rays of the sun and by torrential downpours during the rains, these laterite-based soils were soon leached out, forming water-filled cracks and potholes which female mosquitoes intent on laying eggs found irresistible.[208] Decades after the initial destruction of forest cover had first permitted the crevasses to form, insects were still hatching more soon-to-be-vectors intent on blood meals drawn from indigenous peoples or the rare white who happened by.

On the pretext that Africans were the world's prime carriers of lethal disease (as in the 1900 segregation decrees), western administrators systematically destroyed indigenous traders' western-style businesses, and brought in Lebanese, Syrians and other Middle Easterners to replace them. Also convinced that Africans had a permanent mental age of ten, British colonial authority balked at establishing any industrial plant that would provide them with useful technological or scientific skills. Working towards an even more devastating long-term impact, Christian missions persuaded Africans that everything in their historical cultures was worthless and that everything on offer by enlightened Europeans was good, including the concept of the Nation State.[209]

Then in the late 1920s, after Europe had torn itself apart in nationalistic global war, a new truth finally emerged. This was recognition that every year great numbers of colonialists were either dying or being invalided home, many of them victims of malaria, and that this situation was likely to be permanent. Added to the role played by West African diseases were mindsets among the Europeans themselves. A medical officer reported:

> There appears to be a growing tendency among some European residents to underrate the value of quinine as a prophylactic against malaria. They

> become imbued with the idea that certain ailments, such as loss of memory, neuritis, dyspepsia, black-water fever, [and general ill health] are caused by its use. This idea is, to a certain extent, *fostered by some medical men in England. . . .*[210]

Thus by the year 1928, when the Cairo conference on Tropical Medicine convened with Cuba's W. H. Hoffmann in attendance, even obtuse white men looking for a comfy place to live had come to accept that, relative to the rapidly improving disease environment in European homelands and the USA, West Africa was positively unhealthy. So it was that Hoffmann was able to declare that "in West Africa, the excessive mortality, due to epidemics, is keeping away all foreign immigration, *making impossible any colonization*."[211] This settler-free situation stood in marked contrast to the settler-dominated worlds of Algeria, the Kenyan highlands, the Rhodesias and South Africa.[212]

In 1960, at the time of independence, the number of whites permanently settled in Nigeria was minuscule—fewer than one per thousand. In the half-century since then, whatever its manifold problems, the Nigerian region has *at least* not had to confront the mass displacement of its own peoples by hordes of immigrant aliens. Yet, as is well known, in recent years it has come under the sway of forms of Development imposed by giant multinationals. Cutting their coats according to the cloth, these faceless corporations use West Africans as their resident agents and exploitation-site police.

Linking late twentieth-century Development and the development forms which anticipated it eighty or ninety years earlier are two categories of tiny creatures which follow Darwin's laws of evolution. One consists of the diverse forms of malaria *plasmodia* which have become immune to modern prophylactics. The other creatures are the mosquito hosts which, immunized as well, survive sophisticated chemical sprays. As prime actors in what is now a pan-West African disease environment, they are the living legacy of the early colonial Development schemes which first brought this terrible phenomenon into being.

Writing in 1905, Baillaud asked: "Has the importance of [Development] . . . been sufficiently considered? I am afraid that it has remained unnoticed. I am obliged to say that, for myself, I am entirely unable to have an opinion of the consequences thereof."[213] Writing on the eve of the centennial of the 1897 conquest, the present author cannot but share this sentiment.

7 Afterword: To the Epidemiologic Transition?

The last half-century has seen the triumphal emergence of medicine as a fully scientific discipline of proven effectiveness in curing and preventing life-threatening diseases. Yet it has *also* seen the emergence of a widening gap in the provisioning (and non-provisioning) of effective health services for the privileged few and the underprivileged many. In his analysis of 1995, the Director-General of the World Health Organization attributed the "health catastrophe" that is staring the majority of the world's peoples in the face to "extreme poverty." To this can be added four other evils: overpopulation, consumerism/development, nationalism and ignorance.[1] Let me examine some meanings.

Ignorance falls into two categories: indigenous and foreign. The indigenous sort can be exemplified by the continuing strength of the medieval/nineteenth-century high imperial leprosy Construct. Here, the stigma still attached to the physical condition (Hansen's disease) discourages sufferers from reporting into clinics in time to prevent permanent loss of nerves, fingers, toes and nose. For a variety of reasons, Construct leprosy remains widely supported by foreigners.[2] So too does the Construct which holds that Africans are not very prone to yellow fever. At a time when white racism in the US and UK continues strong, it is perhaps unrealistic to expect that educated people staffing the media and university departments of history will relegate this mischievous Construct to the museum of obsolete ideas.[3]

In sorting through the complexities of the current world health situation, a useful starter is provided by Abdel Omran, the Cairene epidemiologist who coined the term "the epidemiologic transition." Omran contrasted the old-style "Age of Pestilence and Famine" with the "Age of Degenerative and Man-Made Disease" in which annual mortality was well below twenty per thousand.[4] Following on from this, between 1960 and 1994 in the world's economically advanced North life expectancy at birth rose from the mid-sixties to the mid- to late seventies. Elsewhere, in all but the world's thirty poorest countries (mostly in sub-Saharan Africa), average life expectancy rose from around forty-six to around sixty-three.[5]

Among medical professionals, honors have tilted back and forth between those who say that *medical expertise* can claim full marks for increasing human longevity, and vehement dissenters like Thomas McKeown who (writing of England) claimed that improvements in standards of living were the real cause of improved life-chances.[6] There is something to be said for both sides as well as for the "sanitarian" position that lies somewhere in between.[7] No one can doubt that the WHO campaign which eradicated smallpox from the face of the earth in 1977 was a victory for medicine and for humankind. Nevertheless in the viral world out there, niches emptied are soon refilled. Today, in a South freed from smallpox as leading cause of childhood deaths, malaria, diarrheal diseases and acute respiratory infections have stepped in to fill the gap as chief child killers.[8]

Yet despite massive mortalities, global population has been increasing at a horrendous rate.[9] In 1750 planet earth hosted roughly 720 million people. By 1900 (when Omran's epidemiologic transition was beginning to take off in the North) population stood at 1,600 million; by 1950 it had risen to 2,500 million. Doubling in only thirty-six years, by 1986 human numbers had increased to 5,000 million. According to WHO figures, in 1995 the world population stood at 5,700 million. Some of the impetus for this unprecedented rise was due to smallpox eradication and medical interventions. However, other causal factors must be considered as well.

Through painstaking reconstruction of the demographic histories of localized societies, scholars have begun to reveal the rich diversity of human reproductive strategies in times past. Depending on each local group's perceptions of man/land ratios, the extended family's commitment to long-term survival, women's rights to control their own bodies, and other variables, homeostatic controls were brought to bear that prevented the creation of inappropriate offspring. Among these controls were late marriage, enforced celibacy, abortifacients, abortion and infanticide.[10] Michael Walzer's category of "moral types" (1994) permits one to argue that these techniques were an essential and *morally acceptable* element in a localistic "thick culture."[11]

Inasmuch as it concerns the South and changing parental perceptions of what is appropriate, the current crisis of overpopulation is linked with the collapse of localism and the emergence of statism. Both phenomena were triggered by European colonialism, rather than arising from the "animal-like proclivities" of indigenous peoples themselves, as some western Development experts I have talked to claim. Moving from the well-known to the less familiar, we can begin with the observation that within the European homelands whence colonialism came, the mission of the eighteenth-century Enlightenment was to bring under *secular* control intellectualizing activities earlier monopolized by the "universal" church. Whatever its failings, this universal church had at least recognized that its own values did not hold in the neighboring world of Islam. Emerging from this switch from regional "universalism" to global universalism in time for application in British India, then in imperialized Africa and the island Pacific, was the conviction that *all* humankind was part of a continuum stretching from the most backward to the most perfect sort. These ideas held that Europe alone represented Civilization; every other cultural grouping was a primitive form which might never actually achieve a fully civilized condition. Accompanying this exemplary bigotry went the flawed notion that there was a single "human nature," which in its finest, and of course European, form depended on untrammelled human reason to overcome the barriers of superstition and custom.

In bringing these ideas to bear on the imperialized world pre- and post-1960, it important to realize that *there never really was a colonial divide* between colonizers (a category which included people like Lord Cromer's white-skinned menials and messengers as well as Cromer himself), and the peoples who were colonized. Instead, within a generation of conquest, local collaborators had emerged who saw their family's way forward was through learning and imitating European ways. Already fuelled by Enlightenment "truths," change was much furthered in the late nineteenth century by the reinvention of the concept of the State. Following what they took to be the "logic of history" identified by H. W. F. Hegel, imperialists in Africa consolidated the once-discrete territories of hundreds of different ethnic groups and created large colonies or proto-states. Serving as the nerve center of a proto-state like "Nigeria" was a small, highly authoritarian European bureaucracy serviced by locally recruited lower-level clerks.

Within the early colonial context (that of India preceding that of Africa by more than a century), indigenous ruling elites arose. Very often conversant with what the Colonial Masters termed "traditional" culture (unchanged since time immemorial), emerging elites set up secret societies and parties dedicated to opposing colonialism. Yet such was the taint of exposure to the West that these nationalists generally saw to it that their own sons were educated in western-style schools. Studies there would be followed by a few years' stay at a university in Europe. Both agencies inculcated these sons with an inner compulsion to out-European the Europeans.

Yet there is more to the tragedy than this. In areas of human activity involving morals and manners there was usually a considerable time lag between what intellectuals in Europe were thinking, and the composite thoughts that formed in the minds of colonized educated sons. This lag often meant that in taking over control of the State (at the time of Independence) these sons accepted as their behavioral guide the standards the Colonial Masters had exhibited in the 1920s and 1930s when they were at their most unreflexive and most arrogant.[12]

Nationalists' acceptance of the ideology of the colonial state (and its single ruling elite who brooked no opposition) had direct links with the collapse of homeostatic controls on population growth after independence. In the first instance, there was a hemorrhage of leadership away from local communities (with their parochial concerns) towards the capital city with its lush new fields of patronage. Having voted with their feet, most members of the new elite came to despise the rural bumpkins they had left behind. Reciprocating these ill-feelings, most local people became convinced that the central government was a giant swindle and that they must look to themselves for long-term family survival.

Adjusting their ideas about family to the new realities, rural peoples judged that personal security in old age could only be assured if they had two or more surviving sons to keep them in food and shelter. Using their perceptions of the risks of death in childhood and young adulthood, parents quite sensibly produced more babies than their *own* ancestors would have thought appropriate only three or four generations back. From this proliferating number of humankind, 12.2 million children under the age of five living in the world's South died in the single year 1993.[13]

Many interrelated factors have been credited with insuring that timely intervention has not been available to these dying children. Unfortunately, among these are the ideals which career-conscious medical doctors in the South insisted were those of Robert Koch. Coming out of this discipleship (doubtless alien to Koch himself) was a line of thought which held that *proper* medical doctors should be specialists in scientific exotica such as bone marrow transplants or heart surgery. Accepting this as their norm, many medically trained men practiced in a capital city hospital with state-of-the-art operating theaters and laboratories. Not far from the hospital was the Club. Just down the road was the airport with weekly services to the great cities of Europe and North America. Meanwhile in rural areas, modern medical facilities remained few and far between.[14]

In Latin America, very similar situations came to exist. Here the historic pace-setters were Major Gorgas and Theodore Roosevelt, the turn-of-the-century larger-than-life heroes who cleared Havana and the Panama Canal Zone of the yellow fever and malaria which threatened North American interests. Then, in the wake of World War I from which the nation states of Western Europe had to be rescued by their American cousins, the Rockefeller Foundation (USA) went into the funding and direction of health campaigns overseas. Based on the licitly garnered wealth of the Standard Oil Company, the Foundation had already undertaken a massive hookworm abolition campaign in the southern states of the American union with the stated aim of upgrading worker efficiency.[15]

Armando Solórzano's study, "Sowing the Seeds of Neo-Imperialism: The Rockefeller Foundation's Yellow Fever Campaign in Mexico," and Marcos Cueto's "'Sanitation from Above': Yellow Fever and Foreign Intervention in Peru, 1919–1922" investigate the role of Koch-inspired American doctors in clearing large tracts of Latin America of disease while at the same time furthering the centralization of medicine.[16] Solórzano reported that:

> The solutions offered by the Rockefeller Foundation were based on a "scientific medicine" that neglected the social and economic origins of the diseases. The Mexican people started looking toward vaccinations, labo-

ratories, and institutional medicine as the solutions to their deteriorated health conditions.[17]

Writing in 1966 from a knowledge base of Kenyan rural health needs, Maurice King of Britain devised what he called a "medical primer." Not being sympathetic to the "traditional" practitioners to whom most Kenyans turned, King accepted the desirability of western-style "medicalization." Starting from this orthodox position, he went on however to make the revolutionary suggestion that the way forward was to forget high-science career ideals and to establish instead a *modus vivendi* between locally based medical doctors (expat or African) and semi-skilled, western-trained auxiliaries.

Maurice King stressed that: "Medical care in developing countries differs sharply from medical care in industrial ones" and that "the main determinate [of disease] is poverty rather than a warm climate." He also insisted that "the medical care of the common man is immensely worthwhile" and that "medicine is still a major vehicle of compassion, of charity in its true sense."[18] With its admirable mix of old-fashioned moralism and post-Independence optimism, King's was a voice crying in the wilderness. Had it not been for events in China, globe-straddling Development agents would have ignored it entirely.

Containing within its 1949 borders nearly a quarter of all humankind, China was controlled by a Communist leadership who were determined that their land should again become the cultural mentor of what mandarin elites had always regarded as *the* civilized world. Within a few years of their coming to power, the Communists redeemed their country's reputation as "the sick man of Asia" by all but abolishing plague, cholera, smallpox and syphilis. These (perceptual) feats were achieved by combining the medical wisdom of the common people with what the leadership considered was best in low-tech western medicine. Massive campaigns to provide communes with supplies of clean water, sewerage and sanitation were combined with propaganda teaching rural people about elementary personal hygiene. All this seemed to be to good effect. By the late 1950s enthusiastic China-watchers were telling the West of the marvelously effective work being carried out by "bare-footed doctors."[19]

Though much of what actually transpired in the new-made Celestial Kingdom remained opaque, doubtless some things *were* achieved. Starting with a population in 1949 in which average life expectancy at birth was perhaps thirty-five years, by 1957 life expectancy had risen to (a perceptual) fifty-seven, and by 1990 to around seventy. This contrasts favorably with the life expectancy at birth of only 60.3 found today in Dr Abdel Omran's Egypt.

Success in low-tech medicine in China could not pass unnoticed by top people in the West. Terrified that underprivileged peoples everywhere would regard the Asian Communist monster as their guide, western leaders recognized that they *had to be seen* to be outpacing the Chinese as crusaders against disease. In this spirit, in 1965 US President Lyndon Johnson launched a high-tech campaign to abolish malaria, yellow fever and cholera from the face of the earth. US pharmaceutical companies and research labs praised this act of statesmanship.[20] Yet a decade on, huge numbers of Third World peoples were still dying from infectious diseases which Kochian science was, in theory, able to control.

In 1978, meeting in Alma Ata in the then USSR, agents of the World Health Organization agreed that the time had come to turn this situation around. In a sensational declaration, they called for a change of emphasis from high-tech medicine to Primary Health Care (PHC). In 1979 the WHO formally endorsed this policy and called for Health for All by the Year 2000.[21] Since the WHO's high command consisted largely of medical doctors bound to the Kochian paradigm, this represented a considerable volte-face. Some staff may have remained in their heart of hearts less than fully committed to the new ideal.[22] Nevertheless, some individual countries went ahead with the PHC program, and so enabled their peoples to enter the second or third phase of Dr Abdel Omran's Epidemiologic Transition with life expectancies at birth lengthening into the sixties.

At root, primary health care was concerned with the *prevention* of disease; only if funds permitted did it concern itself with actual curing. Frequently cited as example of countries and states with low Gross National Products which gave high priority to PHC were China, Cuba, Costa Rica, Sri Lanka, and Kerala State (India). In the free world perception two of these were social pariahs: Communist China and Communist Cuba (where in 1990 life expectancy was 75.4 and 94 percent of the population were literate). Two other poor but relatively healthy states were in neutral South Asia: Sri Lanka (old Ceylon) and Kerala State. The latter was a curious mixed enclave of Christianity and non-violent Marxism located south of Bombay. Both here and in Sri Lanka local people had long been concerned about their health and had provided a regular clientele to practitioners of Ayurvédic medicine. This tradition had survived the British occupation, and after the 1970s it encouraged rural people to cooperate on easy terms with PHC program workers.[23]

Yet PHC ideas about the roles that should be assigned to inoculation and vaccination remained ambivalent, depending on the country of origin, social strata and ideological commitment of the workers involved. Given real world conditions, most of the materials required were imported from the West. Some PHC workers publicly asked whether any program which made itself dependent on western imports was not a Trojan horse concealing self-seeking agents of Development.

In the USA and Europe, pharmaceutical companies claimed they were willing to carry out what they saw as *necessary, new, high-level research* on vaccines, provided that government regulations allowed them to make a fair profit. Encouraging the companies in their professedly disinterested efforts were the career bureaucrats in the World Health Organization Global Program for Vaccines and Immunization, most of whom were medically trained in the tradition of Koch. Thus motivated, the pharmaceutical companies developed effective vaccines against measles, polio, tetanus and diphtheria which were used globally to wondrous effect. Yet in the case of disease threats which were largely regional (the South) rather than Global, research funding remained sparse. Overall, less than 3 percent of available funding was used for the tropical diseases still threatening the Third World. Queried about this, a former general manager of the Ciba-Geigy pharmaceutical company in Switzerland admitted that research funding was low because most Third World patients were too poor to make the market for the relevant drugs "interesting."[24]

One of the tragedies of the former colonial world was that in most newly independent nation states *military men* either became heads of government or the *de facto* powers behind the thrones of democratically elected puppets. Trained to appreciate the mass destructive potential of expensive western-manufactured weapons while studying at Sandhurst or at Fort Benning, once in power these soldier boys eagerly purchased jet airplanes and submarines, anti-personnel mines, anti-riot gear, and the sophisticated equipment needed to torture prisoners perceived as subversives. For their part, arms manufacturers in the West—headed by the USA ($145 billion annually), Britain ($45 billion), and France ($40 billion)—used the rhetoric of the Cold War (then the threat of regional small-scale bush wars) to justify sales on *credit* to "friendly" Third World states. For them it was all immensely profitable.[25]

Through commissions and slippages it was also immensely profitable for facilitating agents in the recipient nation. However, the situation was rather different for the Treasury/Exchequer of the recipient government. Overburdened with debts incurred through accepting armaments *on credit* (following in the footsteps of sixteenth-century coastal African chiefs confronted with Portuguese traders), Third World countries had to beg the World Bank and the International Monetary Fund for short-term assistance to maintain debt payments to foreign creditors. In Nigeria, in terms of population the single largest nation in black Africa, the national debt in 1990 worked out as 111 percent of the Gross National Product.[26]

With the mid-1980s collapse into world-wide recession, the banking cartels who ran the IMF and World Bank demanded that client states subject their economies to free-market-style structural adjustments before they would be granted more credit to pay off existing debts to foreign creditors. Using Chicago School and Texas economics (which have always been non-holistic and non-humanistic), the IMF and World Bank insisted that any community who used a public service had to pay for it. This meant that such primary health care programs as had managed to pull themselves into existence (following Alma Ata), were left with much-depleted funding.

Typically, in Burkina Faso during the years 1983–90, when population grew by 15 percent, the health budget was cut by 26 percent.[27]

Structural Adjustment Programs (SAPs) also led to curtailment of funding for education. This bore directly on the issue of overpopulation. At the level of theory it has long been suggested that Third World parents would undergo the traumas of pregnancy and birth less often if they could be assured that the babies and young children they already had would survive to maturity. At the Cairo Conference on Population in 1994, reports were made of the huge impact that education for girls could have on the resolution of this problem. It was revealed that girls who had been taught about personal and infant hygiene at the primary level were having fewer and healthier children. It was also shown that education provided young women with the ability to have more power and control over their own lives, an ability which was a necessary precondition for the democratization of the world, a stated western goal.[28]

It might seem that by effectively closing down local schools and PHC facilities, SAPs directly contravened elementary humanitarian and democratic principles. Yet in keeping with the Orwellian *Nineteen Eighty-Four* party slogan, "Ignorance is Strength," western health economists denied that there was any solid epidemiological data which unequivocally demonstrated links between rising mortality rates and the rapid deterioration of quality of life.[29] Given what Christopher Lasch has told us about the betrayal of democracy by multinationalized elites, this is hardly surprising.[30]

Coming from a different direction was another example of what Lasch termed elite betrayal: the American infant formula industry's attempts after 1970 to persuade Third World mothers to feed their infants on their product. Advertising campaigns claiming that (rather than undergoing the animal-like experience of breast-feeding) it was smart and modern to feed baby on formula led to booming sales and corporate shareholder happiness. The American companies defended their free-enterprise stand at a meeting of the World Health Assembly. In the balloting that followed, other than the USA, most nations voted firmly for measures against infant formula. By so doing they risked losing USA funding for WHO. Hoardings advertising formula milk are still commonly found on Cairene streets.[31]

Also challenging what was once the western moral value "thou shall not kill" is the continuing, highly successful American and British corporate campaign to peddle tobacco products in the Third World. Proven beyond a shadow of a scientific doubt in the 1970s to be a *direct* cause of lung cancer and a *contributing* cause of serious heart problems, cigarette smoking is portrayed in Third World advertising as smart, modern and a sure way to increase one's sex appeal.[32] In a scholarly book on mortality not generally given over to moral crusades, Alex Mercer has this to say:

> It has been argued that no other industry kills people on the scale that the tobacco industry does, and unlike other industries which are made to curb

> their activities when the health of workers and consumers is threatened, this industry has actually been allowed to increase its efforts to persuade people to consume its products. Historically, financial advantage for a small minority has often been put before human health. . . . Whether or not this amounts to social murder or social manslaughter, any legal issue would involve a consideration of relevant scientific evidence by those without a vested interest.[33]

We began this "Afterword" with a discussion of the epidemiologic transition until recently unfolding in the developing world and virtually completed in the developed world (since 1996, excluding Russian males). One reason why Westerners are impatient with what they take to be the slowness of the transition to stable population in the South may be that they have forgotten that their own forebears also underwent population explosions: England's population of around 50 million in 1991 emerged from a base of only 2 million in 1520. Amnesia also causes them to overlook that on a per capita basis each western person consumes far more of the world's non-renewable energy resources than does the typical denizen of the South.

In 1991 the UK's share of world energy consumption (measured in terms of oil—largely from the Middle East) stood at only 2.5 percent.[34] Somewhat different was the situation in the United States of America. Numbering (in 1990) 263.25 million people, less than 6 percent of world population, the USA consumed what at a conservative estimate was 23.6 percent of world energy production. Yet because private industry and democratically elected heads of state claimed that the average citizen over the age of sixteen had the right to have the use of a car, the USA felt compelled to maintain a foreign policy (in the Middle East, Afghanistan, Mexico) designed to keep this right inviolate. This policy has been wonderfully (tragically) successful. In September 1996, while driving north to visit my Ojibway neighbors, I found the price of gas at Midwestern US pumps ($1.29) remained much the same (in dollar terms) as it was immediately after the Middle Eastern oil crisis of 1973; in actual terms, taking inflation into account, it was much less.

Until the early 1980s, Americans of all classes and creeds (other than Native Americans on Reservations) regarded themselves as the most progressive people in history. Strengthening them in this belief was confidence that their medical doctors (native born or purchased from European centers of excellence) would soon abolish all infectious diseases: it was only a matter of time. Then in 1981 it was reported that a new infectious disease to which specimens of American manhood were not immune was stalking the land. This was the Acquired Immune Deficiency Syndrome (AIDS), later understood to be the penultimate health status of people infected by the Human Immunodeficiency Virus (HIV). In 1992 the WHO estimated that in the decade just past the global dead numbered 1.5 million and that up to 11 million people were HIV positive. But by 1996 the estimated number had increased to 14–15 million, with the warning that by the year 2000 HIV prevalence would probably be around 20 million.[35]

Several aspects of the HIV/AIDs epidemic ensured that it received blanket media coverage. For a start, though hundreds of millions of research dollars were devoted to it, as of this writing science has failed to devise a preventive vaccine or a cure. This has led to accusations that scientists are incompetent braggarts, parading under false colors. Then too it seemed that HIV was heavily concentrated in two closely intertwined parts of the world, Africa and the USA (victim and beneficiary of the earlier compulsory migration of slaves). Though not denying that this epidemic is a serious health threat (especially amongst heterosexual Africans and homosexual Euro-Americans) some people wondered if the World Health Organization had gone a bit over the top by spending (as in 1993) nearly a third of its annual budget on this *single* disease. In that year, as a cause of death of children under the age of five world-wide, HIV-related mortality accounted for only 0.6 percent of the total.[36]

A related disease occurrence, at present not of great concern to the Media, has been the recent development of forms of tuberculosis resistant to the multiple drug therapy (MDT). As is well known, Robert Koch, the effective creator of modern scientific medicine, discovered the tubercle bacillus causal agent in 1882, then hit upon a TB cure he called "tuberculin." However some time later, rival scientists found that Koch's "tuberculin" was itself lethal. The discovery in the 1950s of multiple drug therapy enabled scientists to believe they had finally worked clear of the Koch débâcle. But with the emergence of MDT-resistant strains, the whole issue has emerged again, stigmatizing, painful and pressing.[37]

Drug-resistant TB touched another raw nerve. By its presence among the impoverished new poor in American, British and Russian cities the disease demonstrated that the Omran age of "pestilence and famine" can return. In the USA, many inner-city TB victims were social dropouts who had fought in Vietnam and later found it impossible to settle down to normal civilian routines. Other common victims were former patients of mental hospitals who had been discharged into "community care" to live (and die) on inner-city streets. Still others were elderly folks who had become street people because their pensions didn't run to the provision of shelter, clothing and food.[38] With the privatization of US welfare services in the autumn of 1996, the number of street people dying from TB can be expected to expand exponentially.

For medical research scientists, another lesson in humility has been malaria. As suggested earlier, before Development began 500 years ago, it seems unlikely that malaria had ever been a problem across the whole of the tropical world. Then beginning in the 1970s scientists were shocked to find that high-tech tools and sprays used to exterminate human-affecting malaria parasites and their mosquito hosts seemed to be encouraging new variants of both creature types to evolve—just as Darwin might have predicted. Today, with more than a million victims in a typical year, malaria is one of the two or three leading causes of death among children in the tropical world.[39]

Usually *not* among the victims of local malaria were the development officers and their consultant friends who were on site for a feasibility study for a new high dam or forest clearance scheme. Determined not to fail their principal clientele, western research laboratories have created expensive prophylactic drugs and sprays which render a site safe during the fortnight or so while a feasibility study is underway, or longer while expat engineers are supervising construction work. What have *not* been developed, however, are inexpensive, long-term effective techniques that indigenous poor peoples can use to save themselves and their children from malaria and the need to produce large families.[40]

Meanwhile on the west bank of the Nile almost within sight of where I write, the great limestone Sphinx now threatened with corrosive pollution from nearby cars and buses continues to gaze imperturbably into space (and into the second-floor eating hall of a nearby Pizza Hut restaurant). When, 4,500 years ago, the Sphinx was first chipped clear of the surrounding stone, average life expectancy for the better-off of the Pharaoh's subjects was forty or forty-five years. This was virtually the same as that expected in rural English surroundings in 1835 when young Alexander Kinglake rode out to consult the Sphinx.

Today, thanks to the epidemiologic transition pinpointed by Egypt's Abdel Omran, this has changed. Globally, among the short-lived multitudes, living largely in the South, there is an explosion in human numbers. This can be contrasted with the explosive increase in the consumption of non-renewable resources by the long-lived *few* living mostly in the North. Standing in the footprints of Kinglake before the world's oldest oracle, one can ask whether this gross imbalance will be allowed to continue? To this question the Sphinx gives no answer.

Notes

Introduction

1. (Italics in original) Alexander William Kinglake, *Eothen* (London, Longman, Green, 1940), 169, 173.
2. Geoffrey Lean, "One Western Life is Worth 15 in the Third World, Says UN Report," *Independent on Sunday*, 23 July 1995. Follow-up: "Green Economist Faces Picket," *The Times Higher Education Supplement* 24 November 1995, 3. Kinglake's musings while standing before the Sphinx—"and still that sleepless rock will lie watching and watching the works of the new busy race [the conquerors of Egypt and India]" (*Eothen*, 198)—was quoted with approval in 1896 by the on-site Development agent for Egypt, W. E. Garstin, Under-Secretary of State for Public Works: R. H. Brown, *History of the Barrages at the Head of the Nile Delta*, introduction by W. E. Garstin (Cairo, National Printing Department, 1896), x.
3. Roy Porter, "The Patient's View: Doing Medical History from Below," *Theory and Society* XIV (1995), 175–98; Anne Digby, *Making a Medical Living* (Cambridge, Cambridge University Press, 1994), 302–10; Andrew Wear, "Interfaces: Perceptions of Health and Illness in Early Modern England" in Roy Porter and Andrew Wear, eds, *Problems and Methods in the History of Medicine* (London, Croom Helm, 1987), 230–56; Dorothy Porter and Roy Porter, *Patient's Progress: Doctors and Doctoring in 18th Century England* (Stanford, CA, Stanford University Press, 1989), 208–14; Matthew Ramsey, *Professional and Popular Medicine in France, 1770–1830* (Cambridge, Cambridge University Press, 1988); William Coleman, "Health and Hygiene in the *Encyclopédie*: A Medical Doctrine for the Bourgeoisie," *Journal of the History of Medicine* XXIX (1974), 399–421; Nancy G. Siraisi, *Medieval & Early Renaissance Medicine* (Chicago, University of Chicago Press, 1990), 120–23, 136–37; David Gentilcore, "Contesting Illness in Early Modern Naples: *Miracolati*, Physicians and the Congregation of Rites," *Past and Present* CXLVIII (1995), 115, 124–25; Carlo M. Cipolla, *Miasmas and Disease: Public Health and the Environment in the Pre-Industrial Age*, trans. Elizabeth Potter (London, Yale University Press, 1992); Charles E. Rosenberg, "The Therapeutic Revolution: Medicines, Meanings, and Social Change in Nineteenth Century America," in his *The Therapeutic Revolution: Essays in the Social History of American Medicine* (University Park, University of Pennsylvania Press, 1979), 3–12,

21–22; Steven M. Stowe, "Seeing Themselves at Work: Physicians and the Case Narrative in the Mid-Nineteenth-Century American South," *American Historical Review* CI no. 1 (February 1996), 43–46.

4. "Robert Koch," *Dictionary of Scientific Biography*, ed. Charles Gillispie (New York, Charles Scribner's Sons, 1981), 420–35. In the world of fiction, reflecting public opinion in the era when medicalization was finally rushing forward, Koch is seen as the model scientific doctor: Sinclair Lewis, *Arrowsmith* (New York, Harcourt Brace & World, 1925). See also: Roslynn D. Haynes, *From Faust to Strangelove: Representations of the Scientist in Western Literature* (Baltimore, MD, Johns Hopkins University Press, 1995) and Gerald L. Geison, *The Private Science of Louis Pasteur* (Princeton, NJ, Princeton University Press, 1995).

5. For examples of overt hostility to the paradigmatic insights of Koch (arrived at in India in 1884) by senior members of the scientific research team at the Office of the Sanitary Commission of the Government of India and the Army Sanitary Commission itself see: *Parliamentary Papers* 1894 LX [Cd 7514], 79, 103, 162, 202; *P.P.* 1898 LXIV [Cd 8688], 180; *P.P.* 1899 LXVI (part II) [Cd 9549], 218, 227, 234, 251; *P.P.* 1900 LVIII [Cd 397], 257; *P.P.* 1906 LXXXII [Cd 2766], 149.

6. Sir Charles Bruce, GCMG, "Tropical Medicine as Instrument of Empire," *Journal of Tropical Medicine and Hygiene* XI (2 November 1908), 334; Nancy Stepan, *The Idea of Race in Science: Great Britain 1800–1960* (London, Macmillan, 1982); Nancy Stepan, *Beginnings of Brazilian Science: Oswaldo Cruz, Medical Research and Policy, 1890–1920* (New York, Science History Publications, 1976); Seymour Drescher, "The Ending of the Slave Trade and the Evolution of European Scientific Racism," in Joseph E. Inikori and Stanley L. Engerman, eds, *The Atlantic Slave Trade: Effects on Economies, Societies and People in Africa, the Americas, and Europe* (Durham, NC, Duke University Press, 1992); John Farley, *Bilharzia: A History of Imperial Tropical Medicine* (Cambridge, Cambridge University Press, 1991); Michael Worboys, "The Emergence of Tropical Medicine: A Study in the Establishment of a Scientific Specialty," in G. Lemaine *et al.*, eds, *Perspectives on the Emergence of Scientific Disciplines* (The Hague, Mouton, 1976), 89. See also: Roy MacLeod and Milton Lewis, eds, *Disease, Medicine and Empire: Perspectives on Western Medicine and the Experience of European Expansion* (London, Routledge, 1988) and Armando Solórzano, "Sowing the Seeds of Neo-Imperialism: The Rockefeller Foundation's Yellow Fever Campaign in Mexico," *International Journal of Health Services*, XXII no. 3 (1992), 529–54.

7. For a overview of the globalization of history after 1492 see: Jerry H. Bentley, "Cross-Cultural Interaction and Periodization in World History," *American Historical Review* CI no. 3 (June 1996), 749–70; for "gentlemanly capitalism" see: P. J. Cain and A. G. Hopkins, *British Imperialism: Innovation and Expansion, 1688–1914*, (London, Longman, 1993); for credit relationships: Joseph C. Miller, *Way of Death: Merchant Capitalism and the Angolan Slave Trade 1730–1830* (London, James Currey, 1988), 664–69; Fernand Braudel, *The Perspective of the World*, trans. Siân

Reynolds (London, Collins, 1984), 38, 44; for consumerism: Ralph Austen and Woodruff D. Smith, "Private Tooth Decay as Public Economic Virtue: The Slave-Sugar Triangle, Consumerism, and European Industrialization," in Inikori and Engerman, *The Atlantic Slave Trade,* 183–203; T. H. Breen, "'Baubles of Britain': The American and Consumer Revolutions of the Eighteenth Century," *Past and Present* CXIX (1988), 73–104.

8. William McNeill, *Plagues and Peoples* (London, Doubleday, 1976); Alfred W. Crosby, *The Columbian Exchange: Biological and Cultural Consequences of 1492* (Westport, CT, Greenwood Press, 1972); Alfred W. Crosby, *Ecological Imperialism: The Biological Expansion of Europe, 900–1900* (Cambridge, Cambridge University Press, 1986); Mark Nathan Cohen, *Health and the Rise of Civilization* (New Haven, CT, Yale University Press, 1989).

9. See Chapter 3, "Smallpox in the New World and in the Old: From Holocaust to Eradication, 1518 to 1977".

10. See Chapter 2, "Dark Hidden Meanings: Leprosy and Lepers in the Medieval West and in the Tropical World under the European Imperium" and Chapter 6, "Yellow Fever, Malaria and Development: Atlantic Africa and the New World 1647 to 1928." An example of a disease crisis which in most polities elicited little novel medical or political response is the 1918 influenza epidemic which killed at least 20 million people world-wide: Alfred Crosby, *America's Forgotten Pandemic: The Influenza of 1918* (Cambridge, Cambridge University Press, 1989). However in recently British-colonized Yoruba land in the Nigeria regions, the death of 250,000 people from influenza led to the establishment of locally managed Aladora faith-healing churches: John Peel, *Aladora* (Oxford, Oxford University Press, 1968).

11. Sir Isaiah Berlin, *The Crooked Timber of Humanity* (New York, Alfred A. Knopf, 1991); Christopher Lasch, *The Revolt of the Elites and the Betrayal of Democracy* (New York, W. W. Norton, 1995), 93; Edward Said, *Culture and Imperialism* (London, Chatto & Windus, 1993); Bhirkhu Paretkh, "Superior People: The Narrowness of Liberalism from Mill to Rawls," *Times Literary Supplement*, 25 February 1994, 11. In some quarters, when talking about the negative aspects of the Enlightenment it has become fashionable to use the term "the Enlightenment Project".

12. McNeill, *Plagues and Peoples.* For warnings against inappropriate disease determinism see: Bill Luckin, "States and Epidemic Threats," *Bulletin of the Society for the Social History of Medicine* XXXIV (1984), 25–27.

13. For an early notice of the distortion of research funding in favor of plague (which was causing public panic) away from a disease which killed far more people (in this case cholera) see *Parliamentary Papers* 1906 LXXXII [Cd 2766], 149. See also: Rajnarayan Chandavarkar, "Plague Panic and Epidemic Politics in India, 1896–1914," in Terence Ranger and Paul Slack, eds, *Epidemics and Ideas: Essays on the Historical Perception of Pestilence* (Cambridge, Cambridge University Press, 1992), 203–40.

14. This point was also made in *The World Health Report 1996, Fighting Disease, Fostering Development: Report of the Director-General* (Geneva, World

Health Organization, 1996), 106–7, 110. See also p. 367 fn 39.

15. The *World Health Report 1996* records that "Countries in the [Eastern Mediterranean] Region believe that it is time to recall that ethical values in medical practice need to be reinforced in today's world where mostly technical and economic considerations prevail." *World Health Report 1996*, 97. On the direct correlation between relative social equality, quality of life and longevity, see Richard Wilkinson, *Unhealthy Societies, The Afflictions of Inequality* (London, Routledge, 1996).

1 *The Human Response to Plague in Western Europe and the Middle East, 1347 to 1844*

1. For a general introduction: Jean-Noël Biraben, *Les hommes et la peste en France et dans les pays européens et méditerranéens: Tome I: La peste dans l'histoire* (Paris, Mouton, 1975), and *Tome II: Les hommes face à la peste* (Paris, Mouton, 1976). For the Middle East see Michael W. Dols, *The Black Death in the Middle East* (Princeton, NJ, Princeton University Press, 1977). The 1347–53 visitation is termed "the black death" and later visitations of what is presumed to have been the same disease are known as "plague" or "pestilence." The cycle of visitations which began in 1347 and ended in 1844 is the *second pandemic*; the first pandemic (also coming out of central Asia), is generally termed "Justinian's Plague"; it struck the West in 541 CE and lasted until 775.
2. Quoted in Ann Montgomery Campbell, *The Black Death and Men of Learning* (New York, AMS Press, 1966), 52.
3. David Herlihy and Christiane Klapisch-Zuber, *Tuscans and their Families: A Study of the Florentine Catasto of 1427* (New Haven, CT, Yale University Press, 1985), 73–78.
4. Dols, *Black Death*, 230–31; Albert Hourani, *A History of the Arab People* (London, Faber & Faber, 1991), 213; Biraben, *Tome I*, 105–11; Emmanuel Le Roy Ladurie, *The Peasants of Languedoc*, trans. John Day (Urbana, University of Illinois Press, 1974), 1–66; Harry Miskimin, *The Economy of Later Renaissance Europe 1460–1600* (Cambridge, Cambridge University Press, 1977), 20–21; Paul Slack, *The Impact of Plague in Tudor and Stuart England* (London, Routledge & Kegan Paul, 1985), 15–17; Roger Mols, "Population in Europe 1500–1700," in Carlo M. Cipolla, ed., *The Fontana Economic History of Europe: The Sixteenth and Seventeenth Centuries* (London, Collins/Fontana, 1974), 38–39; William McNeill, *Plagues and Peoples* (Garden City, NY, Anchor Books, 1976), 150. On plague in mid-seventeenth-century north Italian urban centers see Richard Rapp, *Industry and Economic Decline in Seventeenth-Century Venice* (Cambridge, MA, Harvard University Press, 1976), 22, 42; Carlo M. Cipolla, *Cristofano and the Plague: A Study in the History of Public Health in the Age of Galileo* (London, Collins, 1973), 20; Ann G. Carmichael, "Contagion Theory and Contagion Practice in Fifteenth Century Milan," *Renaissance Quarterly*, XLIV no. 2 (summer 1991), 254; Domenico Selle, *Crisis and Continuity: The Economy of Spanish Lombardy in the Seventeenth Century* (Cambridge, MA,

Harvard University Press, 1979); Eric Cochrane, *Italy 1530–1630*, ed. Julius Kishner (London, Longman, 1988), 280–81; Fernand Braudel, "Putting the Record Straight: The Age of the Genoese," in *Civilization & Capitalism: 15th–18th Century III: The Perspective of the World*, trans. Siân Reynolds (London, Collins/Fontana, 1985), 157–73. In 1722 Daniel Defoe, journalist, novelist and man with an eye to the main chance, published his famous *Journal of the Plague Year*. Defoe's tale of an imagined London in 1665 established itself in the educated English mind as the authoritative account of what a plague crisis necessarily entailed.

5. Turning point identified by Ann G. Carmichael, *Plague and the Poor in Renaissance Florence* (Cambridge, Cambridge University Press, 1986).
6. Andrew B. Appleby, "The Disappearance of Plague: A Continuing Puzzle," *Economic History Review* 2nd series XXXIII no. 2 (May 1980), 161–73; Kari Konkola, "More than a Coincidence? The Arrival of Arsenic and the Disappearance of Plague in Early Modern Europe," *History of Medicine* XLVII no. 2 (1992), 186–209.
7. S. R. Epstein, "Cities, Regions and the Late Medieval Crisis: Sicily and Tuscany Compared," *Past and Present* CXXX (1991), 3–50. For the importance of regional variations: J. M. W. Bean, "The Black Death: The Crisis and its Social and Economic Consequences," in Daniel Williman, ed., *The Black Death: The Impact of the Fourteenth Century Plague* (Binghamton, NY, Center for Medieval and Early Renaissance Studies, 1982), 23–38.
8. Anthony Molho, "Recent Works on the History of Tuscany: Fifteenth to Eighteenth Centuries," *Journal of Modern History* LXII (March 1990), 77.
9. James Longrigg, "Epidemic, Ideas and Classical Athenian Society," in Terence Ranger and Paul Slack, eds, *Epidemics and Ideas: Essays on the Historical Perception of Pestilence* (Cambridge, Cambridge University Press, 1992), 21–44, esp. 34, 39. As Longrigg points out, Chapters 47–57 of Book II of the *History* tell of a "plague" that no author contemporary with Thucydides mentioned and which bestowed immunity on those who survived it: actual bubonic plague bestows no immunity.
10. Quoted in John Larner, *Italy in the Age of Dante and Petrarch 1216–1380* (London, Longman, 1980), 265.
11. Girolamo Fracastoro, an armchair physician and well-connected literary figure in Verona and Rome, wrote a treatise published in 1546 suggesting that plague might be carried by invisible particles bearing contagion; this idea was too far out of the medical mainstream to win acceptance or even to be remembered until the nineteenth century. For an assessment of Fracastoro's contribution by a former World Health Organization official ("obscure, clouded with superstition . . . bore no realistic relation to present knowledge of communicable disease") see: Norman Howard Jones, "Fracastoro and Henle: A Reappraisal of their Contribution to the Concept of Communicable Diseases," *Medical History*, XXI (1977), 68.
12. Quoted in Cipolla, *Cristofano*, 17–18. For the incubation period, I have used the standard public health handbook found on my medical doctor's desk: Abram S. Benenson, *Control of Communicable Diseases in Man*, 15th edition (New York, American

Publication Association, 1990), 326.

13. M. C. Jacob points out that natural philosophers Galileo and Newton contended that their scientific revolution was intended to alter the thinking *only* of people of the better sort; they did not intend to shake the confidence of "the vulgar" in long-established Christian and Aristotelian authority: Margaret C. Jacob, *The Cultural Meaning of the Scientific Revolution* (New York, Alfred A. Knopf, 1988), 3–9, 19–24, 34–35, 87–89, 109–11. For a masterful discussion of the entire movement see: H. Floris Cohen, *The Scientific Revolution: A Historiographical Inquiry* (Chicago, University of Chicago Press, 1994).

14. A brief survey in Dols, *Black Death*, 68–70; McNeill, *Plagues and Peoples*, 21; Henri H. Mollaret, "Le cas de la peste," *Annales de Démographie Historique* (1989), 102; F. F. Cartwright, *A Social History of Medicine* (New York, Longman, 1977), 71, 140–41; M. W. Flinn, "Plague in Europe and the Mediterranean Countries," *Journal of European Economic History* VIII no. 1 (1979), 134–36, 146–47; *Oxford Companion to Medicine*, John Walton, P. Beeson and R. Scott, eds. (New York, Oxford University Press, 1986), 634, 1480.

15. Mollaret, "De la peste," 102–103; Biraben *Tome I*, 16–18; Flinn "Plague," 134–39; John D. Post, "Famine, Mortality and Epidemic Disease in the Process of Modernization," *Economic History Review* 2nd series XXIX no. 1 (1976), 33–34.

16. Biraben, *Tome I*, 86–87; Dr Ahmed Kamel, Ishac Gayed, Mohd. Anwar, eds, "On the Epidemiology and Treatment of Plague in Egypt: The 1940 Epidemic," *Journal of the Egyptian Public Health Association* XVI no. 2 (January 1941), 55.

17. Carmichael, *Plague and Poor*, 94; Biraben, *Tome I*, 130–31; Suzanne Austin Alchon, *Native Society and Disease in Colonial Ecuador* (Cambridge, Cambridge University Press, 1991), 14, 37. Post clinches the case for there being no long-term immunity; "Famine," 34. In the same citation Post also holds that the 80 percent case fatality rate at Novi Bazar in Bosnia in 1814 strongly suggests that there was no "autonomous reduction in the virulence of plague infection" over time since the Novi Bazar figures "do not differ appreciably from the average western-European experience during the 17th century."

18. Mollaret, "De la peste," 102; Dols, *Middle East*, 71–74, 79–83, 213, 226–28. In Europe, only the papal doctor at Avignon, Guy de Chauliac, was sufficiently precise in his empirical observations and data recording to allow modern specialists to distinguish characteristics of bubonic from those of pneumonic forms of plague: Lise Wilkinson, "Review," *Medical History* XXIX (1985), 326. Today, by the timely use of antibiotics, such as tetracycline and streptomycin, the death rate from pneumonic plague can be brought down to nil.

19. Carmichael, *Plague and Poor*, 5–6; Flinn, "Plague," 134–38.

20. Kamel *et al.*, "Plague in Egypt," 53–4.

21. Flinn, "Plague," 143–48; Biraben, *Tome II*, 85–185.

22. Luis García-Ballester, "Changes in the *Regimina Sanitatis*: The Role of the Jewish Physicians," in Sheila Campbell, Bert Hall and David Klausner, eds, *Health, Disease and Healing in Medieval Culture* (New York, St Martin's Press, 1992), 120–31. Ann G. Carmichael, "Plague Legislation

in the Italian Renaissance," *Bulletin of the History of Medicine*, LVII (1983), 508–11.

23. The six Non-Naturals derived from Galen were (1) climate, (2) motion and rest, (3) diet, (4) sleeping patterns, (5) evacuation and sexuality, (6) afflictions of the soul: García-Ballester, "Regimina Sanitatis," 121. See also Nancy G. Siraisi, *Medieval & Early Renaissance Medicine: An Introduction to Knowledge and Practice* (Chicago, University of Chicago Press, 1990), 101, 120–23. For a listing of the same Non-Naturals in medieval Muslim Yünäni medicine: Ismail H. Abdalla, "Diffusion of Islamic Medicine into Hausaland," in Steven Feierman and John M. Janzen, eds, *The Social Basis of Health & Healing in Africa* (Berkeley, University of California Press, 1992), 182. For the continuing role of the six "Non-Naturals" see Roy Porter, "The Patient in England, *c.* 1660–*c.* 1800," in Andrew Wear, ed., *Medicine in Society: Historical Essays* (Cambridge, Cambridge University Press, 1992), 99. In the eighteenth-century West, these ideas came under heavy pressure during the search for the natural history of each specific disease (nosology), following the program laid down by Thomas Sydenham (d. 1689): Guenter Risse, "Medicine in the Age of Enlightenment," in Wear, *Medicine in Society*, 167–68.

24. By the 1380s the divine arrows of disease were often taken to refer to the arrows associated with St Sebastian, a martyred Christian and Roman centurion who had been stripped naked and shot dead by a squad of archers. St Roch, the second of the two plague saints, was a well-born fourteenth-century indigene of the French hexagon who worked among the plague-stricken before he himself picked up the disease, fell out with a nasty crowd and met his death. St Roch is generally depicted as a pilgrim in late medieval dress: Biraben, *Tome II*, 78–79.

25. Carmichael, *Plague and Poor*, 98–99, 108–10; John Henderson, "Epidemics in Renaissance Florence: Medical Theory and Government Responses," in Neithard Bulst and Robert Delort, eds, *Maladie et société (XIIe–XVIIIe siècles)* (Paris, Editions du CNRS, 1989) 165–67; William Bowsky, "The Impact of the Black Death upon Sienese Government and Society," *Speculum* XXXIX (1964), 1–34.

26. Among the rich and powerful, the conflict between instincts of self-preservation and the need to maintain discipline among the vulgar sometimes led to contradictory behavior. In Naples early in the plague of 1656, the cardinal-archbishop reputedly forbade his parish priests to leave; however, the cardinal himself fled to a safe rural haven (the convent of Sant Elmo) and did not return until the plague had departed: Jean Delumeau, *La Peur en Occident: XIVe–XVIIIe siècles: une cité assiégée* (Paris, Fayard, 1978), 125. In the world of literature, the classic account of how golden youth of both sexes amused themselves in 1348 after fleeing from plague-stricken Florence is Boccaccio's *Decameron*.

27. Quoted in Richard C. Trexler, *Public Life in Renaissance Florence* (New York, Academic Press, 1980), 362.

28. Denys Hay, *The Church in Italy in the Fifteenth Century* (Cambridge, Cambridge University Press, 1977); 64; Richard Kieckhefer, *Magic in the Middle Ages* (Cambridge, Cambridge University Press, 1989), 56–68; Aron Gurevich, *Medieval*

Popular Culture: Problems of Belief and Perception*, trans. János M. Bak and Paul A. Hollingworth (Cambridge, Cambridge University Press, 1990), 176ff.; S. J. Watts, *A Social History of Western Europe 1450–1720: Tensions and Solidarities among Rural People* (London, Hutchinson University Library, 1984), 164–73.

29. R. I. Moore, *The Formation of a Persecuting Society* (Oxford, Basil Blackwell, 1987), 27–45.

30. Biraben, *Tome I*, 60–61, 377. A month before the massacre the Bishop of Strasbourg had presided over a gathering of local magnates who passed a resolution agreeing that the Jews had been poisoning local wells. Pope Clement VI's personal physician held that the plague could be contracted *visually*, which was perhaps why the Pope was worried about demons in mirrors: Campbell, *Men of Learning*, 60–61.

31. Biraben, *Tome II*, 68.

32. Quoted in Richard Palmer, "The Church, Leprosy and Plague in Medieval and Early Modern Europe," in W. J. Shiels, ed., *The Church and Healing* (Oxford, Basil Blackwell, 1982), 96.

33. Palmer, "The Church," 97; Carlo Cipolla, *Public Health and the Medical Profession in the Renaissance* (Cambridge, Cambridge University Press, 1976), 36–37. In cities where kinship networks included both priests and men of magisterial rank, clerics often tended to look the other way while their relatives on boards of health closed down chapels and banned processions, citing contagion.

34. Roger French, "The Arrival of the French Disease in Leipzig," in Bulst and Delort, eds, *Maladie et société*, 136–37; Siraisi, *Medieval*, 189; Campbell, *Men of Learning*, 40. In contrast with Latin Christians, educated late fourteenth-century Muslims such as Ibn Khaldun held that belief in astrology was incompatible with belief in Islam: Daniel Panzac, *La Peste dans l'Empire Ottoman 1700–1850* (Paris, Éditions Peters, 1985), 188–89.

35. García-Ballester, "*Regimina Sanitatis*," 121; Siraisi, *Medieval*, 65–77. In the development of a university teaching program, England lagged behind the Continent: the first to be established was at Oxford in 1303. During the remainder of the century the number of medical students was small, with most combining the study of medicine with theology: Mark Zier, "The Healing Power of the Hebrew Tongue: An Example from Late 13th Century England," in Sheila Campbell, Bert Hall and David Klausner, eds, *Health, Disease and Healing in Medieval Culture* (New York, St Martin's Press, 1992), 113.

36. Harold J. Cook, "The New Philosophy and Medicine in Seventeenth Century England," in David C. Lindberg and Robert S. Westman, eds, *Reappraisals of the Scientific Revolution* (Cambridge, Cambridge University Press, 1990), 397–436.

37. Quoted in Cook, "Philosophy," 406–407.

38. For negative comments on empirics by Guy de Chauliac (the pope's personal physician at Avignon in 1348) see Siraisi, *Medieval*, 35. For other comments on "practitioners educated at the university and those trained outside" see Katharine Park, "Medicine and Society in Medieval Europe, 500–1500," in Wear, *Medicine in Society*, 79–80. "According to the Hippocratic corpus, 'Things . . . that are holy are revealed only to men who are holy. The profane may not learn them until they have been initiated into the mysteries of

science.'" (i.e. natural philosophy): quoted in William Eamon, "From the Secrets of Nature to Public Knowledge," in Lindberg and Westman, *Reappraisals of the Scientific Revolution*, 333–34.

39. Quoted in Cook, "Philosophy," 409.

40. García-Ballester, "*Regimina Sanitatis*," 122–24; Cook, "Philosophy," 410–11; Siraisi, *Medieval*, 84–85, 97–107. Galen seems to have had no first-hand knowledge of bubonic plague. He fled from Rome just before a major epidemic broke out, but claimed that the disease in question could be easily cured (at that time there was no cure for plague). He mentioned an eruption which appeared all over the body, sometimes ulcerous but always dry, and that patients sometimes spat up blood. It would seem then that Galen's "plague" was more closely related to typhus fever or to smallpox than to bubonic plague.

41. Vivian Nutton, "The Seeds of Disease: An Explanation of Contagion and Infection from the Greeks to the Renaissance," *Medical History* XXVII (1983), 15; for similar accounts of disease still current in the early nineteenth century see Charles Rosenberg, "Explaining Epidemics," in his *Explaining Epidemics and Other Studies in the History of Medicine* (Cambridge, Cambridge University Press, 1992), 295.

42. García-Ballester, "*Regimina Sanitatis*," 120–22; Carmichael, *Plague and Poor*, 27. According to A. Digby, "this caring, rather than curing role was the stuff of everyday doctoring" until the early twentieth century: Anne Digby, *Making a Medical Living*, (Cambridge, Cambridge University Press, 1994), 310; see also 5–6, 302–12.

43. Quoted in Cipolla, *Public Health*, 77.

44. Quoted in Carmichael, *Plague and Poor*, 97.

45. Quoted in Cipolla, *Public Health*, 108; for analogous arguments see: E. E. Evans-Pritchard, *Witchcraft, Oracles and Magic among the Azande* (Oxford, Clarendon Press, 1937). As part of their two-pronged attack on Galenic/Hippocratic medicine, the Swiss/German magus/scientist Paracelsus (d. 1541) and his followers accused Galen of having used the practical assistance of empirics in order to achieve cures and to leave himself time to spin airy-fairy theories. Paracelsus himself held that cunning women and empirics probably knew as much about *curing* disease as did learned physicians: Charles Webster, "Science and Medicine in Academic Studies before 1640," in his *The Great Instauration: Science, Medicine and Reform, 1626–1660* (London, Duckworth, 1975), 248.

46. Quoted in Irma Naso, "Les Hommes et les epidémies dans l'Italie de la fin du Moyen Age: les réactions et les moyens de défense entre peur et méfiance," in Bulst and Delort, *Maladie et société*, 311.

47. Siraisi, *Medieval*, 42–43. For comments on several score treatises on plague written before 1400 interpreted in the light of post-Kochian knowledge: Larner, *Italy*, 258; these contrast with a more objective assessment by Siraisi, *Medieval*, 128–29.

48. Robert Muchembled, *Culture populaire et culture des élites dans la France moderne, XVe–XVIIIe siècles* (Paris, Flammarion, 1978).

49. Biraben, *Tome II*, 164–67.

50. The thesis set forth by Carmichael, *Plague and Poor*, 127–28.

51. George Holmes, *Europe: Hierarchy and Revolt 1320–1450*

(London, Fontana, 1975), 192–93, 311–12.

52. George Holmes, *The Florentine Enlightenment 1400–1450* (London, Weidenfeld & Nicholson, 1969); Ronald Weissman, *Ritual Brotherhood in Renaissance Florence* (New York, Academic Press, 1982); Ronald Witt, "The *Crisis* after Forty Years," *American Historical Review* CI no. 1 (1996), 117–18.

53. Bronislaw Geremek, *Truands et misérables dans l'Europe modern, 1350–1600* (Paris, 1980).

54. Quoted in Carmichael, "Plague Legislation," 522.

55. Carmichael, *Plague and Poor*, 100–1; Henderson, "Epidemics in Renaissance Florence," 170, 172; Slack, *Impact*, 211, 303–309; Giulia Calvi, *Histories of a Plague Year: The Social and Imaginary in Baroque Florence*, trans. Dario Biocca and Bryant Ragan Jr (Berkeley, University of California Press, 1989), 8. In fact, bubonic plague was *not* contagious. Slack points out that the contempt with which the rich regarded the poor was not necessarily reciprocated by the hatred of the rich by the poor; Paul Slack, "Responses to Plague in Early Modern Europe: The Implications of Public Health," *Social Research* LV no. 3 (1988), 448.

56. Carmichael, *Plague and Poor*, 116–26; Carmichael, "Milan," 255; Palmer, "The Church," 94; Slack, *Impact*, 1–6; Giulia Calvi, "The Florentine Plague of 1630–33: Social behavior and symbolic action," in Bulst and Delort, *Maladie et société*, 333; Robert Favreau, *La ville de Poitiers à la fin du Moyen Age: une capitale regionale* I (Poitiers, 1978), 572.

57. Paul Slack, "The Response to Plague in Early Modern England: Public Policies and their Consequences," in John Walter and Roger Schofield, eds, *Famine, Disease and the Social Order in Early Modern Society* (Cambridge, Cambridge University Press, 1991), 167.

58. "Progetto di controllo e di mediazione sociale" quoted in Molho, "Tuscany," 70.

59. Quoted in Cipolla, Cristofano, 89–90.

60. Biraben, *Tome II*, 103–105; Slack, *Impact*, 45–47; Carmichael, "Milan," 252–53; Ole Peter Grell, "Plague in Elizabethan and Stuart London: The Dutch Response," *Medical History* XXXIV (1990), 425.

61. Delumeau, *La Peur*, 115 (my translation).

62. Quoted in Slack, *Impact*, 75.

63. Per-Gunnar Ottosson, "Fear of the Plague and the Burial of Plague Victims in Sweden 1710–1711," in Bulst and Delort, *Maladie et société*, 376–92. For the unique success of Swedish authority in compelling adults to learn the fundamentals of the Christian faith (licenses to marry were only granted those who could read a text from Scripture): Geoffrey Parker, "Success and Failure during the First Century of the Reformation," *Past and Present* CXXXVI (1992), 77–79.

64. Naso, "Entre peur et méfiance," 324–25.

65. Calvi, "Florentine Plague of 1630–33," 331.

66. Carmichael, *Plague and Poor* and its references. Slack's *Impact*, 6–31 asks questions applicable to all polities.

67. Flinn, "Plague," 142; Slack, "Responses," 181.

68. Brian Pullan, "Plague and perceptions of the poor in early modern Italy," in Ranger and Slack, *Epidemics and Ideas*, 101, 111; Rapp, *Decline . . . in Venice, passim*.

69. Naso, "Entre peur et méfiance," 325; Calvi, "Symbolic Action," 331, 333; Grell, "Stuart London," 425.

70. Slack, "Responses," 183; Pullan, "Plague and Perceptions," 121; Biraben, *Tome II*, 170.
71. Quoted in Cipolla, *Cristofano*, 27.
72. Quoted ibid., 120.
73. Calvi, *Histories*, 196; Slack, *Impact*, 299.
74. Grell, "Stuart London," 424–39; Simon Schama, *The Embarrassment of Riches: An Interpretation of Dutch Culture in the Golden Age* (New York, Alfred Knopf, 1987), 341; David Nicholas, "Town and Countryside: Social, Economic and Political Tensions in Fourteenth Century Flanders," *Comparative Studies in Society and History* X, no. 4 (1968), 458ff. For more on Dutch capitalism in a world setting, see Chapter 6: "Yellow Fever, Malaria and Development."
75. Carmichael, *Plague and Poor*, 111–13.
76. Biraben, *Tome II*, 86–90.
77. Theodore K. Rabb, *The Struggle for Stability in Early Modern Europe* (New York, Oxford University Press, 1975), 116–24. See also E. L. Jones, *The European Miracle: Environments, Economies and Geopolitics in the History of Europe and Asia*, 2nd edition (Cambridge, Cambridge University Press, 1987), 125–26.
78. John Elliott, "A Europe of Composite Monarchies," *Past and Present* CXXXVII (1992), 64–71; William Doyle, "States and their Business' and the "Machinery of Government' in his *The Old European Order, 1660–1800* (Oxford, Oxford University Press, 1978), 211–65. For the German "special case," see: Thomas Robisheaux, *Rural Society and the Search for Order in Early Modern Germany* (Cambridge, Cambridge University Press, 1989), 1–43.
79. Henry Kamen, *Spain in the Later Seventeenth Century 1665–1700* (London, Longman, 1980), 50–53, 167.
80. Flinn, "Plague," 139–44.
81. Biraben, *Tome I*, 230–85; *Tome II*, 85–158; Jean-Pierre Filippini, "Information et stragégie des magistrats de la santé de la Méditerranée face à la peste au XVIIIe siècle," in Bulst and Delort, *Maladie et société*, 207–14. For a report by Nicholas de Nicolay on standard health quarantine measures followed in the Isle of Chios in 1551–53 a decade before it was incorporated into the Ottoman Empire see Panzac, *La Peste*, 299.
82. Gunther E. Rothenberg, "The Austrian Sanitary Cordon and the Control of Bubonic Plague: 1710–1871," *Journal of the History of Medicine* XXVIII (1973), 19; Flinn, "Plague," 143–45; Jones, *European Miracle*, 140–2; Barbara Jelavich, *History of the Balkans: Eighteenth and Nineteenth Centuries* (Cambridge, Cambridge University Press, 1983), 144–48.
83. A. W. Kinglake, *Eothen* (London, Longman, 1935), 1.
84. Panzac, *La Peste*, 516–17. The *OED* reference to the quotation is *Medical Journal I*, 411. For an assertion that "Bubonic plague is a disease of underdeveloped traditional societies" see: Post, "Famine," 35–37.
85. Introductions to the Mamluk regime include Ivan Hrbek, "Egypt, Nubia and the Eastern Deserts," in Roland Oliver, ed., *The Cambridge History of Africa: III: From c. 1050–c. 1600* (Cambridge, Cambridge University Press, 1977), and Robert Irwin, *The Middle East in the Middle Ages: The Early Mamluk Sultanate 1250–1382* (Carbondale, Southern Illinois University Press, 1986). For an assessment of western historians' generally negative interpretation of the Mamluks (negative be-

cause they did not follow the evolutionary pattern of the West), see Jean-Claude Garcin, "The Mamluk Military System and the Blocking of Medieval Moslem Society," in Jean Baechler, John A. Hall and Michael Mann, *Europe and the Rise of Capitalism* (Oxford, Basil Blackwell, 1988), 113–30.

86. Hrbek "Egypt," 53; Dols, *Black Death*, 154–56, 160–62; Janet L. Abu-Lughod, *Cairo: 1001 Years of the City Victorious* (Princeton, Princeton University Press, 1971), 37–8; Irwin, *Middle East*, 146.
87. Dols, *Black Death*, 154–69.
88. Dols, *Black Death*, 162; Irwin, *Middle East*, 141.
89. The situation in Syria at the time of the Black Death was complicated by the violent interplay between the Na'ib of Damascus and the Sultan in Cairo. For rural areas one can posit a scenario as follows; sixty years of peace ending in 1346 with the natural death of a grand old Mamluk Sultan, followed by unrest amongst the propertied on the eve of the Black Death, the arrival of plague jinn, the flight south of survivors, news of hostile Mamluk armies, culminating in north Syrian peasant decisions not to return to their natal villages: Irwin, *Middle East*, 132–44.
90. Hrbek, "Egypt," 48–49. Then as now, the commonplace was brother against brother; brothers united against kinsmen; kinsmen united against the village; the village united against the world.
91. Ibn al-Khatib has been popular with western historians of medicine because of his seemingly progressive ideas about "contagion": L. F. Hirst, *The Conquest of Plague: A Study of the Evolution of Epidemiology* (Oxford, Clarendon Press, 1953), 51; Campbell, *Men of Learning*, 58–59; Dols, *Black Death*, 94. Bubonic plague of course is *not* contagious.
92. Joseph J. Hobbs, *Bedouin Life in the Egyptian Wilderness* (Austin, University of Texas Press, 1989), 24.
93. Hrbek suggests that heavy mortality from plague in the steppes of southern Russia cut down the number of potential recruits for Mamluk service, necessitating a change of recruitment ground to areas further east, the Circassian Mamluks thus replacing the earlier Turkish: Hrbek, "Egypt," 53. See also: Irwin, *Middle East*, 158–59.
94. Robert Irwin, *The Arabian Nights: A Companion Volume* (London, Penguin Press, 1994); Irwin, *Middle East*, 107, 120, 136–37; Hrbek, "Egypt," 40–41; Dols, *Black Death*, 145–48.
95. Hrbek, "Egypt," 47–48; Garcin, "Mamluk Military System," 120–3.
96. Dols, *Black Death*, 188–93; Simon Pepper, "Crusaders' Crags," *Times Literary Supplement* 26 August 1995, 26. Garcin questions whether a European-style bourgeoisie (with its role of self-government) was a necessary attribute of town life. The private endowments—*waqfs*—created by Mamluk emirs provided a large number of amenities—hospitals, schools, mosques, fountains—visible manifestations of vibrant town life: Garcin, "Mamluk Military System," 122.
97. Mamluk sultans and emirs remained patrons of hospitals, public fountains, mosques and school complexes, private palaces in the city center, tombs and mosques in the eastern and southern cemeteries, and their architects retained a spirit of innovation: this is exemplified by the *madrasa* (school) and mausoleum of Al-Ghuri, built fourteen years before the Ottoman takeover.

98. High posts in Chancery in the fourteenth century were however usually reserved for Muslims, particularly for members of the Banu Fadllah extended family group: Irwin, *Middle East*, 131–32.
99. Garcin, "Mamluk Military System," 125–26.
100. Dols, *Black Death*, 181–83: despite much evidence of urban decay in Cairo, Europeans continued to be greatly impressed by Egypt under Islamic rule: Garcin, "Mamluk Military System," 123.
101. It is the former sort whose business records were heaped in the Geniza synagogue in Fustat (Old Cairo). In recent years these have given historians important insights into Mamluk Egyptian trade across the Indian Ocean.
102. For the Ottoman period see Ashin Dad Gupta, *Indian Merchants and the Decline of Surat* c. *1700–1750* (Wiesbaden, Franz Steiner, 1979), 4–5.
103. Abu-Lughod, *City Victorious*, 22–23.
104. Dols, *Black Death*, 109–16, 119–21.
105. Peter Brown, *The World of Late Antiquity: AD 150–750* (New York, W. W. Norton, 1989), 93–4, 100, 143, 186–87; Hrbek, "Egypt," 51.
106. Dols, *Black Death*, 167–8. For the importance of St Anthony and the desert fathers in the creation of the ideology which helped to inform Western ideas about leprosy in the eleventh and twelfth centuries see Chapter 2.
107. Abu-Lughod, *City Victorious*, 58–60; Dols, *Black Death*, 33–34; Peter Gran, "Medical Pluralism in Arab and Egyptian History: An Overview of Class Structures and Philosophies of the Main Phases," *Social Science and Medicine* XIII B (1979), 342–43.
108. Lawrence I. Conrad, "Epidemic Disease in Formal and Popular Thought in Early Islamic Society," in Ranger and Slack, *Epidemics and Ideas*, 77–99.
109. Panzac, *La Peste*, 292.
110. Dols, *Black Death*, 110–21, 297, 335; Panzac, *La Peste*, 291.
111. Jonathan P. Berkey, "Tradition, Innovation and the Social Construction of Knowledge in the Medieval Islamic Near East," *Past and Present* CXXXVI (February 1995), 38–39, 64.
112. Gran, "Medical Pluralism," 342–43; Panzac, *La Peste*, 290; Lawrence I. Conrad, "The Social Structure of Medicine in Medieval Islam," *Social History of Medicine* XXXVII (1985), 11–12.
113. Panzac, *La Peste*, 284 (my translation). The French military doctor Clot Bey made a similar report in the 1830s: LaVerne Kuhnke, *Lives at Risk: Public Health in Nineteenth Century Egypt* (Berkeley, University of California Press, 1990), 74. I am grateful to Professor William McNeill for first bringing the work of Dr Kuhnke to my attention.
114. The Cairene labor shortage also appears to have been one of the reasons for the annual importation of 4–5,000 black Africans: Terence Walz, "The Trade between Egypt and Bilad-a-Sudan 1700–1820," Boston University Graduate School, PhD thesis, submitted 1975. I am grateful to Dr Hugh Vernon-Jackson for bringing this thesis to my attention.
115. Panzac, *La Peste*, 286, (my translation) 306; Conrad, "Social Structure," 13–14; Dols, *Black Death*, 10, 117–18.
116. For the background to the medical situation in the Ottoman heartland see: Rhoads Murphey, "Ottoman Medicine and Transculturalism from the Sixteenth through the Eighteenth Century," *Bulletin of the History*

of Medicine LXVI no. 3 (1992), 376–403.

117. C. A. Bayly notes that "the bulk of Egypt's grain and even some of its cotton was sold not to Europe but to Smyrna and Istanbul, which suggests that demand from *within* the Ottoman Empire still remained considerable." He also quotes figures from the 1790s (just before the Pasha arrived on the scene) to the effect that profits accruing to merchants and tax collectors from pilgrims coming on the haj (pilgrimage) to Mecca and Medina were some £3 million a year, "which stands comparison with contemporary British trade with Bengal. After Muhammad Ali became Protector of the Holy Places, much of this profit found its way into his state coffers": C. A. Bayly, *Imperial Meridian: The British Empire and the World, 1780–1830* (London, Longman, 1989), 232.

118. A convenient summary: "Muhammad Ali and the Egyptians," in Kuhnke, *Lives at Risk*, 17–32.

119. P. J. Cain and A. G. Hopkins, *British Imperialism: Innovation and Expansion, 1688–1914* (London, Longman, 1993), 363. Commenting on Muhammad Ali's success in modernizing Egypt in the face of European opposition, Bernal notes that: "The fact that this episode of modern history is so little known is not at all surprising. It does not fit the paradigm of active European expansion into a passive outside world . . . [in fact Muhammad Ali's was] the greatest Egyptian Empire since the time of Ramesses II": Martin Bernal, *Black Athena: The Afroasiatic Roots of Classical Civilization* I (New Brunswick, NJ, Rutgers University Press, 1987), 249.

120. Greek rebels saw themselves as heirs of the old Byzantine Empire (and Orthodox Church). As late as 1756 in Patrea on Greek Peloponnese, twenty-seven Jewish families accused of spreading plague were bricked into the town wall by Orthodox Greek Christians and left to die of disease and starvation: Panzac, *La Peste*, 310. For modern disease anti-Semitism see Bill Luckin, "States and Epidemic Threats," *Bulletin of the Social History of Medicine* XXXIV (1984), 25–27.

121. Sir Richard F. Burton, *Personal Narrative of a Pilgrimage to Al-Madinah and Meccah*, I (London, Tylston & Edwards, 1893), 13. Less racist than Burton was J. L. Stephens, an American traveller in Egypt in 1835: Lloyd Stephens, *Incidents of Travel in Egypt, Arabia Petraea, and the Holy land*, ed. Victor Wolfgang von Hagen (San Francisco, Chronicle Books, 1991).

122. A. B. Clot Bey, *Mémoires de A. B. Clot Bey*, annoté par Jacques Tagher (Le Caire, L'Institut Français d'Archéologie Orientale, 1949), 285; Amira Sonbol, *The Creation of a Medical Profession in Egypt 1800–1922* (Syracuse, NY, Syracuse University Press, 1992) contrasts the teaching hospital situation under Muhammad Ali with that found under the British after 1882 and finds the latter wanting in elementary skills in public relations. See also F. M. Sandwith, MD, "The History of Kasr el Ainy," in H. P. Keatinge, ed., *Records of the Egyptian Government Faculty of Medicine* (Cairo, Government Press, 1927), 1–19.

123. For factual information on the 1834–36 plague epidemic: Kuhnke, "The Plague Epidemic of 1835: Background and Consequences," in *Lives at Risk*, 69–91.

124. Kuhnke, *Lives at Risk*, 85–86.

125. Bayly, *Imperial Meridian*, 233; Bernal, *Black Athena*, 249.

126. Phrase from Bayly, *Imperial Meridian*, 234.
127. Quoted in Panzac, *La Peste*, 482–83. Conflicting nineteenth-century ideas about contagion (quarantine) and anti-contagion were sorted out by Margaret Pelling, *Cholera, Fever and English Medicine 1825–1865* (Oxford, Oxford University Press, 1978), 1–19.
128. Panzac, *La Peste*, 499–501. This sort of behavior was highly unusual: Egyptian people are by and large slow to anger.
129. Ibid., 500.

2 *Dark Hidden Meanings: Leprosy and Lepers in the Medieval West and in the Tropical World under the European Imperium*

1. Henry Wright, *Leprosy and its Story: Segregation and its Remedy* (London, Parker & Co., 1885), 103–104, 106. See also: Henry Wright, *Leprosy an Imperial Danger* (London, Churchill, 1889). In the New Testament two Lazaruses are mentioned: in John 11: 1–44 the Lazarus of Bethany whom Jesus raised from the dead is the brother of Mary and Martha; in Luke 16: 19–31, Lazarus is the diseased beggar at the rich man's gate. Luke 17: 12–19 contains the parable about Jesus and the ten lepers whom he referred to priests for cure. Re Rubert Boyce, and the possibility of European settlement in India, "The Colonization of Africa," *Journal of the Royal African Society* X no. 40 (July 1911), 397.
2. George Thin, *Leprosy* (London, Percival, 1891), 7.
3. Thin, *Leprosy*, 261. For Calcutta Health Officer Acworth's affirmation of the "Imperial Danger": *Parliamentary Papers* 1895, LXXIII [Cd 7846], 203; H. A. Acworth, 'Leprosy in India," *Journal of Tropical Medicine* II (May 1899), 273. See also Sir Morell Mackenzie, "The Dreadful Revival of Leprosy," *Wood's Medical and Surgical Monographs* V (New York, Wood, 1890).
4. Patrick Feeny, *The Fight against Leprosy* (London, Elek Books, 1964), 75–92. In June 1995 the Pope presided over beatification ceremonies for Damien.
5. Mary Douglas, "Witchcraft and Leprosy: Two Strategies of Exclusion," *Man*, new series, XXVI (December 1991), 723–36; Charles Creighton, *A History of Epidemics in Britain from AD 664 to the Extinction of Plague* (Cambridge, At the University Press, 1891), 69–113; Jonathan Hutchinson, *On Leprosy and Fish-Eating: A Statement of Facts and Explanations* (London, Archibald Constable, 1906), 280–303.
6. Zachary Gussow and George S. Tracy, "Stigma and the Leprosy Phenomenon: The Social History of a Disease in the Nineteenth and Twentieth Centuries," *Bulletin of the History of Medicine* XLIV (1970), 425–49; Megan Vaughan, "Without the Camp: Institutions and Identities in the Colonial History of Leprosy," in her *Curing their Ills: Colonial Power and African Illness* (Cambridge, Polity Press, 1991), 88. See also Rita Smith Kipp, "The Evangelical Uses of Leprosy," *Social Science and Medicine* XXXIX no. 2 (1994) 165–78.
7. *PP* 1878–9 LVI [Cd 2415], 118.
8. Barry R. Bloom and Tore Godal, "Selective Primary Health Care: Strategies for Control of Disease in the Developing World. V. Leprosy," *Reviews of Infectious Disease* V no. 4 (1983), 765–80; W. C. S. Smith, "Leprosy: Elimi-

nation of Leprosy and Prospects for Rehabilitation," *The Lancet*, CCCXLI (9 January 1993), 89.

9. W. Felton Ross, "Leprosy Control: Past, Present and Future," *Proceedings of the 3rd International Workshop of Leprosy Control in Asia* (Taiwan Leprosy Relief Association, 1986), 113–14; Stephen Ell, "Diet and Leprosy in the Medieval West: The Noble Leper," *Janus: Revue Internationale* LXXII (1985), 117; S. Kartikeyan, "The Socio-Cultural Dimension in Leprosy Vaccine Trials," *Leprosy Review* LXI no. 50 (1990).

10. Ernest Muir, "Native Ideas and Practices Regarding Leprosy," *Leprosy Review* VII no. 4 (1936), 193–94.

11. I. Santra, "Survey Reports: Leprosy Survey in the Punjab," *Leprosy in India* III no. 2 (April 1931), 78; K. R. Chatterji, "Survey Reports: Report on Leprosy Survey Work Done at Salbani Police Station, Midnapore, Bengal," *Leprosy in India* IV no. 1 (January, 1932), 22; Kenneth K. Kiple, *The Caribbean Slave: A Biological History* (Cambridge, Cambridge University Press, 1984), 139; Hutchinson, *On Leprosy*: according to the *Dictionary of National Biography 1912–1921*, Hutchinson "adds much to our knowledge [of leprosy] and exposed many fallacies, but his views did not meet with wide acceptance, though he upheld them stoutly to the last."

12. L. M. Irgens, "Leprosy in Norway: An Epidemiology Study Based on a National Patient Registry," *Leprosy Review* LI, Supplement l (1980), 1–130; Acworth, "Leprosy in India," 272; Démétrius Al. Zambaco, *La Lèpre à travers les siècles et les contrées* (Paris, Masson & Cie, 1914), 180–95.

13. A partial exception in which a medical doctor edited the writings of a leper: A. Joshua-Raghavar, *Leprosy in Malaysia, Past, Present and Future*, ed. Dr K. Rajagopalan (A Joshua-Raghavar Sungai Buluh, Selangor, West Malaysia, 1983). Visit to Abou Zaabal courtesy of Dr Adel Abou-Saif of Suez Canal University.

14. Keith Manchester, "Leprosy: The Origin and Development of the Disease in Antiquity," in Danielle Gourevitch, ed., *Maladie et maladies, histoire et conceptualisation* (Geneva, Librairie Droz, 1992), 31–49.

15. F. F. Cartwright, *A Social History of Medicine* (London, Longman, 1977), 26; on the Muslim "Other": Edward Said, *Orientalism* (London: Routledge & Kegan Paul, 1978) and *Culture and Imperialism* (London, Chatto & Windus, 1993).

16. Mirko D. Grmek, *Diseases in the Ancient Greek World*, trans. Mireille Muellner and Leonard Muellner (Baltimore, MD, Johns Hopkins University Press, 1989), 153–76; Manchester, "Leprosy," 40–41. Nutton discusses the "decisive influence on medicine . . . [of] the Alexandrian Library," the principal portion of which was burned by Julius Caesar: Vivian Nutton, "Healers in the Medical Market Place: Towards a Social History of Graeco-Roman Medicine," in Andrew Wear, ed., *Medicine in Society: Historical Essays* (Cambridge, Cambridge University Press, 1992), 31–33. On the fire see Mostafa El-Abbadi, *Life and Fate of the Ancient Library of Alexandria* (Paris, UNESCO/UNDP, 1992) 2nd edition; Christian Meier, *Julius Caesar* (London, HarperCollins, 1995), 410.

17. Giovanni Tabacco, *The Struggle for Power in Medieval Italy* (Cambridge, Cambridge University Press, 1989), 49; Mary

Douglas, *Purity and Danger: An Analysis of the Concepts of Pollution and Taboo* (London, Routledge, 1966).

18. Quoted in R. I. Moore, *The Formation of a Persecuting Society: Power and Deviance in Western Europe 950–1250* (Oxford, Basil Blackwell, 1987), 48.
19. Quoted in A. Moreau-Neret, "L'Isolement des lepreux au Moyen-Age et le problème de 'lepreux errants'," *Fédération des Sociétés d'Histoire et d'Archéologie de l'Aisne: Mémoires* XVI (1970), 33; Thin, *Leprosy*, 27.
20. Mark Whittow, "Ruling the Late Roman and Early Byzantine City: A Continuous History," *Past and Present* CXXIX (November 1990), 3–29; Nutton, "Graeco-Roman," 38ff.; Nancy G. Siraisi, *Medieval & Early Renaissance Medicine* (Chicago, University of Chicago Press, 1990), 10–13; Peter Brown, *The World of Late Antiquity AD 150–750* (New York, W. W. Norton, 1989), 137–48.
21. Richard Hodges and David Whitehouse, *Mohammed, Charlemagne & the Origins of Europe* (Ithaca, NY, Cornell University Press, 1983), 88; Georges Duby, *The Age of the Cathedrals: Art and Society 980–1420*, trans. Eleanor Levieux and Barbara Thompson (Chicago, University of Chicago Press, 1981, 30–31, 34.
22. T. N. Bisson, "The 'Feudal Revolution'," *Past and Present* CXLII (February 1994), 30–4.
23. Katharine Park, "Medicine and Society in Medieval Europe, 500–1500," in Wear, *Medicine in Society*, 67, 72–75: Aron Gurevich, *Medieval Popular Culture: Problems of Belief and Perception* (Cambridge, Cambridge University Press, 1990), 39–78; Paul Fouracre, "Merovingian History and Merovingian Hagiography," *Past and Present* CXXVII (1990), 3–38. Siraisi found that one of the very few health provisioners mentioned in sixth-century texts was the professional, Byzantine-trained *castrator* living at Poitiers; Siraisi, *Medieval*, 10.
24. Godfrey Goodwin, *Islamic Spain* (London, Penguin, 1990), 42–43; Luis García-Ballester, "Changes in the *Regimina Sanitatis*: The Role of the Jewish Physicians," and Mark Zier, "The Healing Power of the Hebrew Tongue: An Example from Late Thirteenth-Century England," both in Sheila Campbell, Bert Hall and David Klausner, eds, *Health, Disease and Healing in Medieval Culture* (New York, St Martin's Press, 1992), 103–31.
25. Quoted in Grmek, *Diseases*, 171 and with slightly different wording, Michael W. Dols, "Leprosy in Medieval Arabic Medicine," *Journal of the History of Medicine* XXXIV (1979), 315. See also R. G. Cochrane and T. F. Davey, eds, *Leprosy in Theory and Practice* (Bristol, John Wright & Sons, 1964), 4.
26. Dols, "Leprosy," 314–33; Dols, "Djudhäm," *The Encyclopedia of Islam*, new edition, supplement (Leiden, E. J. Brill, 1980), 270–74. See also Haidar Abu Ahmed Mohamed, "Leprosy—The Moslem Attitude," *Leprosy Review* LVI (1985), 17–21.
27. Hutchinson, *On Leprosy*, 109. On language: Seth Schwartz, "Language, Power and Identity in Ancient Palestine," *Past and Present* CXLVIII (August 1995), 40–41.
28. H. M. Koelbing and A. Stettler-Schär, "Leprosy, Lepra, Elephantiasis Graecorum—Leprosy in Antiquity," in H. M. Koelbing *et al.*, *Beiträge zur Geschichte der Lepra* (Zurich, Juris Druck, 1972), 101. Dols affirmed in 1979 that "osteoarcheoligical

evidence . . . has produced no indication for leprosy in Biblical Palestine": Dols, "Leprosy," 317.

29. Samuel S. Kottek, *Medicine and Hygiene in the Works of Flavius Josephus* (Leiden, E. J. Brill, 1994), 42–45, 76, 78.
30. On differing interpretations of timing: Françoise Bériac, *Histoire des lépreux au Moyen Age: une société d'exclus* (Paris, Editions Imago, 1988), 38–42; Grmek, *Diseases*, 164–70; Dols, "Leprosy," 326.
31. Moore, *The Formation*, 78; Douglas, "Witchcraft and Leprosy," 723–36.
32. Susan Reynolds, *Kingdoms and Communities in Western Europe 900–1300* (Oxford, Clarendon Press 1984), 12–65; Gerald Harriss, "Political Society and the Growth of Government in Late Medieval England," *Past and Present* CXXXVIII (February 1993), 46–53. For "repute" in seventeenth-century England: Annabel Gregory, "Witchcraft, Politics and 'Good Neighbourhood'," *Past and Present* CXXXIII (November 1991), 31–66.
33. Siraisi, *Medieval*, 57–58; Zier, "Healing Power," 113; Park, "Medicine and Society," 79–80.
34. Danielle Jacquart and Claude Thomasset, *Sexuality and Medicine in the Middle Ages* (Cambridge, Polity Press, 1988), 177 (my italics).
35. Carlo Ginzburg, *Ecstasies: Deciphering the Witches' Sabbath*, trans. Raymond Rosenthal (New York, Penguin, 1991), 63–86.
36. Guy de Chauliac, *La Grande Chirvrgie*, ed. E. Nicaise (Paris, Félix Alcan, 1890), 404ff.
37. Luke Demaitre, "The Description and Diagnosis of Leprosy by Fourteenth Century Physicians," *Bulletin of the History of Medicine* LIX (1985), 327–44; Peter Richards, *The Medieval Leper and his Northern Heirs* (London, D. S. Brewer, Rowman & Littlefield, 1977), 98–99; Moreau-Neret, "L'Isolement," 28.
38. Michael R. McVaugh, *Medicine Before the Plague: Practitioners and their Patients in the Crown of Aragon, 1285–1345* (Cambridge, Cambridge University Press, 1994), 219.
39. Bériac, *Histoire*, 61.
40. Michel Foucault, *Madness and Civilization: A History of Insanity in the Age of Reason*, trans. Richard Howard (London, Tavistock, 1967), 4–5.
41. Park notes that "by the twelfth century—the high-water mark of elite concern with leprosy—about half of all new hospitals were of this kind [leprosaria]": Park, "Medicine and Society," 71.
42. Robert S. Lopez, *The Commercial Revolution of the Middle Ages, 950–1350* (Cambridge, Cambridge University Press, 1971); Georges Duby, *Rural Economy and Country Life in the Medieval West*, trans. Cynthia Postan (Columbia, University of South Carolina Press, 1968); Carlo M. Cipolla, *Before the Industrial Revolution* (New York, Norton, 1976); Janet L. Abu-Lughod, *Before European Hegemony: The World System AD 1250–1350* (Oxford, Oxford University Press, 1989), 135–47.
43. R. W. Southern, *Western Society and the Church in the Middle Ages* (Harmondsworth, Penguin, 1970), 215.
44. Quoted in Bisson, "Feudal Revolution," 42.
45. Jacques Le Goff, *L'Imaginaire médiéval: essais* (Paris, Gallimard, 1985), 145–48; Georges Duby, *The Knight, the Lady and the Priest: The Making of Modern Marriage in Medieval France*, trans. Barbara Bray (Harmondsworth, Penguin, 1983).
46. L. K. Little, *Religious Poverty and the Profit Economy in Medieval Europe* (Ithaca, NY, Cornell

University Press, 1978), 79–80; Giles Constable, "Renewal and Reform in Religious Life: Concepts and Realities," in Robert Benson and G. Constable, eds, *Renaissance and Renewal in the Twelfth Century* (Oxford, Clarendon Press, 1982), 56–57.

47. Little, *Religious Poverty*, 79–80.
48. Quoted in John Larner, *Italy in the Age of Dante and Petrarch 1216–1380* (London, Longman, 1980), 206. St Francis preached before Sultan Al-Kamil in Egypt in 1219.
49. Quoted in Saul Brody, *The Disease of the Soul: Leprosy in Medieval Literature* (Ithaca, NY, Cornell University Press, 1974), 135. The king's prison at Mansoura is now a public museum.
50. Quoted ibid., 127.
51. Gussow and Tracy, "Stigma," 425–49.
52. Marc Pegg, "Le Corps et l'authorité: la lèpre de Baudouin IV," *Annales: Economies, Sociétés, Civilisations* XL no. 2 (1990), 265–87.
53. E. Jeanselme, "Comment l'Europe, au Moyen Age, se protégea contre la lèpres," *Bulletin de la Société Française d'Histoire de la Médecine* XXV (1931), 16; Bériac, *Histoire*, 110.
54. Creighton, *Epidemics*, 107.
55. Marcus Bull, *Knightly Piety and the Lay Response to the First Crusade: The Limousin and Gascony, c. 970–1130* (Oxford, Clarendon Press, 1993), 202–206; Bisson, "Feudal Revolution'; J. H. Mundy, "Hospitals and Leprosaries in Twelfth and Early Thirteenth-Century Toulouse," in John H. Mundy, R. W. Emery and B. N. Nelson, eds, *Essays in Medieval Life and Thought* (New York, Columbia University Press, 1955), 189–91.
56. Simone Mesmin, "Waleran, Count of Meulan and the Leper Hospital of S. Gilles de Pont-Audemer," *Annales de Normandie* XXXII (1982), 18; François-Olivier Touati, "Une Approche de la maladie et du phénomène hospitalier aux XIIe et XIIIe siècles: la léproserie du Grand-Beaulieu à Chartres," *Histoire des Sciences Médicales* XIV no. l (1980), 422; Bisson, "Feudal Revolution," 36.
57. Albert Bourgeois, *Lépreux et maladreries du Pas-de-Calais: (Xe–XVIIIe Siècles)* (Arras, Commission Départementale des Monuments Historique, 1972), XIV, part 2, 35–36; Peter Pooth, "Leprosaria in Medieval West Pomerania," *International Journal of Leprosy* VII (1939), 258; Bériac, *Histoire*, 176.
58. Quoted in Little, *Religious Poverty*, 50. Jacques Le Goff, *Intellectuals in the Middle Ages* (Oxford, Basil Blackwell, 1993) makes virtually no mention of the Jewish contribution.
59. Moore, *The Formation*, 140. See also Brian Stock, *The Implications of Literacy: Written Language and Models of Interpretation in the Eleventh and Twelfth Centuries* (Cambridge, Cambridge University Press, 1983), 90.
60. Zier, "Healing Power" 114–15 (my italics).
61. Park, "Medicine and Society," 76; Siraisi, *Medieval*, 29.
62. Moore, *The Formation*, 99; Kottek, *Medicine and Hygiene*, 43; Ginzburg, *Ecstasies*, 38; Thin, *Leprosy*, 3–4; Mohamed Bey Khalil, ed., *Comptes Rendus*: V, Congrès Internationale de Médecine Tropicale et d'Hygiène, Le Caire, Egypte, Décembre, 1928 (Cairo, Government Printing Office, 1932), 295.
63. Bourgeois, *Lépreux*, 68–69; Bériac, *Histoire*, 72–73; Johs. G. Andersen, *Studies in the Medieval Diagnosis of Leprosy in Denmark: An Osteoarchaeolgical, Historical, and Clinical Study*

(Copenhagen, Useskrift for Laeger, 1969).

64. Keith Manchester and Charlotte Roberts, "The Palaeopathology of Leprosy in Britain: A Review," *World Archaeology* XII no. 2 (1989), 266–67; Michael Farley and Keith Manchester, "The Cemetery of the Leper Hospital of St Margaret, High Wycombe, Buckinghamshire," *Medieval Archaeology* XXXIII (1989), 82–89; Ell, "Diet and Leprosy," 120; Manchester, "Leprosy," 42.
65. For detailed listings of sculptural programs, Etienne Houvet, *Chartres Cathedral* (Nancy-Paris, Les Fils d'E. Spillmann, 1961); see also David Marcombe and Keith Manchester, "The Melton Mowbray 'Leper Head': An Historical and Medical Investigation," *Medical History* XXXIV (1990), 86–91; for an unsubstantiated claim about Colmar, see: Shulamith Shahar, "Des Lépreux pas comme les autres: L'Order de Saint-Lazare dans le Royaume Latin de Jérusalem," *Revue Historique* CCLXVII (1982), 39.
66. Hutchinson, *On Leprosy*, 284; Peter Richards, *Medieval Leper*, 129–36.
67. Bériac, *Histoire*, 202.
68. Gerald Strauss, *Law, Resistance, and the State: The Opposition to Roman Law in Reformation Germany* (Princeton, Princeton University Press, 1986); John Langbein, *Prosecuting Crime in the Renaissance: England, Germany, France* (Cambridge, MA, Harvard University Press, 1974).
69. De Chauliac, *La Grande Chirvrgie*, 404; Rotha Mary Clay, *The Medieval Hospitals of England* (London, Methuen, 1909), 61.
70. Quoted in Clay, *Hospitals*, 62.
71. Quoted in Creighton, *Epidemics*, 105.
72. Foucault, *Madness*, 4. See also A. S. Lyons and R. J. Petrucelli, *Medicine. An Illustrated History* (New York, Abrahams, 1978), 345, 388.
73. Creighton, *Epidemics*, 69–113; Hutchinson, *On Leprosy*, 280–303.
74. Moreau-Neret, "L'Isolement," 33.
75. Richards, *Medieval Leper*, 131–32.
76. Emannual Le Roy Ladurie, *Montaillou: The Promised Land of Error*, trans. B. Bray (New York, G. Braziller, 1978), 322.
77. Jeanselme, "Comment l'Europe," 8–27.
78. Bériac, *Histoire*, 202; Moreau-Neret, "L'Isolement," 31–33.
79. Richard Mortimer, "The Prior of Butley and the Lepers of West Somerton," *Bulletin of the Institute of Historical Research* LIII no. 127 (1980), 100.
80. Quoted ibid., 101.
81. For 1321: Malcolm Barber, "Lepers, Jews and Moslems: The Plot to Overthrow Christendom in 1321," *History* LXVI (1981), 1–17; Ginzburg, *Ecstasies*, 33–62; Charles H. Taylor, "French Assemblies and Subsidy in 1321," *Speculum: A Journal of Medieval Studies* XLII no. 2 (1968), 217–44; C. J. Tyerman, "Philip V of France, the Assemblies of 1319–20 and the Crusade," *Bulletin of the Institute of Historical Research* LVII no. 135 (1984), 15–34.
82. Quoted in Barber, "Lepers," 14.
83. McVaugh, *Medicine*, 220.
84. Bourgeois, *Lépreux*, 68; McVaugh, *Medicine*, 220.
85. Quoted in Le Roy Ladurie, *Montaillou*, 145.
86. Bériac, *Histoire*, 201; Ginzburg, *Ecstacies*, 49–53; John B. Friedman, "'He hath a Thousand Slayn this Pestilence': The Iconography of the Plague in the Late Middle Ages," in Francis X. Newman, ed., *Social Unrest in the Late Middle Ages* (Binghamton, NY, Medieval &

Renaissance Texts & Studies, 1986), 87.

87. Euan Cameron, *The European Reformation* (Oxford, Clarendon Press, 1991), 13; S. J. Watts. "The Supernatural and the Rural World," in *A Social History of Western Europe 1450–1720* (London, Hutchinson University Library, 1984), 163–211; John Bossy, *Christianity in the West* (Oxford, Oxford University Press, 1985), 1–87. Examples of the proliferation of lazar chapels in Farley and Manchester, "The Cemetery," 88.

88. Ginzburg *Ecstasies*; Norman Cohn, *Europe's Inner Demons* (London, Chatto, 1975); Richard Kieckhefer, *European Witch Trials: Their Foundations in Popular and Learned Culture, 1300–1500* (London, Routledge, 1976); Ann Hoeppner-Moran, Georgetown University, personal communication, March 1994; Demaitre, "Description and Diagnosis"; Richards, *Medieval Leper*, 98–99; Moreau-Neret, "L'Isolement," 34.

89. Creighton, *Epidemics*, 107; William McNeill, *Plagues and Peoples* (Garden City, NY, Anchor, 1976), 157.

90. Douglas, "Witchcraft and Leprosy," 725, 735; Stephen R. Ell, "Three Times, Three Places, Three Authors and One Perspective on Leprosy in Medieval and Early Modern Europe," *International Journal of Leprosy* LVII no. 4 (December 1989), 825–33.

91. Roger Chartier, *The Cultural Origins of the French Revolution*, trans. Lydia G. Cochrane (Durham, NC, Duke University Press, 1991), 113–14. Arlette Farge and Jacques Revel, *Rules of Rebellion: Child Abductions in Paris in 1750* trans. Claudia Miéville (Cambridge, Polity Press 1992).

92. P. J. Cain and A. G. Hopkins, *British Imperialism: Innovation and Expansion, 1688–1914* (London, Longman, 1993), 141 *passim.*

93. A. W. Crosby, "Hawaiian Depopulation as a Model for the Amerindian Experience," in Terence Ranger and Paul Slack, eds, *Epidemics and Ideas: Essays on the Historical Perception of Pestilence* (Cambridge, Cambridge University Press, 1992), 175–201. The 1900 census listed 29,799 Hawaiians; the 1930 only 22,636: N. E. Wayson, "Leprosy in Hawaii," *Leprosy Review* III no. 1 (January 1932), 12. By 1980 a turn-around had occurred, inspired by an Hawaiian ethnic consciousness movement. See also, Marshall Sahlins, *How "Natives" Think, About Captain Cook for Example* (Chicago, University of Chicago Press, 1995).

94. Quoted in David E. Stannard, *American Holocaust: Columbus and the Conquest of the New World* (Oxford, Oxford University Press, 1992), 144. See also: Richard Henry Dana, *Two Years Before the Mast*, (first published Boston, 1840; New York, Penguin Books, 1948), 239.

95. Quoted in Ralph S. Kuykendall, *The Hawaiian Kingdom, 1854–1874: Twenty Critical Years* (Honolulu, University of Hawaii Press, 1953), 72.

96. Ronald Takaki, *Pau Hanu: Plantation Life and Labor in Hawaii, 1835–1920* (Honolulu, University of Hawaii Press, 1983), 100; Gussow and Tracy, "Stigma," 438–41: Hawaiians did not always avoid "scientific medicine" by choice: Dana, *Before the Mast*, 240–41.

97. Quoted in James Cantlie, *Report on the Conditions under which Leprosy Occurs in China, Indo-China, Malaya, the Archipelago, and Oceania. Compiled chiefly during 1894* (London, Macmillan, 1897), 132–33;

Cantlie was editor of The *Journal of Tropical Medicine and Hygiene* from 1898 to 1925.

98. Cantlie, *Report*, 133.
99. Quoted in Kuykendall, *Hawaiian Kingdom*, 73.
100. Quoted in Wayson, "Leprosy in Hawaii," 14–15; Acworth, "Leprosy in India," 270.
101. For this and the next two paragraphs see Edward Joesting, *Kauai: The Separate Kingdom* (Honolulu, University of Hawaii Press and Kauai Museum Association, 1984), 235–39.
102. Charles S. Judd, Jr., "Leprosy in Hawaii, 1889–1976," *Hawaii Medical Journal* LXIII (1984), 328.
103. Gussow and Tracy make clear that "The outbreak of leprosy in Hawai'i was a signal event in shaping modern Western attitudes towards the disease": "Stigma," 432. See also Harm Johannes Schneider, *Leprosy and other Health Problems in Haraghe, Ethiopia* (City University of Groningen, Haarlem, 1975), 113.
104. Quoted in Cantlie, *Report*, 126–27.
105. Acworth, "Leprosy in India," 171–3; Joshua-Raghavar, *Leprosy in Malaysia*, 53.
106. R. C. Germond, "A Study of the Last Six Years of the Leprosy Campaign in Basutoland," *International Journal of Leprosy* IV (1936), 219–20; John Iliffe, *The African Poor: A History* (Cambridge, Cambridge University Press, 1987), 217; Vaughan, "Without the Camp," 77–78.
107. Maryinez Lyons, "Sleeping Sickness, Colonial Medicine and Imperialism: Some Connections in the Belgian Congo," in Roy MacLeod and Milton Lewis, eds, *Disease, Medicine, and Empire: Perspectives on Western Medicine and the Experience of European Expansion* (London, Routledge, 1988), 250–51. See also: Steven Feierman and John M. Janzen, "The Decline and Rise of African Population: The Social Context of Health and Disease: Introduction," in Feierman and Janzen, eds, *The Social Basis of Health and Healing in Africa* (Berkeley, University of California Press, 1992), 29; Dr Stanley G. Browne, OBE, "Leprosy," in E. E. Sabben-Clare, D. J. Bradley and K. Kirkwood, eds, *Health in Tropical Africa during the Colonial Period* (Oxford, Clarendon Press, 1980), 75–78; Joseph Conrad, *Heart of Darkness* (1899).
108. Cain and Hopkins, *British Imperialism*, 153–58, 293–95; "Statistics of Kasr El Ainy Hospital, 1900," *Records of the Egyptian Government Faculty of Medicine* (Cairo, Government Press, 1927), 200–201; Dr Naguib Scandar, "Le Lèpre en Egypt," *Comptes Rendus* V, (1932), 296; Robert G. Cochrane, *Leprosy in India: A Survey* (London, World Dominion Press, 1927), 22; Amira el Azhary Sonbol, *The Creation of a Medical Profession in Egypt, 1800–1922* (Syracuse, NY, Syracuse University Press, 1991), 108; Ronald Hyam, *Empire and Sexuality: the British Experience* (Manchester, Manchester University Press, 1990), 132; H. H. Johnson, "Lord Cromer's 'Modern Egypt'," *Journal of the African Society* VII (October 1907), 247. With the introduction of multiple drug therapy in Egypt in 1988, prevalence has dropped to an official 0.8 per 10,000; however, the detection rate continues to rise: Gobara Khalafalla, "The Optimism is Perhaps Justifiable," *World Health Forum* XVII no. 2 (1996), 131.
109. Iliffe, *African Poor*, 227.
110. O. F. Atkey, "Leprosy Control in South Sudan," *International Journal of Leprosy* I (1935), 78; Iliffe, *African Poor*, 220; *Journal*

of Tropical Medicine (September 1898), 55; Cochrane, *Leprosy in India*, 22–25.

111. Beaven Rake *et al.*, *Leprosy in India: Report of the Leprosy Commission in India 1890–91* (Calcutta, Superintendent of Government Printing, India, 1892), 150. After building the case that leprosy was not an "Imperial Danger," requiring compulsory segregation at government expense, the commissioners backtracked and recommended that voluntary segregation be permitted: Khan Bahadur Choksy, MD, "Leprosy Legislation in India," *Lepra* X (1910), 134–41.

112. Rake, *Leprosy Commission Report*, 140; Ernest Muir, "Methods of Campaign against Leprosy in India," *Leprosy Review* III no. 2 (April 1931), 53; V. S. Upadhyay, *Socio-Cultural Implications of Leprosy: An essay in medical anthropology* (Ranchi, Maitryee Publications, 1988), 6; Khalil, *Comptes Rendus* V, 273; Ernest Muir, "Leprosy in Sierra Leone," *Leprosy Review* VII no. 4 (October 1936), 192. Today 70 percent of all lepers are found in the WHO region "South East Asia" (region excludes Pakistan): *The World Health Report 1996: Fighting Disease, Fostering Development* (Geneva, WHO, 1996), 29.

113. Muir, "Methods of Campaign," 55; Barry R. Bloom and Tore Godal, "Selective Primary Health Care: Strategies for Control of Disease in the Developing World: V. Leprosy," *Reviews of Infectious Diseases* IV (July–August 1983), 772; R. Premkumar, "Understanding the Attitude of Multidisciplinary Teams Working in Leprosy," *Leprosy Review* LXV (1994), 74–75; A. D. Power, "A British Empire Leprosarium," *Journal of the Royal African Society* XXXVIII no. 150 (January 1939), 467. For comments suggestive of the continuing difficulty of incorporating leprosy services (with their tradition of dedicated volunteers) into regular regional health services: S. K. Noordeen, "Eliminating Leprosy as a Public Health Problem—Is the Optimism Justified?," *World Health Forum: an International Journal of Health Development* (WHO, Geneva) XVII no. 2 (1996), 117.

114. E. B. van Heyningen, "Agents of Empire: the medical profession in the Cape Colony, 1880–1910," *Medical History* XXXIII (1989), 456.

115. Joshua-Raghavar, *Leprosy in Malaysia*, 54

116. I. Santra, "Reports of Leprosy Survey," *Leprosy in India* II no. 4 (October 1930), 140; Cochrane, *Leprosy in India*, 61; T. G. Mayer, "Leprosy in Nigeria," *Leprosy in India* II no. 4 (October 1930), 132–33.

117. G. Heaton Nicholls, "Empire Settlement in Africa in its Relation to Trade and the Native Races," *Journal of the African Society* XXV no. 98 (January 1926), 109; Iliffe, *African Poor*, 216–17.

118. A. G. de la P., "Lundu, the Leper Isle," *Central Africa* XXVII (1909), 214.

119. Quoted in L. Langauer, "Leprosy in Benin and Warri Provinces of Nigeria," *Leprosy Review* XI no. 1 (January 1940), 97. See also: "Report on Dr. Muir's Tour: Leprosy in Nigeria," *Leprosy Review* XI no. 1 (January 1940), 62; Marc Dawson, "The Social History of Africa in the Future: Medical Related Issues," *African Studies Review* XXX (1987), 83–91; van Heyningen, "Agents of Empire," 468; Charles M. Good, "Pioneer Medical Missions in Colonial Africa," *Social Science and Medicine* XXX no. 1 (1991),

8; John Iliffe, "Leprosy," in his *African Poor*, 214–29; Megan Vaughan, "The Great Dispensary in the Sky: Medical Missionaries," and "Without the Camp: Institutions and Identities in the Colonial History of Leprosy" in her *Curing Their Ills*, 55–99; Terence Ranger, "Godly Medicine: The Ambiguities of Medical Mission in Southeast Tanzania, 1900–1945," in Feierman and Janzen, *Social Basis*, 256–82; Kipp, "Evangelical Uses of Leprosy".

120. M. Elizabeth Duncan, "Leprosy and Procreation—A Historical Review of Social and Clinical Aspects," *Leprosy Review* LVI no. 2 (1985), 160.

121. J. Mérab, *Impressions d'Éthiopie: L'Abyssinie sous Ménélik II* (Paris, H. Libert, 1921), 161 (my translation).

122. H. W., "The Leper's Fate," *Central Africa* no. 110 (February 1892), 28.

123. Quoted in Vaughan, *Curing Their Ills*, 95.

124. Gussow and Tracy, "Stigma," 446; Vaughan, *Curing Their Ills*, 88. See also Marian Ulrich *et al.*, "Leprosy in Women: Characteristics and Repercussions," *Social Science and Medicine* XXXVII no. 4 (1993), 445.

125. H. W., "The Leper's Fate," 28.

126. Ranger, "Godly Medicine'. Ranger notes that by the second and third decades of the twentieth century, "disease was perceived by Africans to be increasing rather than decreasing": Ranger, "Medical Science and Pentecost: The Dilemma of Anglicanism in Africa," in W. J. Shiels, ed., *Studies in Church History*, XIV: *The Church and Healing* (Oxford, Basil Blackwell, 1982), 338.

127. E. Cannon, "The Preparation of Converts for Baptism," *Report on a Conference of Leper Asylum Superintendents and Others* (Cuttack, Orissa Mission Press, 1920), 136.

128. W. C. Irvine, "Christian Teaching and Spiritual Work in the Asylums," ibid., 134–35.

129. Ibid., 134.

130. Frank Oldrieve, *India's Lepers: How to Rid India of Leprosy* (London, Marshall Brothers, 1924), 46–47.

131. "Colonial Medical Reports: No. 24: Southern Nigeria (1905)," *Journal of Tropical Medicine* IX (1906), 61.

132. Quoted in Iliffe, *African Poor*, 218.

133. Rubert Boyce, "The Colonization of Africa," *Journal of the African Society* X no. 40 (1911), 395.

134. Quoted in Robert Strayer, *The Making of Mission Communities in East Africa: Anglicans and Africans in Colonial Kenya, 1875–1935* (London, Heinemann, 1978), 5.

135. Frederick Shelford, "Ten Years' Progress in West Africa," *Journal of the African Society* VI (1906–1907), 348; Margery Perham, ed., *The Diaries of Lord Lugard* III (Evanston, IL, Northwestern University Press, 1959), 19–61.

136. W. P., "The Black Man as Patient," *Central Africa* XX no. 231 (March 1902), 45–47.

137. James Cantlie, "Livingstone College: Address, May 31, 1906," *Journal of Tropical Medicine* IX (16 July 1906), 222 (my italics).

138. Ronald Ross, "Missionaries and the Campaign against Malaria," *Journal of Tropical Medicine and Hygiene* XIII (15 June 1910), 183.

139. "Two Scenes," *Central Africa* XXVII no. 317 (May 1909), 129. For a similar UMCA report from Zanzibar: G. M. Dawson, "A Visit to the Lepers," *Central Africa* no. 531 (March 1927), 43.

140. "Medical Missionaries," *Journal of Tropical Medicine* I (December 1898), 133.

141. Cochrane, *Leprosy in India*, 61;

E. Muir, "Reports," *Leprosy Review* XI no. 1 (January 1940), 5.

142. Sir Rupert Briercliffe, "Leprosy in Nigeria," *Leprosy Review* XI no. 1 (January, 1940), 86; "Leprosy in Nigeria," ibid., 53–54, 67.

143. Justin Willis, "The Nature of a Mission Community: The Universities' Mission to Central Africa in Bonde," *Past and Present* CXL (August 1993), 127–54. On the European background see Strayer, *Making of Mission Communities*; T. O. Beidelman, *Colonial Evangelism: A Socio-historical Study of an East African Mission at the Grassroots* (Bloomington, Indiana University Press, 1982).

144. Willis, "Mission Community," 147. Typical words handed down by a missionary education officer in East Africa in 1912: "religiously, perhaps, all men are brethren: politically the negro will forever be a child": quoted in Strayer, *Making of Mission Communities*, 102.

145. A. C. Howard, "Leprosy in Nigeria," *International Journal of Leprosy* IV (1936), 76; Browne (director of leprosy research at Uzuakoli 1959–1966), "Leprosy," 71ff.

146. "Editorials: Dr. Davey's *Report on Leprosy Control in the Owerri Province, S. Nigeria*," *Leprosy Review* XI no. 1 (January 1940), 122. See also: Ernest Muir, "The Leprosy Situation in Africa," *Journal of the Royal African Society* XXXIX (1940), 142.

147. Muir, "1939 Tour," *Leprosy Review* XI no. 1 (January 1940).

148. H. C. Armstrong, "Account of Visit to Leprosy Institutions in Nigeria," *Leprosy Review* VI no. 3 (July 1935), 157–58. See also, Willis, "Mission Community".

149. Bernard Moiser, "A Description of the Work at the Leprosy Hospital at Ngomahuru, Southern Rhodesia," *Leprosy Review* IV no. 1 (January 1933), 14; Browne, "Leprosy," 72–74.

150. Browne, "Leprosy," 74. See also: E. A. Ayandele, *The Missionary Impact on Modern Nigeria: 1842–1914: A Political and Social Analysis* (London, Longman, 1966), 329; Tim Keegan, "The Crushing of the Eastern Cape: Review of Les Switzer, *Power and Resistance in an African Society: The Ciskei Xhosa and the Making of South Africa* (1994)" in *Times Literary Supplement* 29 April 1994, 25.

151. Review of Hansen's *Leprosy*, *Journal of Tropical Medicine*, 1 (10 November 1895), 176.

152. Cochrane, *Leprosy in India*, 1; Iliffe, *African Poor*, 219.

153. Iliffe, *African Poor*, 225.

154. Cochrane, *Leprosy in India*, 1; Choksy, "Leprosy Legislation," 139.

155. "Report on the Philippine Leprosy Commission," *International Journal of Leprosy* III no. 4 (1935), 392; Khalil, *Comptes Rendus* V, 273; Joshua Raghavar, *Leprosy in Malaysia*, 48; Wayson, "Leprosy in Hawaii". For the continuing legacy of the early twentiety-century Hobbesian approach: Manuel G. Roxas, "Optimism in the Philippines," *World Health Forum* XVII no. 2 (1996), 119. See also Rodney Sullivan, "Cholera and Colonialism in the Philippines, 1899–1903," in MacLeod and Lewis, *Disease, Medicine and Empire*, 284–300, 296.

156. Khalil, *Comptes Rendus* V, 285.

157. Nicholls, "Empire Settlement," 105–16; Muir, "Leprosy in Africa," 138; Randall M. Packard, *White Plague, Black Labour: Tuberculosis and the Political Economy of Health and Disease in South Africa* (London, James Currey, 1989).

158. Joshua-Raghavar, *Leprosy in Malaysia*, 59, 61.

159. Quoted in Vaughan, *Curing Their Ills*, 81.

160. Muir, "Methods of Campaign," 52, 60.
161. Santra, "Reports of Leprosy Survey," 138; Chatterji, "Survey Reports," 22; Santra, "Leprosy Survey in the Punjab," 78, lists as "predisposing causes" that "90% of lepers suffer from syphilis or gonorrhoea."
162. A. C. Stanley Smith, "Leprosy in Kigezi, Uganda Protectorate," *Leprosy Review* II (4) 1931, 72.
163. Quoted in Mérab, *Impressions*, 166. Richard Pankhurst, "The History of Leprosy in Ethiopia to 1935," *Medical History* XXVIII (1984), 57–72; E. Muir, "How Leprosy is Spread in the Indian Village," 64; Cochrane, *Leprosy in India*, 25–26.
164. F. Shelford, "Ten Years," 348. See also the entry "Mohammedanism" in the American publication *The Encyclopedia of Missions* 1st edition 1891, 2nd edition 1904, 484–85.
165. Strayer, *Making of Mission Communites*, 6–7; Anon., "The Conversion of the Moslem World: A Suggestion," *Central Africa* XLV no. 53 (February 1927), 33; Nicholls, "Empire Settlement," 116.
166. Schneider, *Leprosy*, 112: Dols, entry for "Leprosy," *Encyclopedia of Islam*; Mohamed, "Leprosy—the Moslem Attitude," 19.
167. Mayer, "Leprosy in Nigeria," 133; Howard, "Leprosy in Nigeria," 77–78. For the situation in the North in 1910–11: R. R. Kuczynski, *Demographic Survey of the British Colonial Empire* I, *West Africa* (Oxford, Royal Institute of International Affairs, Oxford University Press, 1948), 738–39.
168. W. F. Ross, "Leprosy Control," 12; S. K. Noordeen, B. Lopez and T. Sundaresan, "Estimated Number of Leprosy Cases in the World," *Leprosy Review* LXIII (3) 1992, 282–87. In 1993, in ninety countries, "there were 2.3 million patients registered for treatment (*known prevalence*) of which only 1.1 million cases were on [multiple drug therapy]. The estimated number of new cases (*incidence*) is 900,000 a year." Feenstra carefully distinguishes between *prevalence* (registered cases, which are dropping rapidly in number because of the quick turnaround MDT permits, and *incidence*—the number of new cases each year—which seems *not* to be dropping much since MDT came into being in 1982: D. Feenstra, "Will there be a need for Leprosy Control Services in the 21st Century?" *Leprosy Review*, LXV (1994), 298. See also: Paul C. Y. Chen, "Bringing Leprosy into the Open," *World Health Forum* IX (1988), 323–25. Because of the collapse of health services in Third World countries due to structural adjustment policies it is likely that leprosy will be around at least for another generation: Sheena Asthana, "Economic Crisis, Adjustment and the Impact on Health," in David R. Phillips and Yola Verhasselt, eds, *Heath and Development* (London, Routledge, 1994), 50–64. In an attempt to counter this, the Sasakawa Foundation of Japan pledged to supply MDT drugs to all leprosy-endemic countries for five years: WHO, *Leprosy News* IV no. l (April 1995).
169. Upadhyay, *Socio-Cultural Implications*, 103.

3 *Smallpox in the New World and in the Old: From Holocaust to Eradication, 1518 to 1977*

1. For the Establishment position: Douglas H. Ubelaker, "Patterns of Demographic Change in the Americas," *Human Biology* LXIV no. 3 (June 1992); John

W. Verano and Douglas H. Ubelaker, eds, *Disease and Demography in the Americas* (Washington, DC, Smithsonian Institution Press, 1992); Clark Spencer Larsen and George R. Milner, eds, *In the Wake of Contact: Biological Responses to Conquest* (New York, Wiley-Liss, 1994). For representative cultural relativists: Henry F. Dobyns, *Their Number Became Thinned: Native American Population Dynamics in Eastern North America* (Knoxville, University of Tennessee Press, 1983); W. George Lovell, " 'Heavy Shadows and Black Night': Disease and Depopulation in Colonial Spanish America," *Annals of the Association of American Geographers* LXXXII no. 3 (1992). For the Smithsonian Institution's confrontational attitude towards contemporary Native Americans: Donald J. Ortner, "Skeletal Paleopathology: Probabilities, Possibilities, and Impossibilities," in Verano and Ubelaker, *Disease and Demography*, 12–13; David William Cohen, *The Combing of History* (Chicago, University of Chicago Press, 1994), 4ff.

2. On question posing: Donald Joralemon, "New World Depopulation and the Case of Disease," *Journal of Anthropological Research* XXXVIII (1982); Lovell, " 'Heavy Shadows and Black Night' "; Russell Thornton, Tim Miller and Jonathan Warren; "American Indian Population Recovery Following Smallpox Epidemics," *American Anthropologist* XCIII (1991), 38–41.

3. "Smallpox was the captain of the men of death in [the New World biological war], typhus fever the first lieutenant, and measles the second lieutenant. . . . They were the forerunners of civilization, the companions of Christianity, the friends of the invader": P. M. Ashburn, MD (1947), quoted in Joralemon, "The Case of Disease," 112.

4. Murrin reminds us that *had they but kept up alive and in breeding form*, the Native American population of 1492 would have "outnumbered all European immigrants to 1820 by a ratio of perhaps twenty-five to one and all the Africans who arrived by maybe nine to one": John M. Murrin, "Beneficiaries of Catastrophe: The English Colonies in America," in Eric Foner, ed., *The New American History* (Philadelphia, Temple University Press, 1990), 7.

5. For China see Chapter 4 (syphilis); for India, Chapter 5 (cholera). Ubelaker asserts that pre-Columbian New World people were in fact troubled by "Tuberculosis, treponemal disease, respiratory disease, and parasitism [which] joined with other infectious diseases to produce high infant mortality and significant health problems throughout much of the New World" and warns against a "Rousseauist image of a huge number of American Indians living in harmony in a disease free paradise"; Ubelaker, "Patterns of Demographic Change," 364–65.

6. Alex Mercer, *Disease Mortality and Population in Transition* (Leicester, Leicester University Press, 1990), 70. Carmichael and Silverstein date the change in virulence in England and probably on the Continent to the mid-seventeenth century: Ann G. Carmichael and Arthur M. Silverstein, "Smallpox in Europe before the Seventeenth Century: Virulent Killer or Benign Disease?", *Journal of the History of Medicine* XLII (1987), 161; Hardy, however, holds that gradually increasing virulence did not peak until the *mid-nineteenth* century, and that earlier strains

"in England and perhaps in Europe" were relatively mild: Anne Hardy, "Smallpox in London: Factors in the Decline of the Disease in the Nineteenth Century," *Medical History* XXVII (1983), 113.

7. Deborah Brunton, "Smallpox Inoculation and Demographic Trends in Eighteenth Century Scotland," *Medical History* XXXVI (1992), 409; J. R. Smith, *The Speckled Monster: Smallpox in England 1670–1970, with Particular Reference to Essex* (Chelmsford, Essex Record Office, 1987), 173.
8. Smith, *Speckled Monster*, 179–80. The classic medically informed account is C. W. Dixon, *Smallpox* (London, J. and A. Churchill, 1962).
9. Russell Thornton, J. Warren and T. Miller, "Depopulation in the Southeast after 1492," in Verano and Ubelaker, *Disease and Demography*, 191.
10. Quoted in Joralemon, "The Case of Disease," 118.
11. Hanns J. Prem, "Disease Outbreaks in Central Mexico during the Sixteenth Century," in Noble David Cook and W. George Lovell, *"Secret Judgments of God": Old World Disease in Colonial Spanish America* (Norman, University of Oklahoma Press, 1991), 31–33; Cook and Lovell, "Unravelling the Web of Disease," in *"Secret Judgments"*, 213–43; Guenter Risse, "Medicine in New Spain," in Ronald L. Numbers, ed., *Medicine in the New World: New Spain, New France, and New England* (Knoxville, University of Tennessee Press, 1987), 27; Carmichael and Silverstein, "Smallpox in Europe," 151–54; Raymond A. Anselment, "Smallpox in Seventeenth Century English Literature: Reality and the Metamorphosis of Wit," *Medical History* XXXIII (1989), 75. Joralemon lists diseases confused with smallpox at different stages: "The Case of Disease," 120. The problem of diagnosing multiple-disease crises was made more difficult after the influential British clinician John Hunter (1728–93) announced that "nature" sent only one disease enemy at any one time and that no one could suffer from two diseases simultaneously: Yves-Marie Bercé, *Le Chaudron et la lancette: croyances populaires et médecine préventive (1798–1830)* (Paris, Presses de la Renaissance, 1984), 245.
12. Suzanne Austin Alchon, *Native Society and Disease in Colonial Ecuador* (Cambridge, Cambridge University Press, 1991), 24; Cook and Lovell, *"Secret Judgments"*, 213.
13. Quoted in Ronald Wright, *Stolen Continents: The Indian Story* (London, Pimlico, 1993), 19–21, 30–32. See also: Inga Clendinnen, "The Cost of Courage in Aztec Society," *Past and Present* CVII (1985), 44–6. In 1506, Pope Julius II gave orders that Old St Peter's be torn down, creating another zone of desolation in what had been the built-up area of the medieval city.
14. Quoted in David E. Stannard, *American Holocaust: Columbus and the Conquest of the New World* (New York, Oxford University Press, 1992), 7–8.
15. David Henige, "When Did Smallpox Reach the New World (And Why Does It Matter)?," in Paul E. Lovejoy, ed., *Africans in Bondage: Studies in Slavery and the Slave Trade: Essays in Honor of Philip D. Curtin* (Madison, African Studies Program, University of Wisconsin Press, 1986), 11–26.
16. Henige, "Why Does It Matter?" 17; Francisco Guerra, "The Earliest American Epidemic: The Influenza of 1493," *Social Sci-*

ence History XII (1988), 305–25; Samuel M. Wilson, *Hispaniola: Caribbean Chiefdoms in the Age of Columbus* (Tuscaloosa, University of Alabama Press, 1990), 2, 95–96, 135; Stannard, *American Holocaust*, 47–9.

17. Henige, "Why Does It Matter?" 17; Hugh Thomas, *Conquest: Montezuma, Cortés, and the Fall of Old Mexico* (New York, Simon & Schuster, 1993), xii; Wright, *Stolen Continents*, 44–47.
18. Bernardino de Sahagún, *Florentine Codex: General History of the Things of New Spain: Book 12—The Conquest of Mexico*, trans. Arthur J. O. Anderson and Charles E. Dibble (Salt Lake City, University of Utah Press, 1955), 81.
19. Quoted in Stannard, *American Holocaust*, 79.
20. Quoted ibid. According to Elliott, Cortés in old age retirement in his town-house in Madrid was the center of "an 'academy' holding regular discussions on matters of humanist and religious concerns." The man was much admired by the Franciscans who wrote of him "in their histories of the Conquest as the man chosen of God to prepare the way for the evangelization of mankind": J. H. Elliott, *Spain and its World 1500–1700: Selected Essays* (London, Yale University Press, 1989), 41. In his brilliant summing up of the findings of the international conference, "America in European Consciousness 1493–1750" at the John Carter Brown Library, Providence, Rhode Island, USA, 9 June 1991, Sir John managed to avoid mention of the little unpleasantnesses which the Spanish and the Portuguese brought to the New World; talk revised as: "Final Reflections: The Old World and the New Revisited," in Karen Ordahl Kupperman, ed., *America in European Consciousness 1493–1750* (Chapel Hill, University of North Carolina Press, 1995).
21. On Aztec religious sacrifice: Clendinnen, "The Cost of Courage," 44–89.
22. Serge Gruzinski, *The Conquest of Mexico: The Incorporation of Indian Societies into the Western World, 16th–18th Centuries*, trans. Eileen Corrigan (Cambridge, Polity Press, 1993), 81; James Lockhart, *The Nahuas after the Conquest: A Social and Cultural History of the Indians of Central Mexico, Sixteenth through Eighteenth Centuries* (Stanford, CA, Stanford University Press, 1992), 112–16.
23. Lovell, "'Heavy Shadows and Black Night'," 435–7; Woodrow Borah, "Introduction" in Cook and Lovell, "*Secret Judgments*", 15; Wright, *Stolen Continents*, 64–83.
24. Hardy, "Smallpox in London," 111–12; Ann G. Carmichael, "Infection, Hidden Hunger, and History," *Journal of Interdisciplinary History* XIV no. 2 (Autumn 1983), 255; Mercer, *Disease Mortality*, 46; Frank Fenner, *Smallpox and its Eradication* (Geneva, WHO, 1988), 229; Anselment, "Metamorphosis of Wit," 74–79; Charles Creighton, *History of Epidemics in Britain*, 2nd edition (London, Frank Cass, 1965), 615.
25. Clara Sue Kidwell, "Aztec and European Medicine in the New World, 1521–1600," in Lola Romanucci-Ross, D. Moerman and L. Tancredi, *The Anthropology of Medicine: From Culture to Method* (New York, Praeger, 1982), 23; Borah, "Introduction" in "*Secret Judgments*," 13. See also Alfredo López Austin, *The Human Body and Ideology: Concepts of the Ancient Nahuas*, trans. T. and B. Ortiz de Montellano (Salt Lake City, University of Utah Press, 1988), I,

Chapters 5–6; Risse, "Medicine in New Spain," 51. On European notions about empirics, see Chapter 1, "Plague."

26. Quoted in Stannard, *American Holocaust*, 89, quoting from the standard work, John Hemming, *The Conquest of the Incas* (1970) (New York, Harcourt Brace Jovanovich, 1970), 372.
27. Wright, *Stolen Continents*, 185.
28. Noble D. Cook, *Demographic Collapse: Indian Peru, 1520–1620* (Cambridge, Cambridge University Press, 1981), 60–1.
29. Ann Ramenofsky, *Vectors of Death: The Archaeology of European Contact* (Albuquerque, University of New Mexico Press, 1987).
30. Henry F. Dobyns, "More Methodological Perspectives on Historical Demography," *Ethnohistory* XXXVI no. 3 (Summer 1989) 288–89; Wright, *Stolen Continents*, 123–24.
31. Quoted in Wright, *Stolen Continents*, 123.
32. Quoted in Andrew Delbanco, *The Puritan Ordeal* (Cambridge, MA, Harvard University Press, 1989), 106. On identification of this disease see: Timothy L. Bratton, "The Identity of the New England Indian Epidemic of 1616–1619," *Bulletin of the History of Medicine* LXII (1988), 375–83. See also: Catherine C. Carlson, George J. Armelagos and Ann L. Magennis, "Impact of Disease on the Precontact and Early Historic Populations of New England and the Maritimes," in Verano and Ubelaker, *Disease and Demography*, 148, 150.
33. Quoted in Bratton, "Identity of . . . 1616–1619", 38.
34. Quoted in Alfred W. Crosby, *Ecological Imperialism: The Biological Expansion of Europe, 900–1900* (Cambridge, Cambridge University Press, 1986), 208; 950 of the 1,000 Native Americans around Hartford died of smallpox that same winter: Carolyn Merchant, *Ecological Revolutions; Nature, Gender, and Science in New England* (Chapel Hill, University of North Carolina Press, 1989), 90.
35. Cook and Lovell, "*Secret Judgments*"; Dauril Alden and Joseph C. Miller, "Out of Africa: The Slave Trade and the Transmission of Smallpox to Brazil, 1560–1831," *Journal of Interdisciplinary History* XVIII no. 2 (Autumn 1987), 199; Stannard, *American Holocaust*, 91–93; Claude Lévi-Strauss, "The River of Sorrows," *The Times Higher Education Supplement*, 1 September 1995, 15–17.
36. Quoted in Crosby, *Ecological Imperialism*, 215. In addressing the question of Native American susceptibility to Old World diseases, such as smallpox, the American upper South historian K. Kiple holds: "in part [their pre-1492] epidemiological exemption occurred because most Indian populations *had not attained a sufficient density* to sustain many of the diseases in question. . . . The major reason, however, stemmed from the isolation of America from a world that in establishing *higher and higher levels of civilization* (and consequently dense urban populations) had inadvertently stimulated higher and higher levels of parasite activity as well" (my italics); Kenneth F. Kiple, *The Caribbean Slave: A Biological History* (New York, Cambridge University Press, 1984), 10. Kiple contributed to the Smithsonian Institution publication listed in note 1.
37. The fiction of Native Americans as *homunculi* was the subject of a famous essay *Democrates Alter O Secundus, Sive de Justis Belli Causis Apud Indos* written *c.* 1542 by theologian Juan Ginés de

Sepúlveda, the stay-at-home defender of the right of Spanish colonists to rule over aboriginals in any way they saw fit. Juan de Matienzo, a Spanish jurist actually out in Peru in 1567 (where aboriginals were dying all around from epidemic disease and slave labor), regarded indigenous people as "animals who do not even feel reason, but are ruled by their passions": quoted in H. C. Porter, *The Inconstant Savage: England and the North American Indian, 1500–1660* (London, Duckworth, 1979), 167. See also: Elliott, *Spain and its World*, 49.

38. Porter, *Inconstant Savage*, 157; Irving Rouse, *The Tainos: Rise and Decline of the People Who Greeted Columbus* (New Haven, CT, Yale University Press, 1993).

39. Quoted in Thomas, *Conquest*, xii. Marcus Aurelius' *Meditations* were first set up in print in 1558, which brought them to a wider public.

40. Angus MacKay, *Spain in the Middle Ages: From Frontier to Empire, 1000–1500* (Basingstoke, Macmillan, 1977), 121–97; Henry Kamen, *Inquisition and Society in Spain in the Sixteenth and Seventeenth Century* (Bloomington, Indiana University Press, 1985), 161–97.

41. Quoted in Henry Kamen, *Spain 1469–1714: A Society of Conflict* 2nd edition (London, Longman, 1991), 18.

42. Ida Altman, "A New World in the Old: Local Society and Spanish Emigration to the Indies," in Ida Altman and James Horn, eds, *"To Make America": European Emigration in the Early Modern Period* (Berkeley, University of California Press, 1991), 31.

43. Porter, *Inconstant Savage*, 160; Kamen, *Spain 1469–1714*, 38–44; Jonathan I. Israel, *European Jewry in the Age of Mercantilism 1550–1750*, revised edition (Oxford, Clarendon Press, 1991), 3–4.

44. Thomas, *Conquest*, 359.

45. Bartholomé de Las Casas, *History of the Indies*, trans. J. Collard (New York, Harper & Row, 1971), 94 (my italics). As is well known, in creating the "Black Legend" which stressed Spanish sadism and greed, for didactic reasons Las Casas all but neglected to mention the impact of disease in depopulating the Americas: Cook and Lovell, *"Secret Judgments"*, 241.

46. Kamen, *Spain 1469–1714*, 18. The classic study is Tzvetan Todorov, *The Conquest of America*, trans. Richard Howard (New York, Harper Torchbook, 1992), first published in Paris in 1982 and dedicated "to the memory of a Mayan woman devoured by dogs" for the amusement of the Spanish.

47. Quoted in Porter, *Inconstant Savage*, 162–63.

48. Quoted in Anthony Pagden, *European Encounters with the New World: From Renaissance to Romanticism* (New Haven, CT, Yale University Press, 1993), 67; Pagden seems to accept Oviedo's benevolent self-image at face value. For a reading of Oviedo as literate terrorist see Porter, *Inconstant Savage*, 161–66; Porter's printing history (Toledo, 1526) agrees with that of Francisco Guerra, "The Dispute over Syphilis: Europe versus America," *Clio Medica* XII no. 1 (1978), 44, 46.

49. Quoted in Todorov, *Conquest*, 150–1.

50. Quoted in David Englander *et al.*, *Culture and Belief in Europe 1450–1600* (Oxford, Basil Blackwell, 1990), 323. Sepúlveda never travelled to America to study Aztec customs for himself, yet arrived at conclusions not much different from those of Oviedo, who according to

Pagden, sailed back and forth across the Atlantic four times; Pagden, *European Encounters*, 58.

51. Porter, *Inconstant Savage*, 160; Anthony Pagden, "Dispossessing the Barbarian: The Language of Spanish Thomism and the Debate over the Property Rights of the American Indians," in A. Pagden, ed., *The Languages of Political Theory in Early Modern Europe*, (Cambridge, Cambridge University Press, 1987), 79–98. On Hobbes, Locke and the English, see: C. B. MacPherson, *The Political Theory of Possessive Individualism* (Oxford, Clarendon Press, 1962).
52. Altman and Horn, "*To Make America*", 2.
53. "The devil stalked the America of the sixteenth century": Elliott, *Spain and its World*, 59. One of the characteristics of people who think in binary terms—"Us" and "The Other"—is that all outsiders are lumped together as one undifferentiated "Other." This parochialism necessarily masks the cultural diversity of the real world: on this see Edward W. Said, *Culture and Imperialism* (London, Chatto & Windus, 1993), 23–24 and *passim*.
54. Gerónimoi de Mendieta, Franciscan, quoted in Stannard, *American Holocaust*, 219.
55. Quoted ibid. 114.
56. James Axtell, *The European and the Indian: Essays in the Ethnohistory of Colonial North America* (New York, Oxford University Press, 1981); John Demos, *The Unredeemed Captive* (New York, Alfred A. Knopf, 1994); Jack P. Greene, *Imperatives, Behaviors, and Identities: Essays in Early American Cultural History* (Charlottesville, University Press of Virginia, 1992), 1–11.
57. Quoted in John Keane, *Thomas Paine: A Political Life* (London, Bloomsbury, 1995), 150. Keane reminds us that in the Declaration of Independence, Native Americans were denounced as "merciless Indian savages" whom George III set against honest settler colonists.
58. Norman Gelb, ed., *Jonathan Carver's Travels Through America 1766–1768: An Eighteenth-Century Explorer's Account of Uncharted America* (New York, John Wiley & Sons, 1994), 209–10. See also, Frank Shuffleton, "Thomas Jefferson: Race, Culture and the Failure of the Anthropological Method," in Frank Shuffleton, ed., *A Mixed Race: Ethnicity in Early America* (New York, Oxford University Press, 1993), 265–68.
59. Fenner quotes the written exchange between Amherst and the local commander: "Amherst: 'Could it not be contrived to send smallpox among these disaffected tribes of Indians? We must on this occasion use every stratagem in our power to reduce them'.

    Local commander: 'I will try to inoculate the * * * * with some blankets that may fall in their hands, and take care not to get the disease myself'": Frank Fenner, *The History of Smallpox and its Spread around the World* (Geneva, WHO, 1988), 239.
60. Quoted in D. Peter MacLeod, "Microbes and Muskets: Smallpox and the Participation of the Amerindian Allies of New France in the Seven Years' War," *Ethnohistory*, XXXI no. 1 (Winter 1992), 49–50.
61. Wright, *Stolen Continents*, 211–21; John C. Hudson, *Making the Corn Belt: A Geographical History of Middle-Western Agriculture* (Bloomington, University of Indiana Press, 1994); Hugh Brogan, *The Pelican History of the United States of America* (London, Pelican, 1986), 55–70.
62. Quoted in Carolyn Gilman, *The*

Grand Portage Story (St Paul, Minnesota Historical Society Press, 1992), 63, 145.

63. Michael K. Trimble, "The 1832 Inoculation Program on the Missouri River," in Verano and Ubelaker, *Disease and Demography*, 257–65; Richard H. Frost, "The Pueblo Indian Smallpox Epidemic in New Mexico, 1898–1899," *Bulletin of the History of Medicine* LXIV (1990), 417–18; Robert Boyd, "Population Decline from Two Epidemics on the Northwest Coast," in Verano and Ubelaker, *Disease and Demography*, 251.

64. Ralph W. Nicholas, "The Goddess Sitala and Epidemic Smallpox in Bengal," *Journal of Asian Studies* XLI no. 1 (1981), 2, 25–27. Indigenous Indian practice in the eighteenth century can be contrasted with later ideas of the British occupying force. In the 1870s, the Army Sanitation Commission regarded the isolation of the sick as merely a "theoretical measure" and held to the "practical" wisdom of giving smallpox patients access to "pure air and pure water" in order to prevent their illness from becoming really serious. *Parliamentary Papers* 1876 LVI [Cd 1615], 39; *P.P.* 1878 LIX [Cd 2142], 139.

65. Frost, "Pueblo," 440–45.

66. Joralemon, "The Case of Disease," 114.

67. Sahagún, *Florentine Codex*, 81.

68. Quoted in Crosby, *Ecological Imperialism*, 202.

69. Frost, "Pueblo," 436.

70. Todd L. Savitt, *Medicine and Slavery: The Diseases and Health Care of Blacks in Antebellum Virginia* (Urbana, University of Illinois Press, 1978), 220–21.

71. Georges Vigarello, *Concepts of Cleanliness: Changing Attitudes in France since the Middle Ages*, trans. Jean Birrell (Cambridge, Cambridge University Press, 1988). According to Pagden, "for the Muslim washing was a significant part of ritual devotion and hence an integral part of an alien, and hostile system of beliefs": Pagden, *European Encounters*, 186. It is said that the body of the leading opponent of Granada Muslims, Queen Isabella, was bathed on only three occasions: once just after her birth, once on the night before she married Ferdinand, and once after she had died and was being tidied up for burial. Who then is "alien" and to whom?

72. Gruzinski, *Conquest of Mexico*, 84; James Axtell, *Beyond 1492: Encounters in Colonial North America* (Oxford, Oxford University Press, 1992), 105, 196; Dobyns, *Their Number Became Thinned*, 16.

73. Quoted in Axtell, *Beyond 1492*, 145; see also Carver, ed. Gleb *Travels*, 180; Sahagún, *Florentine Codex*, 81.

74. Joralemon, "The Case of Disease," 119; Suzanne Austin Alchon, "Disease, Population, and Health in Eighteenth Century Quito," in Cook and Lovell, "*Secret Judgments*", 159, 161, 179; S. J. Watts with Susan J. Watts, *From Border to Middle Shire: Northumberland 1586–1625* (Leicester, Leicester University Press, 1974), 68.

75. Nancy M. Farriss, *Maya Society under Colonial Rule: The Collective Enterprise of Survival* (Princeton, NJ, Princeton University Press, 1984), 78–95; on taxpayer revolts in Spain: Kamen, *Spain 1469–1714*, 223–31.

76. Lockhart, *Nahuas* 44–5; Mark A. Burkholder and Lyman L. Johnson, *Colonial Latin America* (New York, Oxford University Press, 1990), 102–103; Joralemon, "The Case of Disease," 110.

77. Alchon, *Ecuador*, 50–52.

78. Daniel T. Reff, "Contact Shock in Northwestern New Spain, 1518–1764," in Verano and

Ubelaker, *Disease and Demography*, 268. See also Robert H. Jackson, *Indian Population Decline: The Missions of Northwestern New Spain, 1687–1840* (Albuquerque, University of New Mexico Press, 1994).

79. Printed by H. Cline in the *Hispanic American Historical Review* in 1964 and reprinted by Englander, *Culture*, 344–46, 351.

80. Gruzinski, *Conquest of Mexico*, 80–89.

81. Ibid., 87; Clendinnen, "The Cost of Courage," 50; Wright, *Stolen Continents*, 244. On the general role of "predisposing causes" see Chapter 5, "Cholera." On accommodation to Spanish rule in Peru see: Kenneth Mills, "The Limits of Religious Coercion in Mid-Colonial Peru," *Past and Present* CXLV (November 1994), 84–121.

82. Prem, "Disease Outbreaks in Central Mexico", 38–42; Wright, *Stolen Continents*, 152–53.

83. Farriss, *Maya Society*, 278–79; Richard Henry Dana, *Two Years Before the Mast* (New York, Penguin, 1948), 79–81.

84. Thornton *et al.*, "American Indian Population Recovery," 38–41; Reff, "Contact Shock," 269. See also Lévi-Strauss, "River of Sorrows", 15–17; Dean R. Snow, "Disease and Population Decline in the Northeast," in Verano and Ubelaker, *Disease and Demography*, 185. See also Burkholder and Johnson, *Latin America*, 101, 102, 107; Axtell, *Beyond 1492*, 237.

85. Robin Price, "State Church Charity and Smallpox: An Epidemic Crisis in the City of Mexico 1797–98," *Journal of the Royal Society of Medicine* LXXV (May 1982), 365–66.

86. Quoted in S. F. Cook, "The Smallpox Epidemic of 1797 in Mexico," *Bulletin of the History of Medicine* VII no. 6 (June, 1939), 962.

87. Quoted in Fernando Casanueva, "Smallpox and War in Southern Chile in the Late Eighteenth Century," in Cook and Lovell, *"Secret Judgments"*, 197, 198, 208.

88. Casanueva, "Smallpox and War," 207–208.

89. Pagden expresses a contrary view which some might hold to be neoscholastic: "the European moral concern with groups which European culture has exploited, oppressed or destroyed seems often to be grounded in a corresponding sentimentalization of the 'other'. We all, it seems, need to salvage some notion of ourselves as potentially benevolent agents, to persuade ourselves that European civilization is not quite so rapacious and destructive of those who do not serve its ends as it so obviously appears to be. To achieve that objective, the critics of colonialism have tended to construct 'others' quite as false as those invented by their opponents": Pagden, *European Encounters*, 186–87. On the image of the West created by Pagden's "others" see: Rhoda E. Howard, "Occidentalism, Human Rights, and the Obligations of Western Scholars," *Canadian Journal of African Studies/La Revue Canadienne des Etudes Africanes* XXIX, no. 1 (1995), 110–26.

90. Henige asserts that even the self-appointed protector of the Indians, Las Casas, early in his American career, advocated bringing in black slaves from Africa "to do the work that had been done by Indians": Henige, "Why Does It Matter?" 23. Re: the problem of finding labor for the vast Louisiana province purchased by President Thomas Jefferson, Thomas Paine suggested to T. J. that he devise a system of assisted emigration for Africans who would come in

as *free* tenant-farmers; Keane, *Paine*, 508–509.

91. James C. Boyajian, *Portuguese Trade in Asia under the Habsburgs, 1580–1640* (Baltimore, MD, Johns Hopkins University Press, 1993). During the 1560s–80s, a hundred New Christians were burnt, and scores more arrested in Goa by the Inquisition: ibid., 72; A. J. R. Russell-Wood, *A World on the Move: the Portuguese in Africa, Asia, and America, 1415–1808* (London, Carcanet, 1992), 107–109. For a vitriolic Scottish literary attack on "The Other," in this case the Portuguese world empire and the "vile" Portuguese settlers sent to the New World in the sixteenth century: Arthur H. Williamson, "Scots, Indians and Empire: The Scottish Politics of Civilization 1519–1609," *Past and Present* CL (February 1996), 76–81.

92. Joseph C. Miller, *Way of Death: Merchant Capitalism and the Angolan Slave Trade 1730–1830* (London, James Currey, 1988), 673–4; Philip D. Curtin, *The Rise and Fall of the Plantation Complex; Essays in Atlantic History* (New York, Cambridge University Press, 1990), 18–28, 81–85; John Thornton, *Africa and Africans in the Making of the Atlantic World, 1400–1680* (Cambridge, Cambridge University Press, 1992), 74–78.

93. Joseph E. Inikori and Stanley L. Engerman, eds, *The Atlantic Slave Trade: Effects on Economies, Societies, and Peoples in Africa, the Americas, and Europe* (Durham, NC, Duke University Press, 1992), 6.

94. Prem lists contemporary or nearly contemporary sources for this tale, including accounts by López de Gómara, Díaz del Castillo (a companion of Cortés in 1521), Motolinía (Franciscan baptizer of pagans beginning in 1525), Mendieta (d. 1604), Munoz Camargo, and Bernardino de Sahagún, Franciscan author of the *General History of the Things of New Spain*: Prem, "Disease Outbreaks in Central Mexico," 24. See also: Alfred Crosby, *The Columbian Exchange: Biological Consequences of 1492* (Westport CT, Greenwood Press, 1972), 49; Alden and Miller, "Out of Africa," 214.

95. *Parliamentary Papers* 1895, LXXIII [Cd 7846], 112, 192.

96. Herbert Klein, *The Middle Passage* (Princeton, Princeton University Press, 1978), 8. See also: Larry Stewart, "The Edge of Utility: Slaves and Smallpox in the Early Eighteenth Century," *Medical History* XXIX (1985), 66; James Walvin, *Black Ivory, A History of British Slavery* (London, Fontana, 1992), 56.

97. Eugenia W. Herbert, "Smallpox Inoculation in Africa," *Journal of African History* XVI, no. 4 (1975), 552–53. For a different assessment of black behavior ashore see: Alden and Miller, "Out of Africa," 195–234.

98. Marc H. Dawson, "Socioeconomic Change and Disease: Smallpox in Colonial Kenya, 1880–1920," in S. Feierman and J. Janzen, eds, *The Social Basis of Health and Healing in Africa* (Berkeley, University of California Press, 1992), 90–93.

99. Gerard Hartwig and K. Patterson, "Introduction," in G. Hartwig and K. David Patterson, eds, *Disease in African History: An Introduction and Case Studies* (Durham, NC, Duke University Press, 1975), 8, 10.

100. Donald R. Hopkins, *Princes and Peasants: Smallpox in History* (Chicago, University of Chicago Press, 1983), 170.

101. Ibid., 200–202. For Yoruba shrines in 1903 see: R. R. Kuczinski, *Demographic Survey of the British Colonial Empire*, I:

West Africa (Oxford, Oxford University Press, 1949), 700.

102. Dawson, "Smallpox," 96.

103. Quoted in Ahmed Bayoumi, "The History and Traditional Treatment of Smallpox in the Sudan," *Journal of Eastern African Research and Development* VI no. 1 (1976), 8. On the eighteenth- and nineteenth-century European fixation with "time immemorial" as an explanation for backwardness among non-western peoples, see Ralph W. Nicholas, "The Goddess Sitala and Epidemic Smallpox in Bengal," *Journal of Asian Studies* XLI no. 1 (November 1981) and innumerable references in the annual sanitation reports submitted to Parliament: choosing one of these at random, "customs that have been in force from time immemorial"; *Parliamentary Papers* 1878 LIX [Cd 2142], 106.

104. Quoted in Herbert, "Smallpox Inoculation," 544.

105. Hopkins, *Princes and Peasants*, 174; Gerald W. Hartwig, "Smallpox in the Sudan," *International Journal of African Historical Studies* XIV no. l (1981), 13–15.

106. Murrin, "Beneficiaries," 11; John J. McCusker and Russell R. Menard, *The Economy of British America 1607–1789* (Chapel Hill, University of North Carolina Press, 1985), 54, 103.

107. Quoted in Stannard, *American Holocaust*, 238. Cotton Mather's tract was *Late Memorable Providences Relating to Witchcrafts and Possessions, Clearly Manifesting, Not only that there are Witches, But that Good Men (as well as Others) May Possibly have their Lives shortened by such Evil Instruments of Satan* (London, 1691).

108. Hopkins, *Princes and Peasants*, 174, corrects the older idea that Onesimus had come from southwestern Libya.

109. Genevieve Miller, "Putting Lady Mary in her Place: A Discussion of Historical Causation," *Bulletin of the History of Medicine* LV (1981), 4; John T. Barrett, "The Inoculation Controversy in Puritan New England," *Bulletin of the History of Medicine* XII (1942), 171. For eighteenth-century confusion about stagnant miasmic air in Turkey *tempo* Lady Montagu, see: Stewart, "The Edge of Utility," 59–60.

110. C. J. Lawrence, "Medicine as Culture: Edinburgh and the Scottish Enlightenment," PhD Thesis, University College, University of London, 1984. Another royal killed by smallpox was Louis XV, the unpopular ruler accused by rioters in 1750 of kidnapping virginal children off the streets so that he could bathe in their blood to cure his "leprosy."

111. Jean-François de Raymond, *Querelle de l'inoculation ou préhistoire de la vaccination* (Paris, Librairie Philosophique J. Vrin, 1982), 85–88; Miller, "Putting Lady Mary," 1–16; Mercer, "Smallpox Epidemics in the Eighteenth Century: The Impact of Immunization Measures," in his *Disease, Mortality*, 46–73.

112. Brunton, "Scotland," 406; Guenter Risse, "Medicine in the age of Enlightenment," in A. Wear, ed., *Medicine in Society* (Cambridge, Cambridge University Press, 1992), 191; Charles Rosenberg, "The Therapeutic Revolution," in his *Explaining Epidemics and Other Studies in the History of Medicine* (Cambridge, Cambridge University Press, 1992), 12–14.

113. Brunton, "Scotland," 414–16; Barrett, "Inoculation Controversy," 174–75.

114. Mercer, *Disease Mortality*, 40, 73, 94; E. A. Wrigley and R. Schofield, *The Population History of England 1541–1871: A Reconstruction* (London, Edward

Arnold, 1981), 417, 453; see also William McNeill, *Plagues and Peoples* (London, Doubleday, 1976), 231. For a useful review of earlier literature: Eric Mercer, "Smallpox and Epidemiological-Demographic Change in Europe: The Role of Vaccination," *Population Studies* XXXIX (1985), 287–307; Michael Anderson, *Population Change in North-Western Europe, 1750–1850* (London, Macmillan Education, 1988), 58–59.

115. Mercer, *Disease Mortality*, 45, 51–52, 54, 181 fn.95.

116. Dorothy Porter and Roy Porter, "The Politics of Prevention: Anti-Vaccinationism and Public Health in Nineteenth-Century England," *Medical History* XXXII (1988), 237, 234, 242 quote Charles Creighton's *Jenner and his Vaccination* (1889) which held that Jenner was "little better than a criminal and money-grabber who had duped . . . the scientific and medical worlds into believing his mythic methods." See also S. A. K. Strahan, *Marriage and Disease: A Study of Heredity and the More Important Family Degenerations* (London, Kegan Paul, Trench, Trübner, 1892), 158.

117. Peter Razzell, *Edward Jenner's Cowpox Vaccine: The History of a Medical Myth* (Firle, Sussex, Caliban Books, 1977), 105–7; Peter Razzell, "Should Remaining Stocks of Smallpox Virus be Destroyed?", *Social History of Medicine* VIII (1995), 305–307.

118. Bercé, *Chaudron et lancette*, 135–38, 299–302.

119. Ibid., 135–39.

120. Quoted in John Z. Bowers, "The Odyssey of Smallpox Vaccination," *Bulletin of the History of Medicine* LV (1981), 19. For late nineteenth-century French peasant resistance to the centralizing State represented by vaccination campaigns: Evelyn Bernette Ackerman, *Health Care in the Parisian Countryside, 1800–1914* (New Brunswick, NJ, Rutgers University Press, 1990), 76, 165–68.

121. Quoted in José G. Rigau-Pérez, "Strategies that Led to the Eradication of Smallpox in Puerto Rico, 1882–1921," *Bulletin of the History of Medicine* LIX (1985), 82.

122. José G. Rigau-Pérez, "Smallpox Epidemics in Puerto Rico during the Prevaccine Era (1518–1803)," *Journal of the History of Medicine* XXXVII no. 4 (1982), 423–38; Rigau-Pérez, "Strategies," 75–78; Bowers, "Odyssey," 26–28.

123. Quoted in Rigau-Pérez, "Strategies," 82 (italics in original): the slogan of course comes from Rudyard Kipling's poem "The White Man's Burden", verse 1 of which reads as follows:

Take up the White Man's burden—
Send forth the best ye breed—
Go bind your sons to exile
To serve your captives' need;
To wait in heavy harness,
On fluttered folk and wild—
Your new-caught, sullen peoples,
Half-devil and half child.

124. Rigau-Pérez, "Strategies," 82, 87.

125. Quoted in Frost, "Pueblo," 440.

126. Ibid., 443–45. For a discussion of the Pueblo, the Hopis and Navajos from the perspective of community and preventative medicine, see Stephen J. Kunitz, *Disease and Social Diversity: The European Impact on the Health of Non-Europeans* (New York, Oxford University Press, 1994), 185–86.

127. Donald A. Henderson, "The History of Smallpox Eradication," in Abraham M. Lilienfeld, ed., *Times, Places, and Persons: Aspects of the History of Epide-*

miology (Baltimore, MD, Johns Hopkins University Press, 1978), 99–108; Hopkins, *Princes and Peasants*, 303–4.

128. Genevieve Miller, "Discussion," in Lilienfeld, *Times, Places and Persons*, 111.
129. Henderson, "Smallpox Eradication," 104–7.
130. *New York Times*, 25 January 1996, A–1, A–5 col. 5: report faxed to me by Donald Hopkins. On earlier high-level discussions see: *Nature* XXIII (December 1993).

4 *The Secret Plague: Syphilis in West Europe and East Asia, 1492 to 1965*

1. Quoted in Lucinda McCray Beier, *Sufferers & Healers: The Experience of Illness in Seventeenth-Century England* (London, Routledge & Kegan Paul, 1987), 137. Graunt held that only 392 out of 229,250 dead (0.0017 percent) were recorded as having died of syphilis.
2. The standard account is Claude Quétel, *History of Syphilis*, trans. Judith Braddock and Brian Pike (Cambridge, Polity Press, 1990). See also: André Basset, "Épidémiologie des tréponématoses: vrais et faux-semblants de la syphilis," in Jean-Pierre Bardet *et al.*, *Peurs et terreurs face à la contagion* (Paris, Fayard, 1988), 362–72, 433–39.
3. Alex Mercer, *Disease, Mortality and Population in Transition: Epidemiological-Demographic Change in England Since the Eighteenth Century as Part of a Global Phenomenon* (Leicester, Leicester University Press, 1990), 40–49; Michael Anderson, *Population Change in North-Western Europe 1750–1850* (London, Macmillan Education, 1988), 43; Anthony S. Wohl, *Endangered Lives: Public Health in Victorian Britain* (London, Methuen, 1983): Wohl, following the conventions of the age he studies, appears to ignore syphilis.
4. S. J. Watts, *A Social History of Western Europe 1450–1720: Tensions and Solidarities among Rural People* (London, Hutchinson University Library, 1984), 58–59, 65–66.
5. Michel Foucault, *Histoire de la sexualité*, Vol. I: *La Volonté du savoir* (Paris, Editions Gallimard, 1976), 121, 194. Sir Francis Bacon: "Knowledge itself is Power," in "Of Heresies" in his *Religious Meditations* (1597).
6. Quoted in David Macey, *The Lives of Michel Foucault* (London, Vintage, 1993), 248.
7. It was Galen's contention that since male and female reproductive organs were essentially identical, no woman could become pregnant unless both she and her male partner ejaculated their seed. Adopting a quite different stance, Aristotle and his many followers held that the woman's role was essentially passive and that the seed ejaculated by the male became a live human fetus. Taking his ideas from the *Timaeus* of Plato, Rabelais held to the theory of women's wandering womb: "an animal, an organ that is not present in men, [and one through which] their whole body is shaken, all their senses transported, all their passions indulged, and all their thoughts confused." Monica H. Green, "Sex and the Medieval Physician," *History and Philosophy of the Life Sciences* XIII no. 2 (1991), 288–89; F. Rabelais, *The Five Books of Gargantua and Pantagruel in the Modern Translation of Jacques LeClerq* (New York, The Modern Library, 1944), 378.

8. For a pioneering suggestion that repressive Enlightenment attitudes towards certain forms of sexuality were merely secularized forms of earlier religious strictures: Théodore Tarczylo, "From Lascivious Erudition to the History of Mentalities," in G. S. Rousseau and Roy Porter, eds, *Sexual Underworlds of the Enlightenment* (Manchester, Manchester University Press, 1987), 40–41.
9. Quoted in Quétel, *Syphilis*, 10.
10. Quoted in Francisco Guerra, "The Dispute over Syphilis: Europe versus America," *Clio Medica* XIII no. 1 (1978), 54.
11. Quoted in Anna Foa, "The New and the Old: The Spread of Syphilis (1494–1530)," trans. Carole C. Gallucci, in Edward Muir and Guido Ruggiero, eds, *Sex & Gender in Historical Perspective* (Baltimore, MD, Johns Hopkins University Press, 1990), 29. See also: Roger French, "The Arrival of the French Disease in Leipzig," in Neithard Bulst and Robert Delort, eds, *Acts du Colloque de Bielefeld, Maladie et Société (XIIe–XVIIIe Siècles)* (Paris, Editions du CNRS, 1989), 133–41.
12. The World Health Report of 1996 lists thirty new infectious diseases recognized *since* 1973: *The World Health Report 1996: Fighting Disease, Fostering Development* (Geneva, WHO, 1996), 112.
13. Basset, "Epidémiologie," 433–39; Mirko D. Grmek, "The Origin and Spread of Syphilis," in his *Diseases in the Ancient Greek World*, trans. Mireille Muellner and Leonard Muellner (Baltimore, MD, Johns Hopkins University Press, 1989), 134–44. For pre-Darwinian awareness of disease change see: James Y. Simpson, "Antiquarian Notice of Leprosy and Leper Hospitals in Scotland and England," *Edinburgh Medical and Surgical Journal* LVII (1841), 302.
14. Megan Vaughan, "Syphilis and Sexuality: The Limits of Colonial Medical Power," in her *Curing their Ills: Colonial Power and African Illness* (Cambridge, Polity Press, 1991), 138; John Orley, "Indigenous Concepts of Disease and Their Interaction with Scientific Medicine," in E. E. Sabben-Clare, D. J. Bradley and K. Kirkwood, eds, *Health in Tropical Africa during the Colonial Period* (Oxford, Clarendon Press, 1980), 130.
15. Quétel, *Syphilis*, 39; Anne Marie Moulin, "L"Ancien et le nouveau: la réponse médicale à l'épidémie de 1493,' in Bulst and Delort, *Maladie et Société*, 125; for Voltaire's gullible acceptance of American origins: Sander L. Gilman, *Sexuality: An Illustrated History* (New York, John Wiley, 1989), 86–87.
16. For readings that ignore niche-filling and Darwin see: Donald J. Ortner, N. Tuross and A. Stix, "Disease in Archaeological New World Populations," *Human Biology* LXIV no. 3 (1992), 339–47; Grmek, "The Origin and Spread," 142; Danielle Jacquart and Claude Thomasset, *Sexuality and Medicine in the Middle Ages*, trans. Matthew Adamson (Cambridge, Polity Press, 1988), 178: Gilman, *Sexuality*, 321; Stanislav Andrewski, *Syphilis, Puritanism and Witch Hunts: Historical Explanations in the Light of Medicine and Psychoanalysis with a Forecast about AIDS* (London, Macmillan, 1989), 210.
17. Frank B. Livingstone, "On the Origin of Syphilis: An Alternative Hypothesis," *Current Anthropology* XXXII no. 5 (December 1991), 587–90. Livingstone and the sources he quotes are impressed by the sudden onslaught of syphilis in America

after the arrival of Europeans, again suggesting that *in America it was an entirely new disease*. See also: Brenda J. Baker and George J. Armelagos, "The Origin and Antiquity of Syphilis: Paleopathological Diagnosis and Interpretation," *Current Anthropology* XXIX no. 5 (December 1988), 732–37.

18. Guerra, "The Dispute over Syphilis," 55. Paracelsus (d. 1541), foe of Galenic medicine, thus may not have been entirely off base when in *c.* 1493 he identified "syphilis" and gonorrhea as one disease.

19. Moulin, "L'Ancien et le nouveau," 130; August Hirsch, *Handbook of Geographical and Historical Pathology*, 2nd edition, trans. Charles Creighton (London, New Sydenham Society, CXII 1985), 64; French, "The Arrival," 136.

20. Guerra, "The Dispute over Syphilis," 46; French, "Arrival of the French Disease," 133–41; Quétel, *Syphilis*, 52.

21. Quoted in Quétel, *Syphilis*, 28; for the conventional approach: Edward Shorter, *Women's Bodies: A Social History of Women's Encounter with Health, Ill Health, and Medicine* (New Brunswick, NJ, Transaction Publishers, 1991), 263–65.

22. Margaret Pelling, "Appearance and Reality: Barber-Surgeons, the Body and Disease," in A. L. Beier and Roger Finlay, eds, *London 1500–1700: The Making of the Metropolis* (London, Longman, 1986), 97–98.

23. John M Riddle, *Contraception and Abortion from the Ancient World to the Renaissance* (Cambridge, MA, Harvard University Press, 1992); Angus McLaren, *A History of Contraception from Antiquity to the Present Day* (Oxford, Basil Blackwell, 1990); Watts, *Social History*, 66–69.

24. Quoted in Quétel, *Syphilis*, 39.

25. For Oviedo, see Chapter 3 on smallpox. Discussing Oviedo, Bartolomé de Las Casas held: "He was one of the greatest enemies the Indians have had and has done them the worst harm, for he was blinder than others in not knowing the truth, perhaps because of his greater cupidity and ambition, qualities and customs which have destroyed the Indies." Quoted in H. C. Porter, *The Inconstant Savage: England and the North American Indian, 1500–1660* (London, Duckworth, 1979), 161.

26. Quoted in Guerra, "The Dispute over Syphilis," 46; also printed by Quétel in *Syphilis*, 35.

27. Quétel, *Syphilis*, 29–32, 34–37; Moulin, "L'Ancien et le nouveau," 129; W. F. Bynum, "Treating the Wages of Sin: Venereal Disease and Specialism in Eighteenth Century Britain," in W. F. Bynum and Roy Porter, eds, *Medical Fringe and Medical Orthodoxy 1750–1850* (London, Croom Helm, 1987), 15–17; Guerra, "The Dispute over Syphilis," 48; Bruce Thomas Boehrer, "Early Modern Syphilis," in John C. Fout, ed., *Forbidden History: The State, Society and the Regulation of Sexuality in Modern Europe* (Chicago, University of Chicago Press, 1992), 27.

28. Boehrer, "Syphilis," 14; Karl Sudhoff, ed., *The Earliest Printed Literature on Syphilis, Being Ten Tractates from the Years 1495–1498* (Florence, Lier, 1925); Natalie Zemon Davis, "Printing and the People: Early Modern France," in Harvey Graff, ed., *Literacy and Social Development in the West* (Cambridge, Cambridge University Press, 1981), 69–95.

29. Quoted in Quétel, *Syphilis*, 19; Quétel reminds us that Grunpeck

lived to the age of eighty-one. See also: Boehrer, "Syphilis," 15–17, 19.

30. Lyndal Roper, "Discipline and Respectability: Prostitution and the Reformation in Augsburg," *History Workshop Journal* XIX (1985), 14.

31. Cardinal Bembo's seminal role in the Italian literary world is established in Brian Richardson, *Print Culture in Renaissance Italy: The Editor and the Vernacular Text, 1470–1600* (Cambridge, Cambridge University Press, 1995).

32. Boehrer, "Syphilis," 20–24; Geoffrey Eatough, *Fracastoro's Syphilis: Introduction, Text, Translation and Notes with a Computer-Generated Word Index* (Liverpool, Francis Cairns, 1984), 1–35. For WHO official, N. Howard-Jones' assessment of Frascatoro see p. 284 fn 11. See also: Vivian Nutton, "The Seeds of Disease: An Explanation of Contagion and Infection from the Greeks to the Renaissance," *Medical History* XXVII (1983), 22–34; Paul W. Ewald, *Evolution of Infectious Disease* (New York, Oxford University Press, 1994), 184.

33. Pelling, "Appearance and Reality," 82–112. Writing in his *London Tradesman* in 1747, R. Campbell claimed that town surgeons still effectively monopolized the cure of "the venereal disease . . . and three Parts in four of their Practice depend upon their Ignorance of this very Distemper which they pretend to cure." Quoted in Bynum, "Wages of Sin," 9.

34. McLaren, *History of Contraception.* See also Hilary Marland, "Introduction", and Marland, "The '*Burgerlijke*' Midwife: The *Stadsvroedvrouw* of Eighteenth-Century Holland," and Merry Wiesner, "The Midwives of South Germany and the Public/Private Dichotomy," in Hilary Marland, ed., *The Art of Midwifery: Early Modern Midwives in Europe* (London, Routledge, 1993), 1–8, 77–94, 192–213. See also: A. Myriam Greilsammer, "The Midwife, the Priest, and the Physician: The Subjugation of Midwives in the Low Counties at the End of the Middle Ages," *Journal of Medieval and Renaissance Studies* XXI (1991), 319.

35. Alain Corbin, "La Grande Peur de la syphilis," in Bardet *et al.*, *Peurs et terreurs*, 333. See also: Roy Porter, "Love, Sex, and Madness in Eighteenth Century England," *Social Research* LIII no. 2 (1986), 235–36.

36. Quoted in Matthew Ramsey, *Professional and Popular Medicine in France, 1770–1830* (Cambridge, Cambridge University Press, 1988), 189. See also: Quétel, *Syphilis*, 86–93.

37. Quoted in Roy Porter, "Quacks and Sex: Pioneering or Anxiety Making?" in his *Health for Sale: Quackery in England 1660–1850* (Manchester, Manchester University Press, 1989), 151.

38. Quétel, *Syphilis*, 29–30, 59–63, 83–86, 116–20.

39. Jacques Rossiaud, *Medieval Prostitution*, trans. Lydia G. Cochrane (Oxford, Basil Blackwell, 1988), 72ff.; Leah Lydia Otis, *Prostitution in Medieval Society: The History of an Urban Institution in Languedoc* (Chicago, University of Chicago Press, 1985).

40. Jacques Rossiaud, "Prostitution, Sex and Society in French Towns in the Fifteenth Century," in Philippe Ariès and André Béjin, eds, *Western Sexuality: Practice and Precept in Past and Present Times* (Oxford, Basil Blackwell, 1985), 76–94.

41. Roper, "Discipline and Respectability," 4–5; Boehrer, "Syphilis", 18–19; Ian W. Archer, *The Pursuit of Stability:*

Social Relations in Elizabethan London (Cambridge, Cambridge University Press, 1991), 211.

42. Roper, "Discipline and Respectability," 5.
43. Rossiaud, *Medieval Prostitution*, 160–65, 178; Otis, *Prostitution . . . in Languedoc*, 42. For overviews see Peter Burke, *Popular Culture in Early Modern Europe* (London, Temple Smith, 1978) and Watts, *Social History*.
44. Ann G. Carmichael, "The Health Status of Florentines in the 15th Century," in Marcel Tetel, R. Witt and R. Goffen, eds, *Life and Death in 15th Century Florence* (Durham, NC, Duke University Press, 1989), 29–31.
45. Quoted in Georges Vigarello, *Concepts of Cleanliness: Changing Attitudes in France since the Middle Ages*, trans. Jean Birrell (Cambridge, Cambridge University Press, 1988), 27.
46. Jeffrey Richards, *Sex, Dissidence and Damnation: Minority Groups in the Middle Ages* (London, Routledge, 1990), 118–19.
47. Quoted in Susan C. Karant-Nunn, "Continuity and Change: Some Effects of the Reformation on the Women of Zwickau," *Sixteenth Century Journal* XII no. 2 (1982), 23–24. See also Roper, "Discipline and Respectability," 15, 18–19; Otis, *Prostitution . . . in Languedoc*, 41.
48. Karant-Nunn, "Continuity and Change," 25.
49. Archer, *Pursuit of Stability*, 211–15, 231–33, 249–54. On the importance of the attack on illicit sex in the making of Protestant reformations in the German lands, the Netherlands and England, see Olwen Hufton, *The Prospect Before Her: A History of Women in Western Europe*, I: *1500–1800* (New York, HarperCollins, 1995).
50. Henry Kamen, *Inquisition and Society in Spain in the Sixteenth and Seventeenth Centuries* (Bloomington, Indiana University Press, 1985), 185, 205. See also: Mary Elizabeth Perry, "Deviant Insiders: Legalized Prostitutes and a Consciousness of Women in Early Modern Seville," *Comparative Studies in Society and History* XXVII no. 1 (1985), 138–58.
51. Church policy, almost from the beginning, had stressed that the man and the woman had freely to give their consent to the union and must not be forced into it by their parents: Watts, *Social History*, 79.
52. Euan Cameron, *The European Reformation* (Oxford, Oxford University Press, 1991), 166–67, 247, 402–405; Watts, *Social History*, 188–200; Lyndal Roper, *The Holy Household: Religion; Morals and Order in Reformation Augsburg* (Oxford, Oxford University Press, 1989).
53. Karant-Nunn, "Continuity and Change," 23–24; Susan Amussen, "Gender, Family and the Social Order, 1560–1725," in Anthony Fletcher and John Stevenson, eds, *Order and Disorder in Early Modern England* (Cambridge, Cambridge University Press, 1985), 203.
54. Quoted in Roper, "Discipline and Respectability," 13–14; see also Quétel, *Syphilis*, 212.
55. Natalie Zemon Davis, "Women in the Crafts in Sixteenth Century Lyon," in Barbara A. Hanawalt, ed., *Women and Work in Preindustrial Europe* (Bloomington, Indiana University Press, 1986), 177. See also Judith Walkowitz, *Prostitution and Victorian Society* (Cambridge, Cambridge University Press, 1980).
56. Thomas Robisheaux, "Peasants and Pastors: Rural Youth Control and the Reformation in Hohenlohe, 1540–1680," *Social History* VI no. 3 (October 1981), 281–300; David Warren Sabean, *Property, Production, and Family*

in Neckarhausen, 1700–1870 (Cambridge, Cambridge University Press, 1990), 247–58, 329–44; Sheilagh C. Ogilvie, "Coming of Age in a Corporate Society: Capitalism, Pietism and Family Authority in Rural Württemberg, 1590–1740," *Continuity and Change* I no. 3 (1986), 279–331; Jean-Louis Flandrin, *Families in Former Times: Kinship, Household and Sexuality*, trans. Richard Southern (Cambridge, Cambridge University Press, 1979); Giovanni Levi, "Reciprocity and the Land Market," in his *Inheriting Power: The Story of an Exorcist*, trans. Lydia G. Cochrane (Chicago, University of Chicago Press, 1988), 66–99.

57. Jean Frédéric Osterwald, *The Nature of Uncleanness Considered* (London, 1708). Osterwald's moral strictures on peasant boy–girl sexual practices were taken over almost word for word and used in criticism of Quebec Native Americans by Antoine Denis Raudot in 1709. This is suggestive of the role of Osterwald in creating the self-image of Europeans, especially those venturing into non-European lands: Antoine Denis Raudot, "Memoir Concerning the Different Indian Nations of North America," Appendix in W. Vernon Kinietz, *The Indians of the Western Great Lakes, 1650–1760* (Ann Arbor, University of Michigan Press, 1965), 367.

58. Michel Foucault, *The History of Sexuality*, III: *The Care of Self*, trans. Robert Hurley (London, Penguin, 1986), 140, 248; Jean Stengers and Anne Van Neck, *Histoire d'une grande peur: la masturbation* (Brussels, Editions d'Université de Bruxelles, 1984), 42–43, 205, 488–9; Rossiaud, *Medieval Prostitution*, 105–106; Roy Porter, "Love, Sex and Medicine: Nicolas Venette and his *Tableau de l'Amour Conjugal*," in Peter Wagner, ed., *Erotica and the Enlightenment* (Frankfurt am Main, Land, 1990), 90–122; Robert Maccubbin, ed., *'Tis Nature's Fault: Unauthorized Sexuality during the Enlightenment* (Cambridge, Cambridge University Press, 1987), 43.

59. Roy Porter, "The Language of Quackery in England, 1660–1800," in Peter Burke and Roy Porter, eds, *The Social History of Language* (Cambridge, Cambridge University Press, 1987), 73–98. See also Porter, *Health for Sale*; Ramsey, *Popular Medicine*.

60. For the publication history of *Onania* see Stengers and Van Neck, *Une Grande Peur*, 49. See also: Robert H. MacDonald, "The Frightful Consequences of Onanism: Notes on the History of a Delusion," *Journal of the History of Ideas* XXVIII (1967); H. Tristram Engelhardt, Jr., "The Disease of Masturbation: Values and the Concepts of Disease," in Arthur Caplan, H. Engelhardt Jr. and J. McCartney, *Concepts of Health and Disease: Interdisciplinary Perspectives* (Reading, MA, Addison-Wesley, 1981), 268; J. Solé, *L'Amour en Occident à l'époque modern* (Paris, Librairie Hachette, 1976); A. D. Harvey, *Sex in Georgian England: Attitudes and Prejudices from the 1720s to the 1820s* (London, Duckworth, 1994), 118–22.

61. Quoted in MacDonald, "Frightful Consequences," 425. Mr Crouch may have been the same distributor whom Roy Porter, in a private communication, listed as publisher/distributor of John Martin's sexual advice book, *Gonosologium Novum: Or a New System of All the Secret Infirmities and Diseases, Natural, Accidental and Venereal in Men and Women* 6th edition (London, 1709).

62. Antoinette Emch-Dériaz, *Tissot:*

Physician of the Enlightenment (Berne, Peter Lang, 1992); S.A.A.D. Tissot, *Onanism or, A Treatise upon the Disorders Produced by Masturbation or, The Dangerous Effects of Secret and Excessive Venery*, trans. A. Hume, MD (London, J. Pridden, 1756), 152. See also: Jeffrey R. Watt, "The Control of Marriage in Reformed Switzerland, 1550–1800," in W. Fred Graham, ed., *Later Calvinism: International Perspectives* (Kirksville, MO, Sixteenth Century Essays & Studies XXII, 1994), 29–53.

63. Stengers and Van Neck, *Un Grande Peur*, 18–19, 156; R. P. Neuman, "Masturbation, Madness, and the Modern Concepts of Childhood and Adolescence," *Journal of Social History* VIII no. 1 (1975), 1–27. Central to the discussion are Lawrence Stone, *The Family, Sex and Marriage in England 1500–1800* (London, Weidenfeld & Nicolson, 1977); Edward Shorter, *The Making of the Modern Family* (London, Collins, 1976). These now are supplemented by Anthony Fletcher, *Gender, Sex and Subordination in England 1500–1800* (London, Yale University Press, 1995). See also Michael Rey, "Parisian Homosexuals Create a Lifestyle, 1700–1750: The Police Archives," in Maccubbin, *'Tis Nature's Fault*, 179–91.

64. Jonathan Hutchinson, "On Circumcision as Preventive of Masturbation," *Archives of Surgery*, II (1890–1891), 268.

65. Michel Foucault, *The Birth of the Clinic: An Archaeology of Medical Perception* (first published 1963), trans. A. M. Sheridan (London, Routledge, 1989): Pavia's clinic is mentioned on 57, 59, 60, 62 and 125.

66. Emch-Dériaz, *Tissot*. See also: Guenter B. Risse, "Medicine in the Age of Enlightenment," in Andrew Wear, ed., *Medicine in Society: Historical Essays* (Cambridge, Cambridge University Press, 1992), 186–87; Matthew Ramsey, "The Popularization of Medicine in France, 1650–1900," in Roy Porter, ed., *The Popularization of Medicine 1650–1850* (London, Routledge, 1992), 109–13.

67. Emch-Dériaz, *Tissot*, 237 (my italics).

68. Emch-Dériaz, *Tissot*; Ramsey, "Popularization," 110.

69. P. du Toit de Mambrini, *De l'Onanisme: ou discours philosophique et moral sur la luxure artificielle et sur tous les crimes relatifs* (Lausanne, Antoine Chapuis, 1760), 6, 171.

70. Quoted in MacDonald, "Frightful Consequences," 425; Tissot, *Onanism*, 152.

71. Tissot, *Onanism*, 83. See also, Porter, "Love, Sex, and Madness," 229.

72. Jean Jacques Rousseau, *Emile, or Education* (first published 1762), trans. Barbara Foxley (London, J. M. Dent & Sons, 1911), 298–99. For the receptivity of "the English" to *Emile* see Linda Colley, *Britons: Forging the Nation 1770–1837* (London, Pimlico, 1992), 239–40, 273–75.

73. Tissot, *Onanism*, 152. Sir Isaiah Berlin showed the Enlightenment for what it was in "The Bent Twig" and other essays in his *The Crooked Timber of Humanity* (New York, Alfred A. Knopf, 1991). Writing after the fall of the Communist bogey in 1989, an event which enabled intellectuals to look critically at the rest of the Western Tradition, Christopher Lasch summed up the new consensus: "The Enlightenment's reason and morality are increasingly seen as a cover for power": C. Lasch, *The Revolt of the Elites and the Betrayal of Democracy* (New York, Norton, 1995), 93.

74. Tissot, *Onanism*, 83.
75. Tissot, *Onanism* 72, 82, 93; see also Emch-Dériaz, *Tissot*, 51–52: Lawrence Stone, "What Foucault Got Wrong," *TLS* 10 March 1995, 4–5.
76. Quoted in Leslie A. Hall, "Forbidden by God, Despised by Men: Masturbation, Medical Warnings, Moral Panic and Manhood in Great Britain, 1850–1950," *Journal of the History of Sexuality* II no. 3 (1992), 370. See also Leslie A. Hall, *Hidden Anxieties: Male Sexuality, 1900–1950* (Cambridge, Polity Press, 1992), 155.
77. Quoted in Hall, "Forbidden," 370. See also: Michael Mason, *The Making of Victorian Sexuality* (Oxford, Oxford University Press, 1994), 73.
78. Henry Maudsley, "Illustrations of a Variety of Insanity," *Journal of Mental Science* July, 1868, quoted in Vieda Skultans, *Madness and Morals: Ideas on Insanity in the Nineteenth Century* (London, Routledge & Kegan Paul, 1975), 90–91; Hutchinson, "On Circumcision," 268; Neuman, "Masturbation," 10; Porter, "Love, Sex and Madness," 227–28; Porter, "Quacks and Sex," 174; Hall, *Hidden Anxieties*, 373; Ronald Hyam, *Empire and Sexuality: The British Experience* (Manchester, Manchester University Press, 1990), 66–67, 76–79; Frank Madden, "Thirty Years of Surgery in Qasr el Aini Hospital, 1898–1928," in Mohamed Bey Khalil, ed., *Comptes Rendus* III (Cairo, Imprimerie Nationale, 1931), 41–42. See also: H. W. Hurt, ed., *Handbook for Boys: Boy Scouts of America* (no place or date of publication but H. Hoover was president [1929–33]): "Conservation: In the body of every boy who has reached his teens, the Creator of the universe has sown a very important fluid. ... Some parts of it find their way into the blood, and through the blood give tone to the muscles, power to the brain, and strength to the nerves. This fluid is the sex fluid. ... Any habit which a boy has that causes this fluid to be discharged from the body tends to weaken his strength, to make him less able to resist disease, and often unfortunately fastens upon him habits which later in life can be broken only with great difficulty. ... To become strong ... one must be pure in thought and clean in habit. This power which I have spoken of must be conserved. ... But remember that to yield means to sacrifice strength and power and manliness". Ibid., 519–20.
79. H. Cohn, *Eye-Diseases from Masturbation: Archives of Ophthalmology* XI (1882), 428–41, quoted in Sandra Dianne Lane, "A Biocultural Study of Trachoma in an Egyptian Hamlet" (doctoral dissertation in medical anthropology, University of California, San Francisco, 1988; Ann Arbor, Michigan University Microfilms, 1988), 119, 206; Stengers and Van Neck, *Une Grande Peur*, 148.
80. Michel Foucault, *Power/Knowledge: Selected Interviews and Other Writings, 1972–1977* (New York, Pantheon, 1980), 36, 108; Neuman, "Masturbation," 12–13; Stengers and Van Neck, *Une Grande Peur*, 157–58; Emch-Dériaz, *Tissot*, 251.
81. Quoted in Hall, "Forbidden," 385.
82. "Review," *Journal of Tropical Medicine and Hygiene* XI (November 1908), 33–34 (my italics).
83. "Hygienic Measures against Syphilis: Harben Lecture No. III," *Journal of Tropical Medicine* VI (2 July 1906), 203 (my italics).
84. Michael Anderson, *Population*

Change in North-Western Europe 1750–1850 (Houndsmill, Basingstoke, Macmillan Education, 1988), 21–26; André Armengaud, "Population in Europe 1700–1914," in Carlo M. Cipolla, ed., *The Fontana Economic History of Europe* (London, Collins/Fontana, 1973), 29–34.

85. This is a conservative estimate: in 1902, the director of the prestigious Pasteur Institute in Paris estimated that there were a million contagious cases of syphilis in France alone: Alain Corbin, *Les Filles de noce: misère sexualle et prostitution (19e et 20e siècles)* (Paris, Aubier Montaigne, 1978), 388.

86. Roderick Floud, K. Wachter and A. Gregory, *Height, Health and History: Nutritional Status in the United Kingdom, 1750–1980* (Cambridge, Cambridge University Press, 1989), 294–95; Mercer, *Disease ... in Transition*, 37–45.

87. Wohl, *Endangered Lives*, 331–33; Hyam, *Empire and Sexuality*, 73–75. For gentlemanly capitalists see P. J. Cain and A. G. Hopkins, *British Imperialism: Innovation and Expansion 1688–1914* (London, Longman, 1993), esp. 105–60.

88. Quoted in Jean-Charles Sournia, *Histoire de l'Alcoolisme* (Paris, Flammarion, 1986), 151. On the impact that the French phobia about low population in the motherland had upon French-ruled territories in North Africa and West Africa (compulsory military service imposed on all able-bodied indigenous males aged twenty and above), see Myron Echenburg, "'Faire du Nègre': Military Aspects of Population Planning in French West Africa, 1920–1940," in Dennis D. Cordell and Joel W. Gregory, eds, *African Population and Capitalism: Historical Perspectives* (Boulder, CO, Westview Press, 1987), 95–108.

89. Quétel, *Syphilis*, 135, 144, 177, 225–26, 325; Armengaud, "Population," 30, 33, 53–54; Eugene Weber, *From Peasants into Frenchmen: The Modernization of Rural France* (Stanford, CA, Stanford University Press, 1976); William Sewell, *Work and Revolution in France: The Language of Labor from the Old Regime to 1848* (Cambridge, Cambridge University Press, 1980).

90. Corbin, "La Grande Peur," 337–48.

91. Corbin, *Filles de noce*, 295–300. On the transformation in the 1860s: Corbin, "La Grande Peur"; Quétel, *Syphilis*, 106–247.

92. Quoted in Quétel, *Syphilis*, 167.

93. S. A. K. Strahan, MD, *Marriage and Disease: A Study of Heredity and the More Important Family Degenerations* (London, Kegan Paul, Trench, Trübner, 1892), 154.

94. Corbin, *Filles de noce*, 387–89; Quétel, *Syphilis*, 165–72; Elizabeth Lomax, "Infantile Syphilis as an Example of Nineteenth Century Belief in the Inheritance of Acquired Characteristics," *Journal of the History of Medicine* XXXIV (1979), 34–35.

95. Corbin, *Filles de noce*, 445–47. Reflecting fashionable paranoia about the coming degeneration of the human race: H. G. Wells, *The Time Machine* (first published 1895) (London, Aerie Books, 1986).

96. Michelle Perrot, "Dames et conflits familiaux," in Philippe Ariès and Georges Duby, *Histoire de la vie privée* (Paris, Seuil, 1985), 270; Jill Harsin, "Syphilis, Wives and Physicians: Medical Ethics and the Family in Late Nineteenth-Century France," *French Historical Studies* XVI no. 1 (Spring 1989), 72–95.

97. Quétel, *Syphilis*, 128–30, 164–

65; Gustave Flaubert, *Voyage en Égypte*, ed. Pierre-Marc de Biase (Paris, Bernard Grasset, 1991), 196–98; English Penguin translation reviewed under the heading "The Bedbugs were the Best Part," *TLS* 4 October 1996, 7. See also Hyam, *Empire and Sexuality*, 2, 19. Flaubert began work on *Saint Anthony* in 1848 (before he visited Cairo), rewrote and enlarged the book in 1856 and rewrote it again for final publication in 1874. For St Anthony put to other uses, see Chapter 3 on leprosy: for Flaubert's scoffing attitude towards medical doctors (i.e. Monsieur Bovary) see *Madame Bovary*, concluding paragraph. See also: Robert A. Nye, "Sex Difference and Male Homosexuality in French Medical Discourse, 1830–1930," *Bulletin of the History of Medicine*, LXIII (1989), 44, 38; Robert A. Nye, *Crime, Madness, and Politics in Modern France: The Medical Concept of National Decline* (Princeton, NJ, Princeton University Press, 1984).

98. Dr Payenneville, "Rapport sur l'organization de la lutte antivénerienne en France," in Mohamed Abdul Khalil, ed., *Comptes Rendus* du Congrès International de Médecine Tropicale et d'Hygiène, Le Caire, Egypt December 1928: V (Cairo, Imprimerie Nationale, 1932), 707.

99. Gregg S. Meyer, "Criminal Punishment for the Transmission of Sexually Transmitted Diseases: Lessons from Syphilis," *Bulletin of the History of Medicine* LXV no. 4 (Winter 1991), 551, 560; Jay Cassel, *The Secret Plague: Venereal Disease in Canada 1838–1939* (Toronto, University of Toronto Press, 1987), 89. For the work of purity crusade hero Prince Morrow, translator of Alfred Fournier's *Syphilis et mariage* into American English—a translator usually approves of the core message of the work he labors on—see Allan Brandt, *No Magic Bullet: A Social History of Venereal Disease in the United States since 1880* (New York, Oxford University Press, 1985). For continuing medical harassment of patients alleged to have syphilis in the USA in the 1940s, see William Styron, "Personal History: A Case of the Great Pox," *New Yorker* 18 September 1995, 62–75.

100. Quoted in Corbin, *Filles de noce*, 392.

101. Colley, *Britons: Forging the Nation*, 238. For an assessment of why many English women who travelled to the Middle East during these years felt disadvantaged compared to Muslim women see Billie Melman, *Women's Orients: English Women and the Middle East, 1718–1918* (London, Macmillan, 1993), 1–22.

102. Eric Trudgill, "Prostitution and Paterfamilias," in H. J. Dyos and M. Wolff, eds, *The Victorian City: Images and Realities* (London, Routledge & Kegan Paul, 1973), 693–705; Hyam, *Empire and Sexuality*, 60, 63.

103. Judith R. Walkowitz, *Prostitution and Victorian Society: Women, Class and the State* (Cambridge, Cambridge University Press, 1980), 42–47, 151–70, 201–13; Richard Davenport-Hines, *Sex, Death and Punishment: Attitudes to Sex and Sexuality in Britain since the Renaissance* (London, Collins, 1990), 53; Wilfrid S. Blunt, *The Secret History of the English Occupation of Egypt* (London, 1907).

104. Quoted in Quétel, *Syphilis*, 235. For a discussion of Butler's "magical appeal" see Walkowitz, *Victorian Society*, 114–18 and her more recent *City of Dreadful Delight: Narratives of Sexual Danger in Late-Victorian London* (Chicago, University of Chi-

cago Press, 1992), 87–93; Peter Gay, *The Bourgeois Experience, Victoria to Freud*, I: *Education of the Senses* (Oxford, Oxford University Press, 1984). See also: George Bernard Shaw, *Mrs Warren's Profession* (stage play) (1894). For Butler's tour in India, Antoinette Burton, *Burdens of History: British Feminists, Indian Women, and Imperial Culture, 1865–1915* (Chapel Hill, University of North Carolina Press, 1994); Hyam, *Empire and Sexuality*, 17–19.

105. Quoted in Walkowitz, *Victorian Society*, 256; David Evans, "Tackling the 'hideous scourge'": 417: the creation of venereal disease centres in early twentieth-century Britain, *Social History of Medicine* V no. 3 (1992), 417.

106. Edward J. Bristow, *Vice and Vigilance: Purity Movements in Britain since 1700* (Dublin, Gill & Macmillan; Lanham, MD, Rowman & Littlefield, 1977), 125–53. On power/knowledge/sadism in Reading Gaol: Oscar Wilde, "Two Letters to the *Daily Chronicle*," in *Complete Works* (London, Collins, 1966), 958–69.

107. Quoted in John M. Eyler, "Poverty, Disease, Responsibility: Arthur Newsholme and the Public Health Dilemmas of British Liberalism," *Milbank Quarterly* LXVII (September 1989), 121–22; Mason, *Victorian Sexuality*; Bristow, *Vice and Vigilance.* Three years after repeal an English jury fined the publisher of an English translation of Émile Zola's *La Terre* (1886) because it hinted that cows copulated; no replacement English translation of this masterpiece appeared for sixty-eight years (until 1954).

108. Though nowadays a small number of women—like those on housing estates near J. Butler's Northumberland birthplace—who want a child but don't want to be burdened with a husband use artificial insemination: Norman Dennis and George Erdoes, *Families without Fatherhood* (London, Institute of Economic Affairs, 1992), 1–127. A future way of reproducing humankind *may* be through cloning.

109. Angus McLaren, "The Sexual Politics of Reproduction in Britain," in John R. Gillis, L. Tilly and D. Levine, *The European Experience of Declining Fertility, 1850–1970: The Quiet Revolution* (Oxford, Basil Blackwell, 1992) argues that working-class women continued to use abortion as a birth-control technique until well into the present century since the decision to use a condom was the man's decision. Michael Mason, writing from a largely middle-class perspective, puts the generalized use of condoms twenty or thirty years earlier, an approach which he claims is "unfashionable"; Mason, *Victorian Sexuality*, 57–64.

110. Marie Carmichael Stopes, *Married Love: A New Contribution to the Solution of Sex Difficulties* (London, A. C. Fifield, 1918), 53, 91. Shortly after her marriage to her third husband (her first two having left her in the virginal condition she was in when she wrote *Married Love*), Stopes founded the birth-control clinics for which she is justly famous. To commemorate the work she did in improving the lives of generations of women, Victor Gollancz republished *Married Love* in December 1995. See also: McLaren, "Sexual Politics," 92; "Stopes, Marie Charlotte Carmichael," *Dictionary of National Biography, 1951–1960*, 930–31.

111. Hyam, *Empire and Sexuality*, 65; Peter Sterns, "Working-Class Women in Britain, 1890–1914," in Martha Vicinus, ed., *Suffer and Be Still: Women in the Victorian Age* (Bloomington, Indiana

University Press, 1972); Patrick Joyce, "Work," in F. M. L. Thompson, ed., *The Cambridge Social History of Britain* II (Cambridge, Cambridge University Press, 1990).

112. Joanna Bourke, "Housewifery in Working-Class England 1860–1914," *Past and Present* CXLIII (May 1994), 167–97.

113. Strahan, *Marriage and Disease*, 158. Testifying to the continuing importance of charlatans and other irregular curers in Britain, in 1917 the Venereal Disease Act finally prohibited non-medically qualified personnel from treating or prescribing for VD; Roger Davidson, "'A Scourge to be Firmly Gripped': The Campaign for VD Controls in Interwar Scotland," *Social History of Medicine* VI no. 2 (1993), 214.

114. Ute Frevert, "The Civilizing Tendency of Hygiene: Working-Class Women under Medical Control in Imperial Germany," in John C. Fout, ed., *German Women in the Nineteenth Century: A Social History* (New York, Holmes & Meier, 1984), 326–27; R. P. Neuman, "Working-Class Birth Control in Wilhelmine Germany," *Comparatives Studies in Society and History* XX no. 3 (July 1975), 422; R. P. Neuman, "The Sexual Question and Social Democracy in Imperial Germany," *Journal of Social History* VII (1974), 280–86. See also Richard Evans, "Prostitution, State and Society in Imperial Germany," *Past and Present* LXX (1976), 122–29.

115. Ludwig Fleck, *The Genesis and Development of a Scientific Fact* (Berlin, 1935) ignored in the West until after World War II. Among Fleck's other important ideas was the inhibiting nature of earlier ideas of syphilis as *Lustseuche*, carnal plague, which led to moral outrage rather than meaningful research; on this see: Gerrit K. Kimsma, "Frames of Reference and the Growth of Medical Knowledge: L. Fleck and M. Foucault," in Henk ten Have, G. Kimsman and S. Spicker, eds, *The Growth of Medical Knowledge* (Dordrecht, Kluwer Academic Publishers, 1990), 45–51; Mary Douglas, *How Institutions Think* (Syracuse, NY, Syracuse University Press, 1986), 12–19. For a contrast between pre-Hitlerian syphilis research and research done in post-war America see James H. Jones, *Bad Blood: The Tuskegee Syphilis Experiment* (New York, The Free Press, 1981), 4.

116. Quétel, *Syphilis*, 252.

117. Evans, "Hideous Scourge", 413–33.

118. Davidson, "VD Controls in Inter-war Scotland," 213–35.

119. Payenneville, "Rapport," 707; Quétel, *Syphilis*, 179–80.

120. Quétel, *Syphilis*, 176–204.

121. Writing his *Mein Kampf* in 1923, Adolf Hitler noted that "Particularly with regard to syphilis, the attitude of the nation and the state can only be designed as total capitulation. . . . The cause lies, primarily, in our prostitution of love. . . . This Jewification of our spiritual life and mammonization of our mating instinct will sooner or later destroy our entire offspring": quoted in Gilman, *Sexuality*, 259.

122. Henri Pequignot, "L'Éclipse des maladies vénériennes en France (1944–1970)," in Bardet *et al.*, *Peurs et terreurs*, 361–62. Quétel, *Syphilis*, 251–55, estimated that in 1986 there were 60 million cases of syphilis worldwide.

123. For a list of mission stations, Robert Cochrane, *Leprosy in the Far East* (London, World Dominion Press, 1929), 23–40. Modern Sino-British relations began when the East India Company met its negative balance of

payments (with the West) by marketing Indian opium in China despite Chinese government disapproval: the First Opium War 1839–42 (to permit free trade in vice) was followed by the Second Opium War of 1858–60 when General Gordon looted and burned down the Summer Palace: Cain and Hopkins, *British Imperialism*, 325, 425.

124. Frank Dikötter, "The Discourse of Race and the Medicalization of Public and Private Space in Modern China (1895–1949)," *History of Science* XXIX part 4 no. 86 (December 1991), 411–20; R. H. van Gulik, *Sexual Life in Ancient China* (Leiden, E. J. Brill, 1961), 311–12.

125. Joseph Needham, "Medicine and Chinese Culture," in his *Clerks and Craftsmen in China and the West: Lectures and Addresses on the History of Science and Technology* (Cambridge, Cambridge University Press, 1970), 263–87; Quétel, *Syphilis*, 51–52.

126. Paul U. Unschuld, "Epistemological Issues and Changing Legitimation: Traditional Chinese Medicine in the Twentieth Century," in Charles Leslie and Allan Young, eds, *Paths to Asian Medical Knowledge* (Berkeley, University of California Press, 1992), 55, 58; Hyam, *Empire and Sexuality*, 59; Christian Henriot, "Prostitution et 'Police des Moeurs' à Shanghai aux XIXe–XXe siècles," in Christian Henriot, ed., *La Femme en Asie Orientale* (Lyon, Université Jean Moulin Lyon III, 1988), 65–67.

127. Unschuld, "Epistemological Issues," 44–61.

128. Ibid., 46, 59. In 1891, Dr George Thin confidently wrote that the Chinese desperately needed to be rescued by medical missionaries: George Thin, *Leprosy* (London, Percival, 1891), 260. Writing at mid-century, Frederic W. Farrar blasted the Chinese because they reduced everything to the "dead level of practical advantage," their arts were "plague-spots" of "utilitarian mediocrity" (i.e. Baconian): quoted in Michael Adas, *Machines as the Measure of Men: Science, Technology and Ideologies of Western Dominance* (Ithaca, NY, Cornell University Press, 1989), 189–90.

129. Quoted in Kerrie L. MacPherson, *A Wilderness of Marshes: The Origins of Public Health in Shanghai, 1843–1893* (Hong Kong, Oxford University Press, 1987), 13.

130. Quoted in Harold Balme, *China and Modern Medicine: A Study in Medical Missionary Development* (London, United Council for Missionary Education, 1921), 5–6.

131. For somewhat similar perceptions by British and British Empire colonialists in northern Nigeria, Kenya, Uganda and Egypt, see: Randall M. Packard and Paul Epstein, "Epidemiologists, Social Scientists, and the Structure of Medical Research on AIDS in Africa," *Social Science and Medicine* XXXIII no. 7 (1990), 772; Madden, "Thirty Years of Surgery," 18–19. In rewriting (in 1922) an article he published in 1904, Madden claimed: "As we go further south towards the Equator, and the disease affects the almost uncivilised black races, its ravages become worse and worse, and the power of resistance, never well developed in these people, seems to be completely broken down by the syphilitic virus": Frank Cole Madden, MD (Melbourne) *The Surgery of Egypt* (Cairo, The Nile Mission Press, 1922), 55.

132. Christian Henriot, "Medicine, V.D. and Prostitution in Pre-Revolutionary China," *Social History of Medicine* V no. 1 (1992), 112.

133. Needham, "Medicine," 287; Mark Elvin, "Female Virtue and the State in China," *Past and Present* CIV (August 1984), 110–52.
134. Elvin, "Female Virtue," 112; Henriot, "Prostitution in à Shanghai," 64–93.
135. Maria Jaschok, *Concubines and Bondservants: A Social History* (London, Zed Books, 1988), 143.
136. Quoted in Davidson, "VD Controls in Inter-war Scotland," 226.
137. *Morbidity and Mortality: Weekly Report* XXXIV no. RR–16 (31 December 1993), 15 (my italics). Writing from Ceylon in 1906, Dr Aldo Castellani questioned whether yaws and venereal syphilis were the same disease (as Jonathan Hutchinson held). Live tests on thirty-two Chinese prisoners had suggested that the two diseases were as "different" as leprosy was from tuberculosis; in this Castellani was supported by Patrick Manson: Aldo Castellani, "Is Yaws Syphilis?" *Journal of Tropical Medicine* IX (1 January 1906), 1–4.
138. Henriot, "Medicine," 110: my reading of Henriot also suggests that they never realized that the reason why western-trained Chinese doctors contributed so little to the published discourse on syphilis, while western doctors published so much, was that the Chinese accurately perceived the role of syphilis and Sinophobia in the making of medicalized white men's image of China.
139. Dikötter, "Discourse of Race," 417–19.
140. Quoted in Joshua S. Horn, *"Away with All Pests . . .": An English Surgeon in People's China* (London, Paul Hamlyn, 1960), 89–90.
141. Quoted ibid., 86; S. M. Hillier and J. A. Jewell, *Health Care and Traditional Medicine in China, 1800–1982* (London, Routledge & Kegan Paul, 1983), 159–61. In 1937 an Asian newspaper reported *re* the slaughter of the sick that "Canton is only putting into practice the suggestions of leading European and American scientists and thinkers. Doomed to certain death, it is better [that the patients be killed quickly]"; anon., "Shooting of Lepers in China," *Leprosy Review* VIII no. 2 (1937), 129–30.
142. Henriot, "Medicine," 119.
143. It seems that *Treponema pallidum* had the last laugh: since 1979 or so syphilis has re-emerged in China.

5 *Cholera and Civilization: Great Britain and India, 1817 to 1920*

1. *Parliamentary Papers* 1902 LXXIV [Cd 1357], 41, 192, 204. Indian figures from David Arnold, "Cholera Mortality in British India, 1817–1947," in Tim Dyson, ed., *India's Historical Demography: Studies in Famine, Disease and Society* (London, Curzon Press, 1989), 263–346. David Arnold, "Cholera and Colonialism in British India," *Past and Present* CXIII (1986), 120, suggests the total from the pre-statistical era 1817–65 was between 10 and 15 million. Adding up guesstimates and later statistics gives, as the low total, 25.75 million and 30.75 as the high. For England: Michael Durey, *The Return of the Plague: British Society and the Cholera 1831–32* (Dublin, Gill and Macmillan Humanities Press, 1979); William McNeill *Plagues and Peoples* (Garden City, NY, Anchor, 1976), 230–46; R. J. Morris, *Cholera 1832: The Social Response to an Epidemic* (London, Croom Helm, 1979). The standard medically informed account is R. Pollitzer, MD, *Chol-*

era (Geneva, World Health Organization, 1959). See also: André Dodin, "Les Persistances du XXe siècle," in Jean-Pierre Bardet *et al.*, *Peurs et terreurs face à la contagion* (Paris, Fayard, 1988), 136–55.

2. The role of human agency and of government conspiracies of silence is a principal theme of Frank M. Snowden, *Naples in the Time of Cholera, 1884–1911* (Cambridge, Cambridge University Press, 1995), 2ff.

3. Thomas R. Metcalf, *Ideologies of the Raj: The New Cambridge History of India* III part 4 (Cambridge, Cambridge University Press, 1994), x; J. B. Foreman, ed., *Complete Works of Oscar Wilde* (London, Collins, 1977), 973.

4. Harrison analyses the social origins of IMS recruits and finds them overwhelmingly lower middle-class, a factor "to which we may perhaps attribute some of the status anxiety and conservatism characteristic of medical officers in this period": Mark Harrison, *Public Health in British India: Anglo-Indian Preventive Medicine 1859–1914* (Cambridge, Cambridge University Press 1994), 29. For the upper classes, "true Britons," see: Linda Colley, *Britons: Forging the Nation 1707–1837* (London, Yale University Press, 1992).

5. Writing of Kipling, who produced "the only literary picture that we possess of nineteenth century Anglo-India," Orwell pointed out that he "never had any grasp of the economic forces underlying imperial expansion . . . [he did] not seem to realise, any more than the average soldier or colonial administrator, that an empire is primarily a money-making concern": George Orwell, "Rudyard Kipling," in Orwell *Selected Essays* (London, Secker & Warburg, 1975), 181–83. For "gentlemanly capitalism" see P. C. Cain and A. G. Hopkins, *British Imperialism: Innovation and Expansion 1688–1914* (London, Longman, 1993), 22ff., 319–24.

6. Charles E. Rosenberg, "Cholera in Nineteenth Century Europe: A Tool for Social and Economic Analysis," *Comparative Studies in Society and History* VIII (1966), 135–62; Bill Luckin, "States and Epidemic Threats," *Society for the Social History of Medicine* XXXIV (June 1984), 26; George Orwell, *Nineteen Eighty-Four: A Novel* (first published 1950) (New York, Signet, 1956), 29.

7. Quoted in Charles E. Rosenberg, *Explaining Epidemics and Other Studies in the History of Medicine* (Cambridge, Cambridge University Press, 1992), 120. See also: P. E. Brown, "John Snow—The Autumn Loiterer," *Bulletin of the History of Medicine* XXXV (1961), 519–28.

8. Paul W. Ewald, *Evolution of Infectious Disease* (Oxford, Oxford University Press, 1994), 23–27, 74–82; Patrice Bourdelais, J.-Y. Raulot and M. Demonet, "La Marche du choléra en France: 1832 et 1854," *Annales: Économies, Sociétés, Civilizations* XXX no. 1 (1978), 137, 142; Snowden, *Naples*, 174; J. E. Nicholson, "Flies and Cholera," *Journal of Tropical Medicine* IX (1 February 1906), 41–43. See also Richard J. Evans, "Blue Funk and Yellow Peril: Cholera and Society in Nineteenth-Century France," *European History Quarterly* XX (1990), 111–19; Richard J. Evans, "Epidemics and Revolutions: Cholera in Nineteenth Century Europe," *Past and Present* CXX (1988), 123–46.

9. Dodin, "Les Persistances," 152; Snowden, *Naples*, 42–43, 116–17; Evans, "Blue Funk," 116;

David Arnold, "Social Crisis and Epidemic Disease in the Famines of Nineteenth-century India," *Social History of Medicine* VI no. 3 (December 1993), 394; Oscar Felsenfeld, "Some Observations on the Cholera (El Tor) Epidemic in 1961–62," *Bulletin of World Health Organization* XXVIII (1963), 289, 291; A. M. Kamal, "Cholera in Egypt," *Journal of the Egyptian Public Health Association*, III (1948), 186.

10. Lawrence I. Conrad, Michael Neve, Vivian Nutton, Roy Porter and Andrew Wear, *The Western Medical Tradition: 800 BC to AD 1800* (Cambridge, Cambridge University Press, 1995), 1–6, 477–94. On medicine as social construction, see also: Roger Cooter, "Anticontagionism and History's Medical Record," in Peter Wright and Andrew Treacher, eds, *The Problem of Medical Knowledge* (Edinburgh, Edinburgh University Press, 1982), 87–108.

11. Christopher Hamlin, "Predisposing Causes and Public Health in Early Nineteenth-Century Medical Thought," *Social History of Medicine* V no. 1 (April 1992), 66; Evans, "Blue Funk," 114–15; Michel Oris, "Choléra et hygiène publique en Belgique: les réactions d'un système social face à une maladie sociale," in Bardet *et al.*, *Peurs et terreurs*, 86–89; Frank M. Snowden, "Cholera in Barletta 1910," *Past and Present* CXXXII (August 1991), 90; François Delaporte, *Disease and Civilization: The Cholera in Paris, 1832*, trans. Arthur Goldhammer (Cambridge MA, MIT Press, 1986), 69; Charles Creighton, *A History of Epidemics in Britain*, II: *From the Extinction of Plague to the Present Time* (Cambridge, At the University Press, 1894), 830–31.

12. *P.P.* 1887 LXIII [Cd 5209], 170; *P.P.* 1899, LXVI Part II [Cd 9549], 257.

13. *P.P.* 1878 LIX [Cd 2142], 39. Random post-Koch examples: *P.P.* 1890 LIV [Cd 6124], 87, 104, 122–23, 132.

14. *Weekly Epidemiological Record* (WHO Geneva) LXVII no. 34, (1992), 253–60; "96 Cholera Cases in 1992 Are Most Since US Began Monitoring," *New York Times*, 11 September 1992, 10.

15. Dodin, "Les Persistances," 153; A. Q. Khan, "Role of Carriers in the Intrafamilial Spread of Cholera," *The Lancet* (4 February 1967), 245–46; M. I. Narkevich *et al.*, "The Seventh Pandemic of Cholera in the USSR 1961–89," *Bulletin of the World Health Organization* LXXI no. 2 (1993), 191–93; Letter, "Cholera and the Environment," *The Lancet* CCCXXXIX (May 1992), 1167–68; F. Vay (of the Suez Quarantine Office), "Bacilli-Carriers and their Part in the Transmission of Infectious Diseases," *Journal of Tropical Medicine and Hygiene* XI (1 August 1908), 233–38; A. A. MacLaren, "Bourgeois Ideology and Victorian Philanthropy: The Contradictions of Cholera," in his *Social Class in Scotland: Past and Present* (Edinburgh, John Donald, 1976), 44; Bernard Vincent, "Le Choléra en Espagne au XIXe siècle," in Bardet *et al.*, *Peurs et terreurs*, 54–55.

16. Patrice Bourdelais, "Cholera: A Victory for Medicine?" in R. Schofield, ed., *The Decline of Mortality in Europe* (Oxford, Clarendon Press, 1991), 138; Evans, "Epidemics and Revolutions," 132–34; Philip D. Curtin, *Death by Migration: Europe's Encounter with the Tropical World in the Nineteenth Century* (Cambridge, Cambridge University Press, 1989), 72–75.

17. In fact cholera did claim some high-ranking victims including in 1832 Casimir Périer, President of the French Council of State. Casual reference to the 1865 edi-

tion of *Burke's Peerage* suggests that younger sons of leading English families out in India not infrequently died cholera: information courtesy Dr Hugh Vernon-Jackson. The most highly placed white victim on the subcontinent was Governor Sir Thomas Munro, who met his death in 1827.

18. On treatment: Snowden, *Naples*, 121–8; Delaporte *Disease and Civilization*, 115–37.
19. Morris, *Cholera*, 122–24; Thierry Eggerick and Michel Poulain, "L'Épidémie de 1866: le cas de la Belgique," in Bardet *et al.*, *Peurs et terreurs*, 56–82.
20. *P.P.* 1878–79 LVI [Cd 2415], 71.
21. Snowden, *Naples*, 112–21; Snowden, "Cholera in Barletta," 88–92; Jonathan Leonard, "Carlos Finlay's Life and the Death of Yellow Jack," *Bulletin of Pan American Health Organization* XXIII no. 4 (1989), 440. For literary interpretations see: Thomas Mann, *Death in Venice* (1911).
22. Beaven Rake *et al.*, *Report of the Leprosy Commission in India, 1890–91* (Calcutta, Printed by the Superintendent of Government Printing, 1892), 80, 83.
23. W. W. Hunter, *Orissa, Or, The Vicissitudes of an Indian Province under Native and British Rule: I* (London, Smith, Elder & Co., 1872), 167.
24. *P.P.* 1889 LVIII [Cd 5851], 109, 125, 183; Mark Harrison, "Quarantine, Pilgrimage, and Colonial Trade: India 1866–1900," *Indian Economic and Social History Review* XXIX no. 2 (1992), 134.
25. For a not untypical statistical report of regional death rates exceeding birth rates: *P.P.* LXV [Cd 1843], 180. C. A. Bayly, *Indian Society and the Making of British India* (Cambridge, Cambridge University Press, 1990), 29, 32; Michelle B. McAlpine, "Famines, Epidemics, and Population Growth: The Case of India," *Journal of Interdisciplinary History* XIV no. 2 (1983), 315; L. Visaria and P. Visaria, "Population, 1757–1947," in D. Kumar, ed., *The Cambridge Economic History of India*, II: *1757–1970* (Cambridge, Cambridge University Press, 1983), 463–532.
26. J. Majeed, "James Mill's 'The History of British India' and Utilitarianism as a Rhetoric of Reform," *Modern Asian Studies* XXIV no. 2 (1990), 209–24; Michael Adas, *Machines as the Measure of Men: Science, Technology, and Ideologies of Western Dominance* (Ithaca, NY, Cornell University Press, 1989), 166–67, 169–72; John Strachey, *India* (London, Kegan Paul, Trench & Co. 1888), 194; William J. Barber, *British Economic Thought and India 1600–1858* (Oxford, Clarendon Press, 1975), 126–76.
27. *P.P.* 1878 LIX [Cd 2142], 155.
28. Revisionists' interpretations introduced by D. A. Washbrook, "Progress and Problems: South Asian Economic and Social History *c.* 1720–1860," *Modern Asian Studies* XXII no. 1 (1988), 57–96.
29. Ashin Das Gupta, *Indian Merchants and the Decline of Surat, c. 1700–1750* (Wiesbaden, Franz Steiner, 1979), 3–19; Ashin Das Gupta and M. N. Pearson, eds, *India and the Indians 1500–1800* (Calcutta, Oxford University Press, 1987); Bayly, *Indian Society*, 36–37.
30. Washbrook, "Progress and Problems," 63–65.
31. Romila Thapar, "Imagined Religious Communities? Ancient History and the Modern Search for a Hindu Identity," *Modern Asian Studies* XXIII no. 2 (1989), 209–19, 120–22; Susan Bayly, *Saints, Goddesses, and Kings: Muslims and Christians in South Indian Society, 1700–1900*

(Cambridge, Cambridge University Press, 1989).

32. Das Gupta, *Indian Merchants*, 3–19; John E. Wills Jr, "European Consumption and Asian Production in the Seventeenth and Eighteenth Centuries," in John Brewer and Roy Porter, eds, *Consumption and the World of Goods* (London, Routledge, 1993), 135–46.

33. Bayly, *Indian Society*, 45–46, 49–53.

34. Quoted in Ralph W. Nicholas, "The Goddess Sitala and Epidemic Smallpox in Bengal," *Journal of Asian Studies* XLI no. 1 (November 1981), 33 (italics mine). See also: John R. McLane, *Land and Local Kingship in Eighteenth Century Bengal* (Cambridge, Cambridge University Press, 1993), 194–96.

35. Kapil Raj, "Knowledge, Power and Modern Science: The Brahmins Strike Back," in Deepak Kumar, ed., *Science and Empire: Essays in Indian Context 1700–1947* (Anamika, Prakashan, 1991), 119; Rudrangshu Mukherjee, "'Satan Let Loose Upon The Earth': The Kanpur Massacres in India in the Revolt of 1857," *Past and Present* CXXVIII (August 1990), 92–116.

36. Ewald, *Evolution*, 80; Aiden Cockburn, *The Evolution and Eradication of Infectious Diseases* (Baltimore, Johns Hopkins University Press, 1963), 155. See also: B. J. Terwiel, "Asiatic Cholera in Siam: Its First Occurrence in the 1820 Epidemic," in Norman G. Owen, ed., *Death and Disease in Southeast Asia: Explorations in Social, Medical and Demographic History* (Singapore, Oxford University Press, 1987), 142.

37. Quoted in O. P. Jaggi, *Epidemics and Other Tropical Diseases* (Delhi, Atma Ram and Sons, 1979), 15.

38. R. Pollitzer, *Cholera* (Geneva, World Health Organization, 1959), 17.

39. Quoted in J. Semmelink, *Geschiedenis der Cholera in Oost-Indië vóór 1817* (Utrecht, C. H. E. Breijer, 1885), 292 (my italics); see also, Anon, "Annesley's Report," *Edinburgh Medical and Surgical Journal* XXXI (1826), 170; Anon, "The Blue Cholera of India," *The Lancet* I (1831–2), 258–59.

40. Quoted in Jaggi, *Epidemics*, 13.

41. K. D. M. Snell, *Annals of the Labouring Poor: Social Change and Agrarian England, 1660–1900* (Cambridge, Cambridge University Press, 1987), 138–227; C. A. Bayly, *Imperial Meridian: The British Empire and the World 1780–1830* (London, Longman, 1989), 80–81, 121–26, 155–60.

42. "Cornwallis," *DNB*; Bayly, *Indian Society*, 65–66, 78; V. G. Kiernan, *The Lords of Human Kind: Black Man, Yellow Man, and White Man in an Age of Empire* (New York, Columbia University Press, 1986); John Hobson, *Imperialism: A Study* (first published 1902) (London, Allen & Unwin, 1938); Ronald Hyam, *Empire and Sexuality: The British Experience* (Manchester, Manchester University Press, 1990), 203.

43. Quoted in Jaggi, *Epidemics*, 18 (my italics).

44. Bayly, *Indian Society*, 76–78, 148–51; Raj, "Brahmins Strike Back," 120–22; G. Viswanatha, *Masks of Conquest: Literary Study & British Rule in India* (New York, Columbia University Press, 1989), 12–52.

45. Wills, "European Consumption and Asian Production," 140. See also: Fernand Braudel, *Civilization and Capitalism: 15th–18th Century* III *The Perspective of the World* trans. Siân Reynolds, (London Collins/Fontana, 1985),

506–7; Arnold Pacy, *Technology in World Civilization* (Oxford, Basil Blackwell, 1990), 120–21.

46. Abbé J. A. Dubois, *Hindu Manners, Customs and Ceremonies*, 3rd edition, trans. Henry K. Beauchamp (Oxford, Clarendon Press, 1906; repr. 1959), 94–95.
47. Bayly, *Imperial Meridian*, 147–48; Bayly, *Indian Society*, 75–76; Adas, *Machines*, 103–104; "Jones," *DNB*; "Colebrooke," *DNB*.
48. Bayly, *Imperial Meridian*, 103, 152, 160–61; Paul Zanker, *Augustus and the Power of Images* (Munich, Becks, 1987); Elizabeth Rawson, "The Expansion of Rome," in John Boardman, J. Griffin and O. Murray, *The Roman World* (Oxford, Oxford University Press, 1988), 45.
49. Bayly, *Imperial Meridian*, 52–53. See also: Steward Gordon, *Marathas, Marauders and State Formation in Eighteenth Century India* (Delhi, Oxford University Press, 1994), who mentions that the British kept the Puna archives locked to prevent researchers from undermining the Millian construct of unchanging India.
50. Washbrook, "Progress and Problems," 79–80; Bayly, *Imperial Society*, 28–32, 95–98.
51. Bayly, *Imperial Society*, 140–47.
52. Bayly, *Imperial Meridian*, 134, 157; W. W. Hunter, *The Indian Empire: Its History, People, and Products* (London, Trübner & Co., 1882), 342.
53. R. E. Enthoven, *The Folklore of Bombay* (Oxford, Clarendon Press, 1924), 258.
54. John W. Cell, "Anglo-Indian Medical Theory and the Origins of Segregation in West Africa," *American Historical Review* XCI no. 2 (1986), 321.
55. Arnold, "Cholera and Colonialism," 130–32; David R. Nalin and Zahidul Haque, "Folk Belief about Cholera among Bengali Muslims and Mogh Buddists in Chittagong, Bangladesh," *Medical Anthropology* I no. 3 (Summer 1977), 55–66; G. O. Oddie, "Hook-Swinging and Popular Religion in South India during the Nineteenth Century," *Indian Economic and Social History Review* XXIII no. 1 (1986), 93–106; I. J. Catanach, "Plague and the Indian Village, 1896–1914," in Peter Robb, ed., *Rural India: Land, Power and Society under British Rule* (London, Curzon Press, 1983), 241.
56. Eggerick and Poulain, "L'Épidémie de 1866," 67–69.
57. Margaret Trawick, "Death and Nurturance in Indian Systems of Healing," in Charles Leslie and Allan Young, eds, *Paths to Asian Medical Knowledge* (Berkeley, University of California Press, 1992), 130; Roger Jeffery, *Politics of Health in India* (Berkeley, University of California Press, 1988), 42–58; Adas, *Machines*, 55–57.
58. J. C. Caldwell, P. H. Reddy and Pat Caldwell, "The Social Component of Mortality Decline: An Investigation in South India Employing Alternative Methodologies," *Population Studies* XXXVII (1983), 191.
59. Adas, *Machines*, 279–80.
60. Adam Smith, *Theory of Moral Sentiments*, ed. D. D. Raphael and A. L. MacFie (Oxford, Clarendon Press, 1976), 239; John Locke, *Some Thoughts Concerning Education* (first published 1693) (Cambridge, At the University Press, 1927), 170–71. See also: Bayly, *Imperial Meridian*, 150–52.
61. Quoted in Jaggi, *Epidemics*, 14 (my italics).
62. Quoted in Arnold, "Cholera and Colonialism," 122.
63. Smith, *Moral Sentiments*, 239.
64. Raj, "Brahmins Strike Back," 119–23; Tapan Raychaudhuri, "Europe in India's Xenology: The Nineteenth Century Record,"

Past and Present CXXXVII (1992), 160–72, 182.

65. Arnold, "Cholera and Colonialism," 151.
66. Quoted in Frank Mort, *Dangerous Sexualities: Medico-Moral Politics in England since 1839* (London, Routledge & Kegan Paul, 1987), 21, taken from James Phillips Kay, *The Moral and Physical Condition of the Working Classes Employed in the Cotton Manufacture in Manchester* 2nd edition (London, 1832). See also: Richard Johnson, "Education Policy and Social Control in Early Victorian England," *Past and Present* XXXIX (1970), 98–99, 100–15, 119; John V. Pickstone, "Ferriar's Fever to Kay's Cholera: Disease and Social Structure in Cottonopolis," *History of Science* XXII (1984), 408.
67. Bayly, *Imperial Meridian*, 100–2, 121–26, 133–63; Snell, *Annals of the Labouring Poor*, 138–227. See also: Eric Hobsbawm and George Rudé, *Captain Swing* (London, Pimlico, 1993); J. L. Hammond and B. Hammond, *The Village Labourer* II (London, Penguin, 1951), 41–128; Colley, *Britons*, 128–29; Pat Thane, "Government and Society in England and Wales, 1750–1914," in F. M. L. Thompson, ed., *The Cambridge Social History of Britain 1750–1950* III (Cambridge, Cambridge University Press, 1990), 2–3, 9–13.
68. A. J. Youngson, *After the Forty-Five: The Economic Impact on the Scottish Highlands* (Edinburgh, Edinburgh University Press, 1973), 176–97; Rosalind Mitchison, "Scotland 1750–1850," in F. M. L. Thompson, *Cambridge Social History of Britain, 1750–1950*, I (Cambridge, Cambridge University Press, 1990), 191–92; C. J. Lawrence, "Medicine as Culture: Edinburgh and the Scottish Enlightenment," PhD Thesis, University College, London, 1984.
69. F. M. L. Thompson, *The Rise of Respectable Society: A Social History of Victorian Britain 1830–1900* (Cambridge, MA, Harvard University Press, 1988), 29–30, 58–61, 63–65; R. J. Morris, *Class, Sect and Party: The Making of the British Middle Class: Leeds 1820–1850* (Manchester, Manchester University Press, 1990); Harold Perkin, *The Making of Modern English Society* (London, Routledge & Kegan Paul, 1969), 196, 214–15, 227; Leonore Davidoff, "The Family in Britain," in F. M. L. Thompson, *The Cambridge Social History of Britain, 1750–1950*, II (Cambridge, Cambridge University Press, 1990), 77–85; H. Cunningham, "Leisure and Culture," ibid., 294–96; Spencer H. Brown, "British Army Surgeons Commissioned 1840–1909 with West Indian/West African Service: A Prosopographical Evaluation," *Medical History* XXXVII (1993), 418. In the making of "modern" class divisions, J. S. Mill (in *On Liberty*, 1859) was aware of fluidity, and used the plural "middle class*es*" (e.g.: "the strong permanent leaven of intolerance . . . which at all times abides in the middle classes of this country"), as well as the term "the middle *class*, who are the ascendant power in the present social and political condition of the kingdom": J. S. Mill, *On Liberty and Other Writings*, ed. Stefan Collini (Cambridge, Cambridge University Press, 1989), 33, 87.
70. W. D. Rubinstein, "The Victorian Middle Classes: Wealth, Occupation, and Geography," in Pat Thane and Antony Sutcliffe, eds, *Essays in Social History* (Oxford, Clarendon Press, 1986), 188–215; Perkin, *Making of*

Modern English Society, 213–15. Exemplifying James Mill's intemperate language: James Mill, *Elements of Political Economy* 3rd edition (London, Henry G. Bohn, 1844), 46–50. On John Stuart Mill's debt to Marcus Aurelius, whom he termed "the highest ethical product of the ancient mind": *On Liberty*, 29, 59; Bayly, *Imperial Meridian*, 103, 152, 160–61. Benjamin Disraeli's descriptions of British society and its keystones—as in *Coningsby* (1844)—were dead on target, but it has been fashionable among professional historians to minimize the importance of Disraeli's fictional writings.

71. Eric Stokes, "The First Century of British Colonial Rule in India: Social Revolution or Social Stagnation?," *Past and Present* LVIII (1973), 147. J. S. Mill's words are appropriate: "Despotism is a legitimate mode of government in dealing with barbarians, provided the end be their improvement. . . . Liberty, as a principle, has no application to any state of things anterior to the time when mankind have become capable of being improved by free and equal discussion. Until then, there is nothing for them but implicit obedience to an Akbar or a Charlemagne, if they are so fortunate to find one": J. S. Mill, *On Liberty*, 13–14. Curiously enough, in striking contrast to the sixteenth-century Spanish imperial experience of which there was rigorous intellectual criticism almost from the very beginning (Bartolomé de Las Casas), in the course of the British conquest and rule of India, there seems to have been no significant criticism until the early twentieth century (Hobson, Edward Thompson, Leonard Woolf).

72. Boyd Hilton, *Age of Atonement: The Influence of Evangelicalism on Social and Economic Thought, 1795–1865* (Oxford, Clarendon, Press, 1988), 78, 100; R. J. Morris, "Clubs, Societies and Associations," in Thompson, *The Cambridge Social History* III, 406–19.

73. Morris, "Clubs," 410; Joan Thirsk, *Economic Policy and Projects: The Development of a Consumer Society in Early Modern England* (Oxford, Oxford University Press, 1978); Brewer and Porter, *Consumption*; Johnson, "Education Policy and Social Control," 104.

74. Patrick Joyce, "Work," in Thompson, ed. *The Cambridge Social History* II, 142–80, 183–84, 346–51; J. Zeitlin and C. Sabel, "Historical Alternatives to Mass Production," *Past and Present* CVIII (1985); Ruth Richardson, *Death, Dissection and the Destitute* (London, Routledge, 1987), 275.

75. E. P. Thompson, "Hunting the Jacobin Fox," *Past and Present* CXLII (February 1994), 94–140. Malthus, in his first edition (1798), mentioned only the "positive checks"—plague, famine, war—then in later editions (apparently after readers had protested against his heartlessness) introduced the "preventative checks" such as birth control: Patricia James, ed., *Malthus, Essay On Population* (first published 1798) (Cambridge University Press, 1989), iv, 207–8.

76. Davidoff, "The Family," in Thompson, *Cambridge Social History* II, 89; Marilyn E. Pooley and Colin G. Pooley, "Health, Society and Environment in Victorian Manchester," in Robert Woods and John Woodward, eds, *Urban Disease and Mortality in Nineteenth-Century England* (London, Batsford, 1984), 149.

77. Hilton, *Age of Atonement*, 78, 100; Morris, "Clubs," 406–19; Evans, "Epidemics and Revolutions," 131–32.

78. Michel Foucault, *The Birth of the Clinic: An Archaeology of Medical Perception*, trans. A. M. Sheridan (London, Routledge, 1976), 192; Delaporte, *Disease and Civilization*, 115–37; Lindsay Granshaw, "The Rise of the Modern Hospital in Britain," in Andrew Wear, ed., *Medicine in Society: Historical Essays* (Cambridge, Cambridge University Press, 1992), 202–205.
79. Richardson, *Death, Dissection*, 95; Durey, *Return of the Plague*, 171–79; Frank McLynn, *Crime & Punishment in Eighteenth-Century England* (Oxford, Oxford University Press, 1991), 271–74; Peter Linebaugh, "The Tyburn Riot against the Surgeons," in Douglas Hay, E. P. Thompson *et al.*, *Albion's Fatal Tree: Crime and Society in Eighteenth Century England* (New York, Pantheon, 1975), 65–117; E. P. Thompson, *Whigs and Hunters* (London, Allen Lane, 1975).
80. Anthony Brundage, *England's "Prussian Minister": Edwin Chadwick and the Politics of Government Growth, 1832–1854* (University Park, Pennsylvania State University Press, 1988), 1–2; Richardson, *Death, Dissection*. For the Auto-Ikon as now restored: *The Observer* 6 December 1992, 22.
81. Creighton, *Epidemics*, 797; Durey, *Return of the Plague*, 170, 195.
82. Richardson, *Death, Dissection*, 175, 228–30; Creighton, *Epidemics*, 828; Morris, *Cholera*, 110.
83. Anon, "Cholera," *The Lancet* I (1831–32), 264; Cooter, "Anticontagionism," 96, 101, 105–6; M. Pelling, *Cholera, Fever and English Medicine, 1825–1865* (Oxford, Oxford University Press 1978), *passim*; Erwin Ackerknecht, "Anticontagionism between 1821 and 1867," *Bulletin of the History of Medicine* XXII (1948), 562–93; *DNB* "Charles Maclean" (*fl.* 1788–1824).
84. Hamlin, "Predisposing Causes," 59–60; Hilton, *Age of Atonement*, 155.
85. David Craigie, "An Account of the Epidemic Cholera of Newburn in January and February 1832," *Edinburgh Medical and Surgical Journal* XXXVII (1832), 356. On cholera-prone miners in Belgium see Eggerick and Poulain, "L'Épidémie de 1866," 89–91.
86. Anon., "Cholera at Sunderland," *Edinburgh Medical and Surgical Journal* XXXVII (1832), 215.
87. MacLaren, "Bourgeois Ideology," 47; Johnson, "Education Policy and Social Control," 105–106; Morris, *Cholera*, 34, 174; Creighton, *Epidemics*, 830–31; Hamlin, "Predisposing Causes," 64; Durey, *Return of the Plague*, 150; Brian Harrison, *Drink and the Victorians: The Temperance Question in England 1815–72* (Stoke-on-Trent, Keele University Press, 1994).
88. Quoted in Richardson, *Death, Dissection*, 227. Dr Henry Gaulter in his *Malignant Cholera in Manchester* (1833) violently opposed this wall-postering campaign, which "[w]ithout any adequate counterbalance of benefit . . . committed the capital offence of setting and keeping at work, through a whole community, that agitation and fear which, as we have seen, rendered the human frame most capable of being acted upon by the cause of cholera": quoted in Morris, *Cholera*, 116.
89. Pelling, *Cholera, Fever*, 7–10, 19–20. For the short-term impact of the Beer Act of 1830 and the aphorism, "The sovereign people are in a beastly state," see Thompson, *Respectable Society*, 312.

90. Morris, *Cholera*, 105.
91. Quoted in Richardson, *Death, Dissection*, 76–77. For the official amnesia in evidence by 1833—analogous to Italian government denials of cholera in Snowden's Naples—see Morris, *Cholera* 197–98; Mort, *Medico-Moral Politics*, 18, 223.
92. Quoted in Hank Ten Have, "Knowledge and Practice in European Medicine: The Case of Infectious Diseases," in Hank Ten Have, G. Kimsma and S. Spicker, eds, *The Growth of Medical Knowledge* (Dordrecht, Kluwer, 1990), 33.
93. Snell, "Social Relations—The Poor Law," in his *Annals of the Labouring Poor*, 104–37.
94. Morris, *Cholera*, 197–98.
95. Snell, "The Poor Law"; Richardson, *Death, Dissection*, xvi, 248, 270; Davidoff, "The Family," 91; Michael Anderson, "Social Implications of Demographic Change," in Thompson, *Cambridge Social History* II, 9–10; Creighton, *Epidemics*, 841, 843. Re: distress as a predisposing cause of cholera: John Burnett, *Idle Hands: The Experience of Unemployment, 1790–1990* (London, Routledge, 1994) notes that among "men 'broken' by worklessness in the 1840s . . . psychological distress, even more than physical ill-health, seems the one aspect of morbidity consistently linked to unemployment": *Times Literary Supplement*, 20 January 1995, 26.
96. J. S. Mill saw a preliminary draft of the report and advised Chadwick to give it a strong binding theme. Chadwick obviously took this advice: Brundage, *England's "Prussian Minister"* 80. See also: Hamlin, "Predisposing Causes," 62–70; Anthony Wohl, *Endangered Lives: Public Health in Victorian Britain* (London, Methuen, 1983), 146–48. 146–48; Pelling, *Cholera, Fever*, 1–19; Colley, *Britons*, 154–55.
97. Pelling, *Cholera, Fever*, 1–32.
98. Mort, *Medico-Moral Politics*, 30. Rival consultant engineers in 1842 had this to say of John Roe and Chadwick: "The truth is evident that [Chadwick] has been content to inform himself in respect of the Metropolitan sewage by special deference to the opinion of one individual, whose object has been to give himself importance by vaunting his own contrivances, by exalting his own commission, exaggerating his own success, and with unbecoming boldness casting unjust reflections on the adjoining commissions, traducing the competency of his brother surveyors of the surrounding jurisdictions": quoted in Gerry Kearns, "Private Property and Public Health Reform in England 1830–70," *Social Science and Medicine* XXVI no. 1 (1988), 192.
99. Kearns, "Private Property," 194–96; J. A. Hassan, "The Growth and Impact of the British Water Industry in the Nineteenth Century," *Economic History Review* 2nd series XXXVIII (1985), 543. For French parallels: William Coleman, *Death is a Social Disease: Public Health and Political Economy in Early Industrial France* (Madison, University of Wisconsin Press, 1982), xvi–xxi, 171–238; Ann F. La Berge, *Mission and Method: The Early Nineteenth-Century French Public Health Movement* (Cambridge, Cambridge University Press, 1994), 184–95, 238–40.
100. Christopher Hamlin, "Muddling in Bumbledom: On the Enormity of Large Sanitary Improvement in Four British Towns, 1855–1885," *Victorian Studies* XXXII no. 1 (Autumn 1988), 55–83; Curtin, *Death by Migration*, 116.
101. "John Snow," *DNB*; "John

Snow," in Gillispie, ed., *Dictionary of Scientific Biography*; Brown, "John Snow"; W. R. Winterton, "The Soho Cholera Epidemic 1854," *History of Medicine* VIII no. 2 (1980), 11–20; Michel Dupâquier and Fred Lewes, "Le Choléra en Angleterre au XIXe siècle: la médecine à l'épreuve de la statistique," *Annales de Démographie Historique*, 1989, 217–21.

102. Hamlin, "Bumbledom," 59, 80. In Manchester, it was reported in 1866 that the Corporation had placed an extra charge on water rates to prevent the widespread adoption of water closets. As late as 1902, 63 percent of the city's privies were not served by water closets, leaving fecal matter lying about until dustmen got around to shifting it: Pooley and Pooley, "Victorian Manchester," 174, 234.

103. Morris, *Cholera*, 200–206; Durey, *Return of the Plague*, 207–12; Snell, "The Poor Law," 133; Richardson, *Death, Dissection*, 268; Creighton, *Epidemics*, 841, 843; Kearns, "Private Property," 194; Brundage, *England's "Prussian Minister"*, 84.

104. Quoted in Durey, *Return of the Plague*, 206. Soon after the cholera epidemic of 1848–49, the Dutch doctor J. de Bosch Kemper held that the aim of "the enlightened" medical few who knew what was best for every member of the population was "to create" through "social surveillance . . . a man who could be master of his own body, who could control his passions and his habits," as in Smith's *Theory of Moral Sentiments*: quoted in Ten Have, *Medical Knowledge*, 33.

105. M. Callcott, "The Challenge of Cholera: The Last Epidemic at Newcastle upon Tyne," *Northern History* XX (1984), 175.

106. Wohl, *Endangered Lives*, 111; Hamlin, "Bumbledom," 61.

107. Kearns, "Private Property"; Gerry Kearns, "Environmental Management in Islington 1830–55," in W. F. Bynum and Roy Porter, eds, *Living and Dying in London, Medical History*: Supplement XI (1991), 122–25; Christopher Hamlin, "Providence and Putrefaction: Victorian Sanitarians and the Natural Theology of Health and Disease," *Victorian Studies* XXVIII no. 3 (Spring 1985), 393. Charles Dickens had pointed out the evils of the Circumlocution Office (the Court of Chancery) in *Bleak House* (1852–53).

108. M. J. Daunton, "Health and Housing in Victorian London," in Bynum and Porter, *Medical History*: Supplement XI, 126–44; Anne Hardy, "Parish Pump to Private Pipes: London's Water Supply in the 19th Century," in Bynum and Porter, *Medical History:* Supplement XI; Anne Hardy, "Public Health and the Expert: The London Medical Officers of Health, 1856–1900," in Roy MacLeod and Milton Lewis, eds, *Government and Expertise: Specialists, Administrators, and Professionals 1860–1919* (Cambridge, Cambridge University Press, 1988), 128–42.

109. Pelling, *Cholera, Fever*, 196; see also Howard Markel, "Cholera, Quarantines and Immigration Restriction: The View from Johns Hopkins, 1892," *Bulletin of the History of Medicine* LXVII (1993).

110. Harrison, "Quarantine," 126; Norman Longmate, *King Cholera: The Biography of a Disease* (London, Hamish Hamilton, 1966), 237. See also: *The Lancet* CCCXXXVIII (18 September 1991), 792; WHO, Geneva, *Weekly Epidemiological Record* LXVI no. 10 (8 March 1991), 69.

111. Quoted in Raychaudhuri, "Europe in India's Xenology," 165.

112. On the reconstituted medical establishment see: Mark Harrison, "The Foundations of Public

Health in India: Crisis and Constraint," in his *Public Health*, 60–98. On the history of Public Works: *P.P.* 1878–79 IX Report from the Select Committee on East India (Public Works); Ian Stone, *Canal Irrigation in British India: Perspectives on Technological Change in a Peasant Economy* (Cambridge, Cambridge University Press, 1984), 13–67.

113. Arnold, "Cholera Mortality," 267–68.

114. *P.P.* 1899 LXVI Part II [Cd 9549], 244; *P.P.* 1902 LXXIV [Cd 1357], 93. On economic and demographic indicators in time of famine, but ignoring policies of government and the Public Works Department, see Tim Dyson "On the Demography of South Asian Famines: Part I," *Population Studies* XLV (1991), 5–25.

115. Charles Blair, *Indian Famines: Containing Remarks on their Management* (Edinburgh, William Blackwood & Sons, 1874), 182–85 (Blair was "executive director, Indian Public Works Department"); David Arnold, *Famine: Social Crisis and Historical Change* (Oxford, Basil Blackwell, 1988) omits all mention of the PWD.

116. *P.P.* 1877 LXV [Cd 1707], 247–48; *Report of Committee on Nutrition* (London, British Medical Association, 1933), 327.

117. Quoted in Ira Klein, "Population Growth and Mortality in British India: Part II: The Demographic Revolution," *Indian Economic and Social History Review* XXVII no. 1 (1990), 37. See also: Michael Worboys, "The Discovery of Colonial Malnutrition between the Wars," in David Arnold, ed., *Imperial Medicine and Indigenous Societies* (Manchester, Manchester University Press, 1988), 208–25; Lenore Manderson, "Health Services and the Legitimization of the British State: British Malaya 1786–1914," *International Journal of Health Services* XVII no. 1 (1987), 108.

118. A. K. Sen, *Poverty and Famines: An Essay on Entitlement and Deprivation* (Oxford, Oxford University Press, 1981), 1–48. See also: N. Twose, *Behind the Weather: Why the Poor Suffer Most: Drought and the Sahel* (Oxford, Oxfam, 1984); John Abraham, "The Causes of Famine," in his *Food and Development: The Political Economy of Hunger and the Modern Diet* (London, Kogan Page, 1991), 90–104.

119. *P.P.* 1881 LXXI, Part III, "Famine Commission", 93 (my italics). Six years earlier, W. Thornton, Secretary for Public Works in the India Office, in a statement of the obvious reported that "Public Works have always formed rather a weak side of Anglo-Indian administration": William Thomas Thornton, *Indian Public Works and Cognate Indian Topics* (London, Macmillan, 1875), 1.

120. *P.P.* 1881 LXXI, Part III, Famine Commission, 106, 128, 164, 175, 199, 216, 220. For the rivalry between engineers (claiming professional knowledge) and district finance officers as to which group of experts was to do what: *P.P.* 1870, LIII, 56.

121. *P.P.* 1881 LXVIII, "Financial Statement," 17.

122. *P.P.* 1878–79 IX, "Report, East India Public Works," 84 (my italics); *P.P.* 1881 LXVIII, "Financial Statement," 17; Cain and Hopkins, *British Imperialism*, 316–50. See also; Patrick K. O'Brien, "The Costs and Benefits of British Imperialism 1846–1914," *Past and Present* CXX (August 1988), 163–200 esp. 187.

123. Quoted in Cain and Hopkins, *British Imperialism*, 341: Mayo was assassinated in 1872.

124. *P.P.* 1895 LXXIII "Moral and

Material Progress," xxii; *P.P.* 1878 LIX [Cd 2142], 3; David Hardiman, "Usury, Dearth and Famine in Western India," *Past and Present* CLII (August 1996), 126, 133, 145–46, 148. On the £95 million Britain invested between 1845 and 1875 see: W. J. Macpherson, "Investment in Indian Railways, 1845–1875," *Economic History Review* 2nd series, VII no. 2 (1955), 177–86.

125. Indicative of time lag, in 1893 (months after the Hamburg crisis) Surgeon-Major J. Lewtas, MB, in the office of the Indian Sanitation Commission, published a paper claiming that in neither India *nor in Europe* had rail travel had any appreciable effect on the progress of cholera: *P.P.* 1895 LXXIII [Cd 7846], 102, 145. For earlier claims see: Max von Pettenkofer, MD, "Cholera," *The Lancet* II (1 November 1884), 769; *P.P.* 1877 LXV [Cd 1843], 182; *P.P.* 1878 LIX [Cd 2142], 26; *P.P.* 1878–79 LVI [Cd 2415], 62; *P.P.* 1890–91 LIX [Cd 6501], 162; *P.P.* 1892 LVIII [Cd 6735], 10. On Hamburg: Pollitzer, *Cholera*, 39; Richard Evans, *Death in Hamburg: Society and Politics in the Cholera Years 1830–1910* (Cambridge, Cambridge University Press, 1987).

126. *P.P.* 1881 LXXI, "Irrigation as Protection against Famine" Part II, 71: *P.P.* 1865 XXXIX, "Irrigation," 549; *P.P.* 1880 LIII [Cd 2737], 3; Peter Harnetty, "Cotton Exports and Indian Agriculture, 1861–1870," *Economic History Review* 2nd series, XXIV no. 1 (1971) 414–29.

127. Sir John Strachey, *India* (London, Kegan Paul, Trench & Co., 1888), 134; *P.P.* 1895 LXXIII, "Material and Moral Progess," xxii; *P.P.* 1905 LVIII, "Material and Moral Progress," 141; Hunter, *Indian Empire*, 419–24. See also: "Richard Strachey," *DNB*. For an extended official history, *P.P.* 1904 LXVI [Cd 1851] "Report on the Indian Irrigation Commission 1901–1903," Part I.

128. Strachey, *India*, 132–33; Klein, "Population Growth and Mortality," 402.

129. *P.P.* 1878 LIX [Cd 2142], 39; *P.P.* 1878–79 LVI [Cd 2415], 33; *P.P.* 1881 LXIX [Cd. 2981], 140; *P.P.* 1895 LXXIII [Cd 7846], 111.

130. For a modern study see Ann Cheesmond and Alan Fenwick, "Human Excretion Behaviour in a Schistosomiasis Endemic Area of the Geizira, Sudan," *Journal of Tropical Medicine and Hygiene* LXXXIV (1981), 101ff.

131. Khwaja Arif Hasan, *The Cultural Frontier of Health in Village India: Case Study of a North India Village* (Bombay, Manaktalas, 1967), 77–79.

132. *P.P.* 1881 LXIX [Cd 2981], 176.

133. On the secure middle-class status enjoyed by engineers in Britain see R. A. Buchanan, "Engineers and Government in Nineteenth-Century Britain," in MacLeod and Lewis, *Government and Expertise*, 41–58.

134. Elizabeth Whitcome, "Development Projects and Environmental Disruption: The Case of Uttar Pradesh, India," *Social Science Information* XI no. 1 (1972), 29–49. For an overview, see her "Irrigation and Railways," in Kumar, *Cambridge Economic History of India II*, 677ff. On Egypt and the legacy left by engineers imported from India: Thierry Ruf, "Histoire hydraulique et agricole et lutte contra la salinisation dans le Delta du Nil," *Sécheresse* VI (1995), 307–17.

135. Provincial sanitary reports sent to head office in Calcutta invariably first listed annual deaths from cholera, reflecting European fears of the disease. Somewhat lower on the list were "fevers," a wide

category of diseases all taken to be caused by miasmas. Opening the records at random, I find that in Bengal in 1885 the overall death rate was 22.74 per thousand, with 15.75 per thousand of these being credited to "fevers." In human terms this worked out at 1,042,142 Bengali fever dead in that single year: *P.P.* 1887 LXIII [Cd 5209], 189, 196.

136. *P.P.* 1904 LXVI [Cd 1851], 103, 123; *P.P.* 1881 LXXI, Part III, "Famine", 444.

137. Hobson, *Imperialism*, 303. In writing about such things, Isaiah Berlin speaks of the mood, "in which men prefer to be ordered about, even if this entails ill-treatment, by members of their own faith or nation or class, to tutelage, however benevolent, on the part of ultimately patronizing superiors from a foreign land or alien class or milieu": Berlin, "The Bent Twig," in *The Crooked Timber of Humanity* (New York, Alfred A. Knopf, 1991), 251.

138. *P.P.* 1900 LVIII [Cd 397], 249, 250. On the priority of political contingency over mere scientific theory (germs) see also: Christopher Hamlin, "Politics and Germ Theories in Victorian Britain: The Metropolitan Water Commissions of 1867–69 and 1892–93," in MacLeod and Lewis, *Government and Expertise*, 110–27.

139. This reverses Arnold's argument that "the government of India, strongly influenced by Cunningham [*sic*], its long standing sanitary commissioner, clung to [an obsolete position]": Arnold, "Cholera and Colonialism," 144. Cuningham himself took offense at the barrage of criticism levelled against him in USA professional journals: *P.P.* 1876 [Cd 1615], 40.

140. Paraphrased by John Chandler Hume, Jr, "Colonialism and Sanitary Medicine: The Development of Preventive Health Policy in the Punjab, 1860 to 1900," *Modern Asian Studies* XX no. 4 (1986), 720. See also: Harrison, *Public Health*, 102–105; *P.P.* 1877 LXV [Cd 1843], 201; *P.P.* 1881 LXIX [Cd 2981], 94, 95, 96, 144, 188.

141. *P.P.* 1890–91 LIX [Cd 6501], 98, 155 (my italics).

142. *P.P.* 1892 XXIV [Cd 6735], 174, 9, 146, 190, 220; *P.P.* 1898 LXIV [Cd 8688], 180; *P.P.* 1899 LXVI Part II [Cd 9549], 218, 277, 234. Exaggerating, Ross (with Muhammad Bux discoverer of the mosquito vector of malaria in 1897) claimed that "sixteen years had elapsed since Robert Koch had discovered the cause of cholera" before scientists in India recognized the discovery *c.* 1896 (in reality twelve years after Koch): Ronald Ross, *Memoirs: With a Full Account of the Great Malaria Problem and its Solution* (London, John Murray, 1923), 184–56.

143. *P.P.* 1895 LXXIII [Cd 7846], 212.

144. Anon, "The Depreciation of the Attractions of the Indian Medical Service and Its Remedies," *Journal of Tropical Medicine* IX (1 March 1906), 38.

145. Quoted in Dubois, *Hindu Manners*, xv.

146. *P.P.* 1878–79 LVI [Cd 2415], 118. See also: Anon, "Plague Administration in India," *Journal of Tropical Medicine and Hygiene* (16 December 1907), 400, C. A. Bayly, "Knowing the Country: Empire and information in India," *Modern Asian Studies* XXVII (1993), 34ff.

147. "The White Man's Burden." See also: Edward Said, *Culture and Imperialism* (London, Chatto & Windus, 1993), 159–96.

148. Anon, "The Training of the Indian Subordinate Medical Service," *Journal of Tropical Medicine*

IX (2 July 1906), 203–204. See also: Manderson, "Health Services and Legitimization," 95. On the nature of the science internalized by Indians trained in England "[its] finality and extremely mathematical, certain nature, far removed from the tentativeness . . . of science at the frontiers" [i.e. another example of "the monstrous worship of fact"]: Raj, "Brahmins Strike Back," 123.

149. Anon, "Training," 204; Anon, "Government Control over Medicine," *Journal of Tropical Medicine and Hygiene* X (16 December 1907), 399–401; Poonam Bala, *Imperialism and Medicine in Bengal: A Socio-Historical Perspective* (New Delhi, Sage Publications, 1991), 81; Pollitzer, *Cholera* 78; Arnold, "Cholera Mortality," 263; Sumit Guha, "Mortality Decline in Early Twentieth-century India: A Preliminary Enquiry," *Indian Economic and Social History Review* XXVIII (4) (1991), 378.

150. Derek Sayer, "British Reactions to the Amritsar Massacre 1919–1920," *Past and Present* CXXXI (May 1991), 134, 152.

151. Pollitzer, *Cholera*, 82; William C. Summers, "Cholera and Plague in India; The Bacteriophage Inquiry of 1927–36," *Journal of the History of Medicine and Allied Sciences* XLVIII (1993), 299–300; Rajnarayan Chandavarkar, "Plague panic and epidemic politics in India, 1896–1914," in Ranger and Slack, *Epidemics and Ideas*, 226.

152. Quoted in Harrison, *Public Health*, 233. For a summary of the Government of India "Report of the Health Survey and Development Committee" (the Bhore Committee) (1946), *see* David Arnold, "The Rise of Western Medicine in India," *The Lancet*, CCCXLVII (19 October 1996), 1075.

153. WHO, Geneva: "Cholera," *Weekly Epidemiological Record*, LXVI no. 10 (8 March 1991); W. E. Van Heyningen and John R. Seal, *Cholera: The American Scientific Experience 1947–80* (Boulder, CO, Westview Press, 1983); *The Lancet* CCCXLV (11 February 1995), 359–61.

6 *Yellow Fever, Malaria and Development: Atlantic Africa and the New World, 1647 to 1928*

1. Patrick Manson, "The Malaria Parasite," *Journal of the African Society* VI no. 23 (April, 1907), 226–27.
2. Quoted in William Coleman, *Yellow Fever in the North: The Methods of Early Epidemiology* (Madison, University of Wisconsin Press, 1987), 5. See also: James D. Goodyear, "The Sugar Connection: A New Perspective on the History of Yellow Fever," *Bulletin of the History of Medicine* LII (1978), 14.
3. Sir Rubert Boyce, "The Distribution and Prevalence of Yellow Fever in West Africa," *Journal of Tropical Medicine and Hygiene* XIII (1 December 1910), 362.
4. George Pinckard, MD, Royal College of Physicians, *Notes on the West Indies Written during the Expedition under the Command of the Late Gen. Sir Ralph Abercromby* III (London, Longman, Hurst, Reis & Orme, 1806), 138.
5. Donald Joralemon, "New World Depopulation and the Case of Disease," *Journal of Anthropological Research* XXXVIII (1982), 111, 127.
6. Roy M. Anderson and Robert M. May, *Infectious Diseases in Humans* (Oxford, Oxford University Press, 1991), 374–418.

7. Edward Said, *Culture and Imperialism* (London, Chatto & Windus, 1993), 69–70, 106–16; Fernand Braudel, *Civilization and Capitalism: 15th–18th Century, III: The Perspective of the World*, trans. Siân Reynolds (London, Collins/Fontana, 1985), 392–93.
8. Joseph C. Miller, *Way of Death: Merchant Capitalism and the Angolan Slave Trade, 1730–1830* (London, James Currey, 1988), 306–307, 674–75, 682.
9. R. J. Morris, "Clubs, Societies and Associations," in F. M. L. Thompson, ed., *The Cambridge Social History of Britain 1750–1950* III (Cambridge, Cambridge University Press, 1990), 409, 433. See Chapter 5, "Cholera."
10. Robert William Fogel, "Afterword: The Moral Problem of Slavery" in his *Without Consent or Contract: The Rise and Fall of American Slavery* (New York, W. W. Norton, 1991), 388–417.
11. Quoted in Basil Davidson, *The Black Man's Burden: Africa and the Curse of the Nation State* (New York, Times Books, 1992), 24.
12. Suzanne Miers and Richard Roberts, eds, *The End of Slavery in Africa* (Madison, University of Wisconsin Press, 1989); Paul E. Lovejoy and Jan S. Hogendorn, *Slow Death for Slavery: The Course of Abolition in Northern Nigeria, 1897–1936* (Cambridge, Cambridge University Press, 1993).
13. Nancy Stepan, *The Idea of Race in Science: Great Britain 1800–1960* (London, Macmillan Press, 1982); Seymour Drescher, "The Ending of the Slave Trade and the Evolution of European Scientific Racism," in Joseph E. Inikori and Stanley L. Engerman, eds, *The Atlantic Slave Trade: Effects on Economies, Societies, and Peoples in Africa, the Americas and Europe* (Durham, NC, Duke University Press, 1992), 361–96.
14. W. H. Hoffmann, "Yellow Fever in Africa from the Epidemiological Standpoint," in Mohamed Bay Khalil, ed., *Proceedings: Congrès International de Médecine Tropicale et d'Hygiène: Le Caire, Egypte, Décembre 1928* V, (Cairo, Government Printing Office, 1932), 920; Coleman, *Yellow Fever in the North*, 14.
15. In India, among top echelon British medical officials, the place-specific idea remained firmly entrenched until after 1898: *Parliamentary Papers* 1899 LXVI pt 1 [Cd 9549], 223; *P.P.* 1899 LXVI pt 2 [Cd 9549], 254.
16. World Health Organization, *Prevention and Control of Yellow Fever in Africa* (Geneva, WHO, 1986), 1; Philip D. Curtin, *Death by Migration: Europe's Encounter with the Tropical World in the Nineteenth Century* (Cambridge, Cambridge University Press, 1989), 132–40; Anderson and May, *Infectious Diseases*, 11; Hoffmann, "Yellow Fever," 917–19; Bruno Latour, *The Pasteurization of France*, trans. Alan Sheridan and John Law (Cambridge, MA, Harvard University Press, 1988), 144.
17. Thomas P. Monath, "Yellow Fever: Victor, Victoria? Conqueror, Conquest? Epidemics and Research in the Last Forty Years and the Prospects for the Future," *American Journal of Tropical Medicine and Hygiene* XLV no. 1 (1991), 27; World Health Organization, *Yellow Fever*, 22; Hoffmann, "Yellow Fever," 917–19.
18. W. C. Gorgas, "Recent Experiences of the United States Army with Regard to Sanitation of Yellow Fever in the Tropics," *Journal of Tropical Medicine* VI (2 February 1903), 49; "Professor Koch's Investigations on Malaria," *British Medical Journal*, 12 May 1900, 1183–84; Thomas E. Skidmore, "Racial Ideas and

Social Policy in Brazil, 1870–1940," in Richard Graham, ed., *The Idea of Race in Latin America, 1870–1940* (Austin, University of Texas Press, 1990), 9.

19. Joralemon, "New World Depopulation," 111–12; R. Hoeppli, *Parasitic Disease in Africa and the Western Hemisphere: Early Documentation and Transmission by the Slave Trade* (Basil, Verlag für Recht und Gesellschaft, 1969), 52–55; Coleman, *Yellow Fever in the North*, 190–93.

20. Hoffmann, "Yellow Fever," 918; Monath, "Yellow Fever," 34.

21. Monath, "Yellow Fever," 30, 32–35; WHO, *Yellow Fever*, 3–5, 25–27; K. M. De Cock *et al.*, "Epidemic Yellow Fever in Eastern Nigeria, 1986," *The Lancet*, 19 March 1988, 630–32.

22. Hoffmann, "Yellow Fever," 915. Sir Rubert Boyce defined West African "endemic" as, "smoldering amongst the natives in very many centres, but not necessarily in all centres . . . [it was not] necessarily endemic in every village or town": "The Discussion on the Distribution and Prevalence of Yellow Fever in West Africa at the Society of Tropical Medicine and Hygiene," *Journal of Tropical Medicine and Hygiene* XIV (1 February 1911), 76.

23. Hoffmann, "Yellow Fever," 919–20; James Cantlie, "The Education and Position of the Sanitarian in the Tropics," *Journal of Tropical Medicine and Hygiene* XVII (15 August 1914), 296; Anderson and May, *Infectious Diseases*, 10, 426–27.

24. WHO, *Yellow Fever*, 18; Monath, "Yellow Fever," 30, 32–35.

25. WHO, *Yellow Fever*, 4–5, 18; De Cock *et al.*, "Epidemic Yellow Fever," 630; Boyce, "Yellow Fever," 358.

26. WHO, *Yellow Fever*, 5; Monath, "Yellow Fever," 29.

27. For criticism of Khaled J. Bloom's *The Mississippi Valley's Great Fever Epidemic of 1878* (Baton Rouge, Louisiana State University Press, 1993) because he "acknowledges none of the current discussion among scholars about issues related to the history of public health, for example the purported resistance of African Americans to yellow fever," see Todd L. Savitt (of East Carolina University) writing in the *American Historical Review* C no. 5 (December 1995), 1698. See also Philip D. Curtin, "The End of the 'White Man's Grave'?: Nineteenth-Century Mortality in West Africa," *Journal of Interdisciplinary History* XXI no. 1 (1990), 63.

28. Jill Dubisch, "Low Country Fevers: Cultural Adaptations to Malaria in Antebellum South Carolina," *Social Science and Medicine* XXI no. 6 (1985), 641–42.

29. Mary J. Dobson, "Mortality Gradients and Disease Exchanges: Comparisons from Old England and Colonial America," *Social History of Medicine* II (1989), 266–67; John Duffy, "The Impact of Malaria on the South," in Todd L. Savitt and James Harvey Young, eds, *Disease and Distinctiveness in the American South* (Knoxville, University of Tennessee Press, 1988), 34.

30. Mark Ridley, "The Microbe's Opportunity," *Times Literary Supplement*, 13 January 1995, 6.

31. Quoted in Karen Kupperman, "Fear of Hot Climates in the Anglo-American Experience," *William and Mary Quarterly* XLI (1984), 237.

32. Duffy, "Impact of Malaria," 29.

33. Frank B. Livingstone, "Anthropological Implications of Sickle

Cell Gene Distribution in West Africa," *American Anthropologist* LX (1958), 549–51; Carol Laderman, "Malaria and Progress: Some Historical and Ecological Considerations," *Social Science and Medicine* IX (1975), 591.

34. I. Hrbek, ed., UNESCO *General History of Africa*, III: *Africa from the Seventh to the Eleventh Century*, abridged edition (London, James Currey, 1992), 81.

35. Walter A. Schroeder, Edwin Munger and D. Powers, "Sickle Cell Anaemia, Genetic Variations, and the Slave Trade to the United States," *Journal of African History* XXXI (1990), 168–69; Joao Lavinha *et al.*, "Importation Route of the Sickle Cell Trait into Portugal: Contribution of Molecular Epidemiology," *Human Biology* LXIV no. 6 (December 1992), 891–901; John M. Janzen, "Health, Religion, and Medicine in Central and Southern African Traditions," in Lawrence E. Sullivan, ed., *Healing and Restoring: Health and Medicine in the World's Religious Traditions* (New York, Macmillan, 1989), 230; Thurstan Shaw, "The Guinea Zone," in Hrbek, *UNESCO . . . Africa*, 228.

36. Anderson and May, *Infectious Diseases*, 374.

37. Livingstone, "Sickle Cell"; Frank B. Livingstone, "The Duffy Blood Groups, Vivax Malaria, and Malaria Selection in Human Populations: A Review," *Human Biology* LVI no. 3 (September 1984), 413–25; Stephen L. Wisenfeld, "Sickle-Cell Trait in Human Biological and Cultural Evolution," *Science* CLVIII (1967), 1134–40 cited in K. David Patterson and Gerald W. Hartwig, "The Disease Factor: An Introductory Overview," in Patterson and Hartwig eds, *Disease in African History* (Durham, NC, Duke University Press, 1978), 6, 21; Laderman, "Malaria," 588.

38. Anderson and May, *Infectious Diseases*, 419, quoting Armstrong (1978) and Forsyth *et al.* (1988); Chris Newbold, Alister Craig and Adrian Hill, "Malaria Genes and Genomes: A YAC, a Map, a TRAP and a STARP," *Wellcome Trust Review* IV (1995), 24–25.

39. Anderson and May, *Infectious Diseases*, 409–19.

40. Stephen Frenkel and John Western, "Pretext or Prophylaxis? Racial Segregation and Malarial Mosquitoes in a British Tropical Colony: Sierra Leone," *Annals of the Association of American Geographers* LXXVIII (June 1988), 216. For the argument used against Indian children (in colonial discourse termed "blacks") see Colonel P. Hehir, IMS, "Prevention of Malaria in the Troops of Our Indian Empire," *Journal of Tropical Medicine and Hygiene* XVII (1 October 1914), 297.

41. Quoted in D. Maier, "Nineteenth-Century Asante Medical Practices," *Comparative Studies in Society and History* XXI (1979), 64.

42. Quoted ibid., 65. See also: H. M. Feinberg, "New Data on European Mortality in West Africa: The Dutch on the Gold Coast, 1719–1760," *Journal of African History* XV no. 3 (1974), 370–71; Anon, "Epidemic Visitations," *Journal of Tropical Medicine and Hygiene* XIII (1 November 1910), 324–28; Hoffmann, "Yellow Fever," 915; Henry Rose Carter, *Yellow Fever: An Epidemiological and Historical Study of Its Place of Origin*, ed. Laura Armistead Carter and Wade Hampton Frost (Baltimore, Williams & Wilkins, 1931), 254.

43. Ralph Austen, *Africa in Economic History* (London, James

Currey, 1987), 91–95; Patterson and Hartwig, *Disease in African History*, 6–7.

44. John Hunwick, "The Early History of the Western Sudan to 1500", in J. F. A. Ajayi and Michael Crowder, eds, *History of West Africa* I, 2nd edition (New York, Columbia University Press, 1976), 145–49; Thirstan Shaw, "The Pre-history of West Africa," in Ajayi and Crowder, *History of West Africa*, 68; T. Lewicki, "Trade and Trade Routes in West Africa," in Hrbek, UNESCO *General History of Africa* III, 190–93, 200–15.

45. James C. Boyajian, *Portuguese Trade in Asia under the Hapsburgs, 1580–1640* (Baltimore, MD, Johns Hopkins University Press, 1993); A. J. R. Russell-Wood, *A World on the Move: The Portuguese in Africa, Asia and America, 1415–1808* (London, Carcanet, 1992), 59; Fernand Braudel, *The Mediterranean and the Mediterranean World in the Age of Philip II* (London, Fontana/Collins, 1976), trans Siân Reynolds; on the Arab technological assistance which made the Portuguese voyages possible: Abbas Hamdani, "An Islamic Background to the Voyages of Discovery," in *The Legacy of Muslim Spain*, ed. Salma Jayyusi (Leiden, E. J. Brill, 1992), 289–95; for Africa: Austen, *Africa*, 85–86; John Thornton, *Africa and Africans in the Making of the Atlantic World, 1400–1680* (Cambridge, Cambridge University Press, 1992), 26–28, 37–39, 44–53, 115–16; George E. Brooks, *Landlords and Strangers: Ecology, Society, and Trade in Western Africa, 1000–1630* (Boulder, CO, Westview Press, 1993), 135; F. Guerra, "Aleixo de Abreu (1568–1630)," *Journal of Tropical Medicine and Hygiene* LXXI (1968), 55–69; Goodyear, "The Sugar Connection," 9.

46. Discussed at length in Miller, *Way of Death*; Lovejoy and Hogendorn, *Slow Death for Slavery*, 682; P. C. Lloyd, *The Political Development of Yoruba Kingdoms in the Eighteenth and Nineteenth Centuries*, Occasional Paper no. 31 (London, Royal Anthropological Institute, 1971); Robin Law, *The Oyo Empire c. 1600–1836: A West African Imperialism in the Era of the Atlantic Slave Trade* (Oxford, Oxford University Press, 1977); M. Gleave, "Hill Settlements and their Abandonment in Western Yorubaland," *Africa* XXXIII (1963), 343–52; M. Gleave and R. M. Prothero, "Population Density and Slave Raiding," *Journal of African History* XII (1971), 319–27.

47. Johannes Menne Postma, *The Dutch in the Atlantic Slave Trade 1600–1815* (Cambridge, Cambridge University Press, 1990), 9, 176; Braudel, *Civilization and Capitalism*, 48; Jonathan I. Israel, *European Jewry in the Age of Mercantilism, 1550–1750* (Oxford, Clarendon Press, 1989), 84–85; Miller, *Way of Death*, 665, 667, 672, 675, 681, 684.

48. J. F. A. Ajayi, *Christian Missions in Nigeria 1841–91* (London, Heinemann, 1965), 53–56, 465; J. Suret-Canale and Boubacar Barry, "The Western Atlantic Coast to 1800," in Ajayi and Crowder, *History of West Africa*, 343; Robert S. Smith, *Kingdoms of the Yoruba* (London, James Currey, reprint 1988), 96; J. Eades, *The Yoruba Today* (Cambridge, Cambridge University Press, 1980); K. M. Buchanan and J. C. Pugh, *Land and People in Nigeria: The Human Geography of Nigeria and its Environmental Background* (London, University of London Press, 1955); Bernard Lewis, "Slaves in Arms," in his *Race and Slavery in the Middle East: An Historical*

Enquiry (New York, Oxford University Press, 1990), 63, 65–66, 68–71, 157–59; Allan Fisher and H. J. Fisher, *Slavery and Muslim Society in Africa: The Institution in Saharan and Sudanic Africa and the Trans-Saharan Trade* (London, C. Hurst 1970); M. Hiskett, "The Image of Slaves in Hausa Literature," in J. S. Willis, ed., *Slaves and Slavery in Muslim Africa* (Totowa, NJ, F. Cass 1985), 106–24; Kwame Anthony Appiah, "The Invention of Africa," in his *In My Father's House: Africa in the Philosophy of Culture* (New York, Oxford University Press, 1992), 3–27.

49. Quoted in Miller, *Way of Death*, 673.

50. Joseph E. Inikori and Stanley L. Engerman, "Introduction: Gainers and Losers in the Atlantic Slave Trade," in Inikori and Engerman, *Atlantic Slave Trade*, 5–6; Philip Curtin, *The Atlantic Slave Trade: A Census* (Madison, University of Wisconsin Press, 1969); Ralph Austen, "The Trans-Saharan Slave Trade: A Tentative Census," in H. A. Gemery and J. S. Hogendorn, eds, *The Uncommon Market: Essays in the Economic History of the Atlantic Slave Trade* (New York, 1979); Paul E. Lovejoy, "The Volume of the Atlantic Slave Trade: A Synthesis," *Journal of African History* XXIII (1982), 473–502.

51. Miller, *Way of Death*, 157–58; H. G. Wells, *The Time Machine* (1895), Chapter 6, "Among the Morlocks"; Anon, "The Death of Dr Stewart," *Journal of Tropical Medicine* IX (1 February 1906), 40–41; Curtin, "End of the 'White Man's Grave'?", 63–88. See also: Amin Maalouf, *Les Croisades vues par les Arabes* (Paris, Editions J'ai Lu, 1983), 55–56.

52. Kenneth F. Kiple and Brian T. Higgins, "Yellow Fever and the Africanization of the Caribbean," in John W. Verano and Douglas H. Ubelaker, eds, *Disease and Demography in the Americas* (Washington, Smithsonian Institution Press, 1992), 237–48; Kenneth Kiple, *The Caribbean Slave: A Biological History* (Cambridge, Cambridge University Press, 1984), 12–22, 161–76; Kenneth F. Kiple, "A Survey of Recent Literature on the Biological Past of the Black," in Kiple, ed., *The African Exchange: Towards a Biological History of Black People* (Durham, NC, Duke University Press, 1987), 8; Kenneth F. Kiple and V. H. King, *Another Dimension to the Black Diaspora* (Cambridge, Cambridge University Press, 1981), 29–49; Donald B. Cooper and Kenneth F. Kiple, "Yellow Fever," in Kenneth F. Kiple, ed., *The Cambridge World History of Disease* (Cambridge, Cambridge University Press, 1993), 1102. For a recent attempt to sidestep the issue of disease determinism: Steven M. Stowe, "Seeing Themselves at Work: Physicians and the Case Narrative in the Mid-Nineteenth Century American South," *American Historical Review* CI no. 1 (February 1996), 57–58.

53. Jack Greene, "Changing Identity in the British West Indies in the Early Modern Era: Barbados as a Case Study," in his *Imperatives, Behaviors, and Identities: Essays in Early American Cultural History* (Charlottesville, University Press of Virginia, 1992), 38; John J. McCusker and Russell R. Menard, *The Economy of British America, 1607–1789* (Chapel Hill, NC, Institute of Early American History and Culture, 1985), 153.

54. Quoted in Greene, *Imperatives*, 19,

55. Quoted ibid., 38 (my italics).

56. McCusker and Menard,

Economy, 153, Greene, *Imperatives*, 38.

57. Ralph A. Austen and Woodruff D. Smith, "Private Tooth Decay as Public Economic Virtue: The Slave-Sugar Triangle, Consumerism, and European Industrialization," in Inikori and Engerman, *Atlantic Slave Trade*, 183–203; McCusker and Menard, *Economy*, 156; Basil Davidson, *The Fortunate Isles: A Study in African Transformation* (London, Hutchinson, 1989), 10, 38–39.

58. Philip D. Curtin, *The Rise and Fall of the Plantation Complex: Essays in Atlantic History* (Cambridge, Cambridge University Press, 1990). See also Jan De Vries, *The Economy of Europe in an Age of Crisis, 1600–1750* (Cambridge, Cambridge University Press, 1976), 137–38.

59. Austen and Smith, "Private Tooth Decay," 193–95; McCusker and Menard, *Economy*, 150; Brian Dietz, "Overseas Trade and Metropolitan Growth," in A. L. Beier and Roger Finlay, eds, *London 1500–1700: The Making of the Metropolis* (London, Longman, 1986), 132; John Chartres, "Food Consumption and Internal Trade," in Beier and Finlay, *London 1500–1700*, 176; D. C. Coleman, *The Economy of England 1459–1750* (Oxford, Oxford University Press, 1977), 118; Daniel Roche, *The People of Paris: An Essay on Popular Culture in the 18th Century*, trans. Marie Evans (Leamington Spa, Berg, 1987), 11.

60. Stuart B. Schwartz, *Reconsidering Brazilian Slavery* (Urbana, University of Illinois Press, 1992), 42–45; Fogel, *Without Consent Or Contract*, 24–25.

61. Greene, *Imperatives*, 33; McCusker and Menard, *Economy*, 152.

62. Quoted in David W. Galenson, "White Servitude and the Growth of Black Slavery in Colonial America," *Journal of Economic History* XLI no. 1 (March 1981), 42. See also: Larry Gragg, "'To Procure Negroes': The English Slave Trade to Barbados, 1627–60," *Slavery and Abolition* XVI no. 1 (April 1995), 70.

63. Mark A. Burkholder and Lyman L. Johnson, *Colonial Latin America* (New York, Oxford University Press, 1990), 121; Goodyear, "The Sugar Connection," 10–17; K. David Patterson, "Yellow Fever Epidemics and Mortality in the United States, 1693–1905," *Social Science and Medicine* XXXIV no. 8 (1992), 855–65. For "time obedience" see: Mark M. Smith, "Time, Slavery and Plantation Capitalism in the Ante-Bellum American South," *Past and Present* CL (February 1996), 142–68.

64. Paraphrased in Greene, *Imperatives*, 22.

65. H. Roy Merrens and George D. Terry, "Dying in Paradise: Malaria, Mortality, and the Perceptual Environment in Colonial South Carolina," *Journal of Southern History* L no. 4 (November 1984), 533–50. See also: Thornton, *Africa and Africans*, 142–48.

66. Eric Mercer, *Disease, Mortality and Population in Transition* (Leicester, University of Leicester Press, 1990), 37, 164; Gloria L. Main, *Tobacco Colony: Life in Early Maryland 1650–1720* (Princeton, Princeton University Press, 1982), 99–102; David Galenson, *Traders, Planters, and Slaves: Market Behavior in Early English America* (Cambridge, Cambridge University Press, 1986), 37. Relevant essays in Thad W. Tate and David L. Ammerman, eds, *The Chesapeake in the Seventeenth Century: Essays on Anglo-American Society* (Chapel Hill, University

of North Carolina Press, 1979), including: James Horn, "Servant Emigration to the Chesapeake in the Seventeenth Century," 51ff.; Carville V. Earle, "Environment and Mortality in Early Virginia," 96ff.; Lois Green Carr and Russell R. Menard, "Immigration and Opportunity: the Freedman in Early Colonial Maryland," 238ff.

67. Joan Thirsk, *Economic Policy and Projects: The Development of a Consumer Society in Early Modern England* (Oxford, Oxford University Press, 1978); Peter Kriedte, Hans Medick and Jürgen Schlumbohm, *Industrialization before Industrialization*, trans. Beate Scheupp (Cambridge, Cambridge University Press, 1981); Hermann Kellenbenz, "Rural Industries in the West from the End of the Middle Ages to the Eighteenth Century," in Peter Earle, ed., *Essays in European Economic History* (Oxford, Oxford University Press, 1974).
68. Greene, *Imperatives*, 26.
69. Postma, *The Dutch*, 126, 280–91; for Osterwald, see Chapter 4, "Syphilis".
70. Greene, *Imperatives*, 22.
71. Quoted ibid., 37.
72. Richard S. Dunn, *Sugar and Slaves: The Rise of the Planter Class in the English West Indies* (Chapel Hill, University of North Carolina Press, 1972), 312.
73. Paraphrased in Greene, *Imperatives*, 37.
74. Fogel, *Without Consent or Contract*, 142–47; J. R. Ward, *British West Indian Slavery, 1750–1834: The Process of Amelioration* (Oxford, Clarendon Press, 1988), 155–56; Kiple, "Survey of Recent Literature," 8.
75. Quoted in B. W. Higman, *Slave Populations of the British Caribbean 1807–1834* (Baltimore, MD, Johns Hopkins University Press, 1988), 264. See also: Todd Savitt, "Slave Health and Southern Distinctiveness," in Savitt and Young, *Disease and Distinctiveness*, 131.
76. Quoted in Jack Eckert, "Every Prospect of a Healthy Summer: The 1839 Outbreak of Yellow Fever in Charleston, South Carolina," *Transactions & Studies of the College of Physicians of Philadelphia: Medicine & History* Series V vol. XIV no. 2 (June 1992), 171.
77. Pinckard, *Notes on the West Indies*, 145.
78. Higman, *Slave Populations*, 266; Raymond Dumett, "Disease and Mortality among Gold Miners of Ghana: Colonial Government and Mining Company Attitudes and Policies, 1900–1938," *Social Science and Medicine* XXXVII (1993), 214.
79. Sidney W. Mintz, *Sweetness and Power: The Place of Sugar in Modern World History* (New York, Viking, 1985), 99–100; Curtin, *Rise and Fall of the Plantation Complex*, 146ff.; Dale W. Tomich, *Slavery in the Circuit of Sugar: Martinique and the World Economy 1830–1848* (Baltimore, MD, Johns Hopkins University Press, 1990), 15–21; Paul Farmer, "Many Masters: The European Domination of Haiti," in his *AIDS and Accusation: Haiti and the Geography of Blame* (Berkeley, University of California Press, 1992), 155.
80. Quoted in Farmer, *Haiti*, 156.
81. James E. McClellan III, "Science, Medicine and French Colonialism in Old-Regime Haiti," in Teresa Meade and Mark Walker, eds, *Science, Medicine and Cultural Imperialism* (London, Macmillan, 1991), 47–48.
82. J. M. Powell, *Bring Out Your Dead: The Great Plague of Yellow Fever in Philadelphia in 1793* (first published 1949) (Philadelphia, University of Pennsylvania Press, 1993), 4–7; Mar-

tin S. Pernick, "Politics, Parties, and Pestilence: Epidemic Yellow Fever in Philadelphia and the Rise of the First Party System," in Judith Walzer Leavitt and Ronald L. Numbers, eds, *Sickness and Health in America: Readings in the History of Medicine and Public Health* 2nd edition, revised (Madison, University of Wisconsin Press, 1985), 241–56. See also: William S. Middleton, "Felix Pascalis-Ouvrière and the Yellow Fever Epidemic of 1797," *Bulletin of the History of Medicine* XXXVIII (1964), 497–515.

83. Robin Blackburn, *The Overthrow of Colonial Slavery, 1776–1848* (London, Verso, 1988), 231–64.
84. David Geggus, "Yellow Fever in the 1790s: The British Army in Occupied Saint Domingue," *Medical History* XXIII (1979), 38–58.
85. Quoted ibid. 57 and Braudel, *Civilization and Capitalism*, 412. See also: Blackburn, *Overthrow*, 247–51; John B. Blake, "Yellow Fever in Eighteenth Century America," *Bulletin of the New York Academy of Medicine* XLIV no. 6 (1968), 676.
86. Quoted in Blackburn, *Overthrow*, 250.
87. Farmer, *Haiti*, 164.
88. Gorgas, "Recent Experiences," 49.
89. M. B. Akpan, "Liberia and Ethiopia, 1880–1914: The Survival of Two African States," in A. Ado Boahen, ed., *UNESCO General History of Africa, VII: Africa under Colonial Domination 1880–1935* (London, Heinemann Education, 1981), 270–73.
90. Drescher, "Ending of the Slave Trade," 372; Ronald Hyam, *Empire and Sexuality: The British Experience* (Manchester, Manchester University Press, 1990), 200; Farmer, *Haiti*, 269; Blackburn, *Overthrow*, 257–58; Said, *Culture and Imperialism*, 309, 338, 349.
91. Blackburn, *Overthrow*, 254.
92. Farmer, *Haiti*, 156–59, 174–75; Eugene D. Genovese, *Roll, Jordan Roll: The World the Slaves Made* (New York, Vintage Books, 1974), 174–75. "In its 190 years of existence, nine of Haiti's 41 heads of state declared themselves heads of state for life, and 29 were assassinated or overthrown": *The Egyptian Gazette*, 2 April 1995, 4. "Few countries in modern times have received so bad a press from foreign observers as Haiti": Sidney W. Mintz, *Caribbean Transformations* (Chicago, Aldine, 1974), 267.
93. American cotton production increased from around 0.7 million bales in 1830, to 1.8 million in 1840 and to 2.7 million bales in 1854; most of this was exported to mills in Great Britain: Fogel, *Without Consent or Contract*, 30. On the dangers of a single crop economy: James O. Breeden, "Disease as a Factor in Southern Distinctiveness," in Savitt and Young, *Disease and Distinctiveness*, 17.
94. McCusker and Menard, *Economy*, 170; Jack Greene, *Pursuits of Happiness: The Social Development of Early Modern British Colonies and the Formation of American Culture* (Chapel Hill, University of North Carolina Press, 1988), 143, 147; Eugene Genovese and Elizabeth Fox-Genovese, "The Fruits of Merchant Capital," in J. William Harris, ed., *Society and Culture in the Slave South* (London, Routledge, 1992), 31; Smith, "Time, Slavery and Plantation Capitalism," 96–97.
95. Fogel, *Without Consent or Contract*; Robert W. Fogel and Stanley L. Engerman, *Time on the Cross: The Economics of American Negro Slavery* (Boston, Little, Brown, 1974); Michael Kammen,

People of Paradox: An Inquiry Concerning the Origins of American Civilization (Ithaca, NY, Cornell University Press, 1972), 247; Greene, *Imperatives*, 1–2. "If ever America undergoes great revolutions, they will be brought about by the presence of the black race on the soil of the United States; that is to say, they will owe their origins, not to the equality, but to the inequality of condition": Alexis de Tocqueville, *Democracy in America* II (New York, Vintage Books, 1945), 270. Harriet Beecher Stowe published her radicalizing *Uncle Tom's Cabin* in 1852.

96. Fogel, *Without Consent or Contract*, 281–387.
97. Jo Ann Carrigan, "Yellow Fever: Scourge of the South," in Savitt and Young, *Disease and Distinctiveness*, 62–63; Todd L. Savitt, "Slave Health," 123; Mirko Grmek, *Disease in the Ancient Greek World*, trans. Mircelle and Leonard Mueller (Baltimore, MD, Johns Hopkins University Press, 1989), 265–66; Livingstone, "The Duffy Blood Groups," 416. "The South is . . . above all, as to the white folk a people with a common resolve indomitably maintained—that it shall be and remain a white man's country": quoted in Breeden, "Disease as a Factor", 4.
98. Patterson, "Yellow Fever," 857–58, 860; Breeden, "Disease as a Factor," 10; Carrigan, "Scourge of the South," 57.
99. Carrigan, "Scourge of the South," 59. "[Yellow fever] was and is generally, propagated by the negroes, especially by the negro children": Carter, *Yellow Fever*, 264.
100. Margaret Humphreys, *Yellow Fever and the South* (New Brunswick, NJ, Rutgers University Press, 1992), 51–52; Shane White and Graham White, "Slave Clothing and African-American Culture in the Eighteenth and Nineteenth Centuries," *Past and Present* CXLVIII (August 1995), 149–86; Elizabeth Fox-Genovese, *Within the Plantation Household: Black and White Women of the Old South* (Chapel Hill, University of North Carolina Press, 1988), 169–72, 318.
101. Ronald Ross, *Memoirs: With a Full Account of The Great Malaria Problem and its Solution* (London, John Murray, 1923), 123; Howard L. Holley, *The History of Medicine in Alabama* (Birmingham, AL, University of Alabama School of Medicine, 1982), 15, 18; Michael Adas, *Machines as the Measure of Men: Science, Technology, and Ideologies of Western Dominance* (Ithaca, NY, Cornell University Press, 1989), 154, 299, 301, 406.
102. Quoted in Kiple and King, *Another Dimension*, 44.
103. Samuel A. Cartwright, MD, "Report on the Diseases and Physical Peculiarities of the Negro Race," in Arthur L. Caplan, H. Engelhardt, J. McCartney, *Concepts of Health and Disease: Interdisciplinary Perspectives* (Reading, MA, Addison-Wesley, 1981), 314. Other Cartwrightian insights were that "black blood" is caused by not engaging in enough exercise "to vitalize and decarbonize their blood" and that "The black blood distributed to the brain chains the mind to ignorance, superstition and barbarism, and bolts the door against civilization, moral culture and religious truth": ibid., 324.
104. Quoted in Carrigan, "Scourge of the South," See also: Stowe, "Physicians and the Case Narrative," 57–58.
105. Quoted in John Duffy, *Sword of Pestilence: The New Orleans Yellow Fever Epidemic of 1853* (Baton Rouge, Louisiana State University Press, 1966), 8 (my italics).

106. Quoted in Hugh Brogan, *The Pelican History of the United States of America* (London, Penguin, 1986), 356.
107. Carter, *Yellow Fever*, 264. See also *Yellow Fever Bureau Bulletin* III no. 3 (1914), 350–57.
108. Mary Kingsley, *West African Studies* (London, Macmillan, 1901). See also Curtin, *Death by Migration*, 67–68.
109. Humphreys, *Yellow Fever*, 7.
110. Duffy, "Impact of Malaria," 51.
111. Quoted in Duffy, *Sword of Pestilence*, 10.
112. Ibid. 167; Carrigan, "Scourge of the South," 60.
113. Quoted in Humphreys, *Yellow Fever*, 23.
114. Ibid. 12; Duffy, *Sword of Pestilence*, 6, 171.
115. Bloom, *Great Yellow Fever Epidemic of 1878*, 230–31; Humphreys, *Yellow Fever*, 50, 100–102; Thomas H. Baker, "Yellowjack: The Yellow Fever Epidemic of 1878 in Memphis Tennessee," *Bulletin of the History of Medicine* XLII (1968), 241–64; J. M. Keating, *The Yellow Fever Epidemic of 1878, in Memphis, Tenn.* (Memphis TN, The Howard Association, 1879); Carrigan, "Scourge of the South," 66–67. "Contrary to expectations, the blacks of Memphis were proving to be painfully liable to this epidemic. Of the 99 yellow fever internments officially recorded on September 10, 35 were black": Bloom, *Great Yellow Fever Epidemic 1878*, 170: see Savitt, Review of Bloom, *American Historical Review* C no. 5 (December 1995), 1698.
116. Baker, "Yellowjack"; Humphreys, *Yellow Fever*, 100; John H. Ellis, *Yellow Fever & Public Health in the New South* (Lexington, University of Kentucky Press, 1992), 158, 160. In the decade ending 1880, capital values in Shelby County (greater Memphis) fell by 22 percent; the number of hands employed in manufacturing fell by 30 percent; brickyards dropped from nine to three; breweries dropped from two to one; tombstone-cutters *increased* from five to six; the percentage of blacks in Shelby County increased from 48 to 56 percent; Bloom, *Great Yellow Fever Epidemic of 1878*, 230.
117. Carrigan, "Scourge of the South," 67–68; Humphreys, *Yellow Fever*, 138, 145.
118. Quoted in Carrigan, "Scourge of the South," 68.
119. Quoted in Humphreys, *Yellow Fever*, 149.
120. Quoted in Bloom, *Great Yellow Fever Epidemic of 1878*, 255.
121. Breeden, "Disease as a Factor," 13.
122. Quoted in Humphreys, *Yellow Fever*, 165.
123. Ibid.
124. Brogan, *History of the United States*, 415.
125. Breeden, "Disease as a Factor," 13–14.
126. Jo-Ann Carrigan, "Mass Communication and Public Health: The 1905 Campaign against Yellow Fever in New Orleans," *Actes Proceedings* I: XXVIIIth International Congress for History of Medicine (Paris, Les Editions de Médecine Pratique, 1983), 234–35.
127. P. J. Cain and A. G. Hopkins, "Brazil," in Cain and Hopkins, *British Imperialism: Innovation and Expansion 1688–1914* (London, Longman, 1993), 298–306.
128. Curtin, *Plantation Complex*, 46–56.
129. Cain and Hopkins, *British Imperialism*, 298; Braudel, *Civilization and Capitalism*, 421; Teresa Meade, "Cultural Imperialism in Old Republic Rio de Janeiro: The Urban Renewal and Public Health Project," in T. Meade and Mark Walker,

eds, *Science, Medicine and Cultural Imperialism* (London, Macmillan, 1991), 95. For British influence in Portuguese Africa see G. Heaton Nicholls, "Empire Settlement in Africa in its Relation to Trade and the Native Races," *Journal of the African Society* XXV no. 48 (January 1926), 111.

130. Burkholder and Johnson, *Colonial Latin America*, 119. See also: Stuart B. Schwartz, *Slaves, Peasants, and Rebels: Reconsidering Brazilian Slavery* (Urbana, University of Illinois Press, 1992).

131. Quoted in Blackburn, *Overthrow*, 414.

132. Cain and Hopkins, *British Imperialism*, 90, 300.

133. G. Couto and C. de Rezende, "Control of Infectious Diseases in Brazil and Especially in Rio de Janeiro," *Yellow Fever Bureau Bulletin* II (1913), 297; Donald B. Cooper, "Brazil's Long Fight against Epidemic Disease, 1849–1917, with Special Emphasis on Yellow Fever," *Bulletin of the New York Academy of Medicine* LI, no. 5 (May 1975), 665.

134. Quoted in Cooper, "Brazil's Long Fight," 672.

135. Nancy Stepan, *Beginnings of Brazilian Science: Oswaldo Cruz, Medical Research and Policy, 1890–1920* (New York, Science History Publications, 1976), 48.

136. Skidmore, "Racial Ideas . . . in Brazil"; George Reid Andrews, "Racial Inequality in Brazil and the United States: A Statistical Comparison," *Journal of Social History* XXVI no. 2 (1992), 233.

137. In contrast, in the United States, the legal status of slavery was attached to any person of mixed blood no matter how small–$\frac{1}{16}$, $\frac{1}{32}$. For the proportion see: Main, *Tobacco Colony*, 127. "While [contemporary] North Americans believe that one single African ancestor is enough to produce an 'African-American', or a 'person of African descent', Brazilians tend to believe that they inherit characteristics from all their forebearers": Peter Fry, "Why Brazil is Different," *Times Literary Supplement* 8 December 1995, 7.

138. Blackburn, *Overthrow*, 381–417.

139. Cooper, "Brazil's Long Fight," 679; Couto and De Rezende, "Control of Infectious Diseases in Brazil," 298; Stepan, *Beginnings*, 59; Ilana Löwy, "Yellow Fever in Rio de Janeiro and the Pasteur Institute Mission (1901–1905): The Transfer of Science to the Periphery," *Medical History* XXXIV (1990), 156.

140. Quoted in Cooper, "Brazil's Long Fight," 679.

141. Couto and De Rezende, "Control of Infectious Diseases in Brazil," 298.

142. Andrews, "Racial Inequality," 233; Carlos E. A. Coimbra, Jr., "Human Factors in the Epidemiology of Malaria in the Brazilian Amazon," *Human Organization* XLVII no. 3 (1988), 257.

143. Anon., "Sanitary Environment a Bar to the Spread of Yellow Fever," *Journal of Tropical Medicine* I (November 1898), 105; "Compilation of Reports on Yellow Fever," ibid. 106.

144. Meade, "Cultural Imperialism," 95–119. For a similar situation in Cairo under Lord Cromer: Janet L. Abu-Lughod, *Cairo: 1001 Years of the City Victorious* (Princeton, NJ, Princeton University Press, 1991), 150–51.

145. Cain and Hopkins, *British Imperialism*, 303–304.

146. Meade, "Cultural Imperialism," 114–16.

147. Löwy, "Pasteur Institute Mission," 160; Stepan, *Beginnings*, 85–91; *Journal of Tropical Medicine and Hygiene* XIV (March 1911), 76.

148. Blackburn, *Overthrow*, 383–417; Braudel, *Civilization and Capitalism*, 440; David Brion Davis,

Slavery and Human Progress (Oxford, Oxford University Press, 1984), 287.

149. Curtin, *Plantation Complex*, 196–97.

150. Juliet Barclay, *Havana: Portrait of a City* (London, Cassell, 1993).

151. Curtin, *Death by Migration*, 131; Davis, *Slavery*, 238, 286; Jack Ericson Eblen, "On the Natural Increase of Slave Populations: The Example of the Cuban Black Population, 1775–1900," in Stanley Engerman and Eugene Genovese, eds, *Race and Slavery in the Western Hemisphere: Quantitative Studies* (Princeton, NJ, Princeton University Press, 1975), 211–45.

152. Jonathan Leonard, "Carlos Finlay's Life and the Death of Yellow Jack," *Bulletin of Pan-American Health Organization* XXIII no. 4 (1989), 446; Löwy, "Pasteur Institute Mission," 146; María Maltilde Suárez and Walewska Lemoine, "From Internalism to Externalism: A Study of Academic Resistance to New Scientific Findings," *History of Science* XXIV (1986), 390, 400.

153. Quoted in Brogan, *History of the United States*, 386.

154. Hoffmann, "Yellow Fever," 915; J. Guiteras, "Endemicity of Yellow Fever," *Yellow Fever Bureau Bulletin* II (1913), 365–74.

155. François Delaporte, *The History of Yellow Fever: An Essay on the Birth of Tropical Medicine* (Cambridge, MA, MIT Press, 1991), 141; "Henry Rose Carter," *Dictionary of American Biography*.

156. Rodney Sullivan, "Cholera and Colonialism in the Philippines, 1899–1903," in Roy MacLeod and Milton Lewis, eds, *Disease, Medicine, and Empire: Perspectives on Western Medicine and the Experience of European Expansion* (London, Routledge, 1988), 284–300; Humphreys, *Yellow Fever*, 146, 210, 214.

157. Quoted in John Farley, *Bilharzia: A History of Imperial Tropical Medicine* (Cambridge, Cambridge University Press, 1991), 39. Kipling published the poem with the title "The White Man's Burden" in 1899.

158. Raymond Buell, ed, *Report on the Commission on Cuban Affairs* (New York, Foreign Policy Association Inc., 1935), 103.

159. Hoffmann, "Yellow Fever," 916; Ronald Ross, "The Progress of Tropical Medicine," *Journal of the African Society* XV (April 1905), 283; Leonard, "Carlos Finlay's, Life," 449; Löwy, "Pasteur Institute Mission," 150, 153–4; Delaporte, *Birth of Tropical Medicine*, 125–46; Margaret Warner, "Hunting the Yellow Fever Germ: The Principle and Practice of Etiological Proof in Late Nineteenth-Century America," *Bulletin of the History of Medicine* LIX (1985), 361–82; Curtin, *Death by Migration*, 132.

160. Joseph A. Le Prince and A. J. Orenstein, *Mosquito Control in Panama: The Eradication of Malaria and Yellow Fever in Cuba and Panama* (New York, The Knickerbocker Press, 1916), 242–3. See also: Gorgas, "Recent Experiences," 49–52.

161. Burkholder and Johnson, *Colonial Latin America*, 91–94.

162. Ibid., 126–27; Ross, "Progress of Tropical Medicine," 288. For fictional insights, Graham Greene, *Getting to Know the General* (New York, Pocket Books/Simon & Schuster, 1984), 14–16.

163. Patrick Manson, "An Exposition of the Mosquito-Malaria Theory and its Recent Developments," *Journal of Tropical Medicine* I (August 1898), 4–8. For the successful eradication of malaria 1901–1903 using Ross's advice: Anon., "The Suppression of Malaria at Ismailia" (Suez Ca-

nal), *Journal of Tropical Medicine* IX, (August 1906), 243–44.

164. "Professor Koch's Investigations on Malaria," *British Medical Journal* (10 February 1900), 326; ibid. (12 May 1900), 1183–84; ibid. (30 June 1900), 1598. See also: Anderson and May, *Infectious Diseases*, 377.

165. Quoted in Gordon Harrison, *Mosquitoes, Malaria and Man: a History of Hostilities since 1880* (New York, Dutton, 1978), 94.

166. Quoted in Rubert W. Boyce, *Mosquito or Man? The Conquest of the Tropical World* (London, John Murray, 1910), 61. In *Instructions for the Prevention of Malarial Fever for the Use of Residents in Malarial Places* known to have been written by Ross ("In a community in which natives form the great bulk of the population, it is obvious that intelligent co-operation on a large scale can hardly be looked for"), Ross expresses similar racialist ideas: *British Medical Journal* I (10 February 1900), 329. See also, Major R. Ross, "The Fight against Malaria: An Industrial Necessity for our African Colonies," *Journal of the African Society* VI (January 1903), 149–51.

167. Anon., "The Death of Dr Stewart," *Journal of Tropical Medicine* IX (1 February 1906), 41.

168. Rubert Boyce, "The Colonization of Africa," *Journal of the African Society* X no. 40 (July 1911), 394–96. See also: Stepan, *Idea of Race . . . 1800–1960*; Drescher, "Ending of the Salve Trade," 361–96; Nicholls, "Empire Settlement," 108.

169. William B. Cohen, "Malaria and French Imperialism," *Journal of African History* XXIV (1983); Ross, "Progress of Tropical Medicine," 277; A. Kassab, "The Colonial Economy: North Africa," in A. Adu Boahen, ed., UNESCO *General History of Africa* VII: *Africa under Colonial Domination 1880–1935* (London, Heinemann Educational, 1985), 420–22, 430–31, 440; Said, *Culture and Imperialism*, 207; Curtin, *Death by Migration*, 132–37. See also: Anne Marcovich, "French Colonial Medicine and Colonial Rule: Algeria and Indochina," in MacLeod and Lewis, *Disease, Medicine, and Empire*, 104–109.

170. Leo Spitzer, "The Mosquito and Segregation in Sierra Leone," *Canadian Journal of African Studies II* no. 1 (Spring 1968), 58–59; Boyce, "The Colonization of Africa," 395.

171. Joseph E. Inikori, "Under-Population in Nineteenth-Century West Africa: The Role of the Export Slave Trade," *African Historical Demography* II (Edinburgh, Center of African Studies University of Edinburgh, 1981), 302; Abdullahi Mahadi and J. E. Inikori, "Population and Capitalist Development in Precolonial West Africa: Kasar Kano in the Nineteenth Century," in Dennis D. Cordell and Joel W. Gregory, eds, *African Population and Capitalism: Historical Perspectives* (Boulder, CO, Westview Press, 1987), 62–73; Patterson and Hartwig, *Disease in African History*, 8–10; Steven Feierman and John M. Janzen, *The Social Basis of Health & Healing in Africa* (Berkeley, University of California Press, 1992), 29–30.

172. Quoted in E. A. Ayandele, *The Missionary Impact on Modern Nigeria* (London, Longman, 1966), 240.

173. Ajahi and Crowder, *History of West Africa*.

174. Cain and Hopkins, *British Imperialism*, 351–62, 381–84; Austen, *Africa*, 109–10, 112–13; Walter Rodney, "The Colonial Economy," in UNESCO *General History of Africa* VII, 335–36; Martin Lynn, " 'The Imperialism

of Free Trade' in West Africa, *c.* 1800–*c.* 1870," *Journal of Imperial and Commonwealth History* XV (1986).

175. Austen, *Africa*, 114, 117; Cain and Hopkins, *British Imperialism*, 383–84; Kingsley, *West African Studies*, 294–95.

176. Emile Baillaud, "The Problem of Agricultural Development in West Africa," *Journal of the African Society* XVIII (January 1906), 206; P. N. Davies, *Sir Alfred Jones: Shipping Entrepreneur Par Excellence* (London 1978); Ross, *Memoirs*, 372–73. For Jones's connections with the Congo Free State (for which he was consul in Liverpool): Maryinez Lyons, "Sleeping Sickness, Colonial Medicine and Imperialism: Some Connections in the Belgian Congo," in MacLeod and Lewis, *Disease, Medicine and Empire*, 247.

177. Frederic Shelford, "Ten Years' Progress in West Africa," *Journal of the African Society* VI (1906), 345; Dumett, "Disease and Mortality among Gold Miners of Ghana," 213–14.

178. Kingsley, *West African Studies*, 283. The Royal African Society and its *Journal* was founded to honor Kingsley: a plaque commemorating her was recently erected in the Simonstown building in which she died while serving as a nurse in the Boer War: *African Affairs: The Journal of the Royal African Society* XCV no. 380 (July 1996), 432.

179. J. D. Hargreaves, "The European Partition of West Africa," in J. F. A. Ajayi and Michael Crowder, eds., *History of West Africa* II (New York, Columbia University Press, 1973), 402–23; G. N. Uzoigwe, "European Partition and Conquest of Africa: An Overview," in UNESCO *General History of Africa VII* 19–44; M. H. Y. Kaniki, "The Colonial Economy: The Former British Zones," in Boahen, UNESCO *General History of Africa VII*, 383. On Chamberlain, "the first politician to notice that Britain faced the threat of industrial decline, and the first to seek to do something about it by using the power of the state": Peter Marsh, *Joseph Chamberlain: Entrepreneur in Politics* (London, Yale University Press, 1994).

180. Quoted in Michael Crowder, *West Africa under Colonial Rule* (London, Hutchinson, 1968), 128.

181. John Flint, *Sir George Goldie and the Making of Nigeria* (London, Oxford University Press, 1960), 304–306; Crowder, *Under Colonial Rule;* William F. S. Miles, "Colonial Hausa Idioms: Towards a West African Ethno-Ethnohistory," *African Studies Review* XXXVI no. 1 (September 1993), 15, 17. Ilorin is the author's African hometown.

182. Michael Worboys, "Manson, Ross and Colonial Medical Policy: Tropical Medicine in London and Liverpool, 1899–1914," in MacLeod and Lewis, *Disease, Medicine, and Empire*, 21–37; Michael Worboys, "The Emergence of Tropical Medicine: A Study in the Establishment of a Scientific Specialty," in Gérard Lemaine *et al.*, *Perspectives on the Emergence of Scientific Disciplines* (The Hague, Mouton, 1976), 85. According to Manson, "In this matter of tropical medicine, Mr. Chamberlain deserves a title far more honourable than that of Imperialist—he is a humanitarian": "Sir P. Manson on the London School of Tropical Medicine," *Journal of Tropical Medicine* VII (1 January 1904), 11.

183. H. E. Annett, J. E. Dutton and J. H. Elliot, *Report on the Malaria Expedition to Nigeria of the Liverpool School of Tropical Medicine and Medical Parasitology* (Liverpool, At the University

Press, 1901); Sir S. R. Christophers, *Report on Housing and Malaria* extract no. 6 (1) from the *Quarterly Bulletin* of the Health Organisation of the League of Nations, II (1933), 431–32; Philip D. Curtin, "Medical Knowledge and Urban Planning in Tropical Africa," *American Historical Review* XC no. 3 (1985), 598ff.; Frenkel and Western, "Pretext or Prophylaxis?', 214–17; John W. Cell, "Anglo-Indian Medical Theory and the Origins of Segregation in West Africa," *American Historical Review* XCI no. 2 (1986), 330–35; Spitzer, "The Mosquito and Segregation," 56; Thomas S. Gale, "Segregation in British West Africa," *Cahiers d'Études Africaines* XX no. 4 (1980), 498.

184. Quoted in Frenkel and Western, "Pretext or Prophylaxis?" 216.

185. Annett *et al.*, "Report," 47; H. E. Annett, "The Work of the Liverpool School of Tropical Medicine," *Journal of the African Society*, I (October 1900), 209.

186. Anon: "The Housing of Europeans on the West Coast of Africa," *Journal of Tropical Medicine and Hygiene* IX (15 December 1906), 376; Curtin, "Medical Knowledge and Urban Planning," 602–3; Donald Denoon, "Temperate Medicine and Settler Capitalism: On the Reception of Western Medical Ideas," in MacLeod and Lewis, *Disease, Medicine, and Empire*, 121–22, 133; The *Oxford English Dictionary* (1908–14) suggests that Patrick Manson, writing in the *British Medical Journal* in 1904, invented the word "segregation."

187. Dr S. W. Thompstone, "Northern Nigeria, Medical Report for 1904," *Journal of Tropical Medicine* IX (February 1906), 12.

188. R. R. Kuczynski, *Demographic Survey of the British Colonial Empire*, I: *West Africa* (Oxford, for the Royal Institute of International Affairs, Oxford University Press, 1948), 684.

189. Thompstone, "Northern Nigeria, Medical Report, 1904," 15; Thompstone, "Northern Nigeria, Medical Report for the Year 1905," *Journal of Tropical Medicine* IX (September 1906), 55, 59; Megan Vaughan, "Syphilis in Colonial East and Central Africa: The Social Construction of an Epidemic," in Terence Ranger and Paul Slack, eds, *Epidemics and Ideas: Essays on the Historical Perception of Pestilence* (Cambridge, Cambridge University Press, 1992), 279–81, 300–302. See also Chapter 4, on syphilis.

190. "Yellow Fever in West Africa," *Yellow Fever Bureau Bulletin* II (1913), 249 (my italics).

191. Frenkel and Western, "Pretext or Prophylaxis?" 217–18; Gale, "Segregation," 505; Curtin, "Medical Knowledge and Urban Planning," 604.

192. Sir Rubert Boyce, "The Distribution and Prevalence of Yellow Fever in West Africa," *Journal of Tropical Medicine and Hygiene* XIII (1 December 1910), 357; Curtin, "Medical Knowledge and Urban Planning," 606. See also: Boyce, "The Colonization of Africa," 394–96.

193. Quoted in "Discussion on Yellow Fever," *Yellow Fever Bureau Bulletin* IV (August 1911), 284–85. See also: Boyce, "Distribution and Prevalence of Yellow Fever," 362; Gale, "Segregation," 498.

194. Shelford, "Ten Years' Progress," 345.

195. "West Africa—Reports on Certain Outbreaks of Yellow Fever in 1910 and 1911," *Yellow Fever Bureau Bulletin* II (1912), 272–74. It was noted that Europeans were allowed in the port of Sekondi only during the hours between 7 a.m. and 5 p.m.: this was based on an analogy between the behavior of malarial mosqui-

toes and yellow fever mosquitoes. It is now known that this analogy is misleading since the latter are most commonly daytime biters: ibid., 377; WHO, *Prevention and Control of Yellow Fever in Africa*, 23. See also: "Yellow Fever in West Africa," *Yellow Fever Bureau Bulletin* IV (August 1911), 129.

196. "The Discussion of the Distribution and Prevalence of Yellow Fever in West Africa at the Society of Tropical Medicine and Hygiene," *Journal of Tropical Medicine and Hygiene* XIV (1 March 1911), 75.

197. Dumett, "Disease and Mortality among Gold Miners of Ghana," 217–18, 229. For yellow fever and the French at Dakar (Senegal) see Daniel R. Headrick, *The Tentacles of Progress: Technology Transfer in the Age of Imperialism, 1850–1940* (New York, Oxford University Press, 1988), 160–67. Between 1900 and 1909 yellow fever epidemics occurred in Togo, Dahomey; there were five epidemics in Senegal: Gale, "Segregation," 409.

198. Boyce, "Distribution and Prevalence: of Yellow Fever," 357.

199. Quoted in Cohen, "Malaria and French Imperialism," 34.

200. Kuczynski, *Demographic Survey*, 701.

201. Baillaud, "Problem of Agricultural Development," 117–29.

202. M. H. Y. Kaniki, "The Colonial Economy: The Former British Zones," UNESCO *General History of Africa* VII, 404–405; C. Caldwell, "The Social Repercussions of Colonial Rule: Demographic Aspects," UNESCO *General History of Africa* VII, 474; Myron Echenberg, "'Faire du Nègre': Military Aspects of Population Planning in French West Africa, 1920–1940," in Cordell and Gregory, *African Population and Capitalism*, 95–108; Roger Tangri, *Politics in Sub-Saharan Africa* (London, James Currey, 1985), 2; Patterson and Hartwig, "The Disease Factor: An Introductory Overview," 13–14.

203. Baillaud, "Problem of Agricultural Development," 127.

204. R. Mansell Prothero, *Migrants and Malaria* (London, Longman, 1965), 1–7, 25–46; Caldwell, "Social Repercussions," 474; Steven Feierman and John M. Janzen, "Decline and Rise of African Population" in their *Social Basis of Health*, 30. See also: Randall M. Packard, "Agricultural Development, Migrant Labour and the Resurgence of Malaria in Swaziland," *Social Science and Medicine* XXII no. 9 (1986), 861–67.

205. Thompstone, "Northern Nigeria, Medical Report, 1905," 15. See also: Nina L. Etkin and Paul J. Ross, "Malaria, Medicine, and Meals: Plant Use among the Hausa and Its Impact on Disease," in Lola Romanucci-Ross, D. Moerman and L. Tancredi, *The Anthropology of Medicine: From Culture to Method* (New York, Praeger, 1982), 252. For the migrant link between coastal malaria and inland places see also: Meredeth Tushen, "Population Growth and the Deterioration of Health: Mainland Tanzania, 1920–1960," in Cordell and Gregory, *African Population and Capitalism*, 193; Marc Dawson, "Health, Nutrition, and Population in Central Kenya, 1890–1945," ibid., 202–3, 205–6; for the Cameroons, see Mark W. DeLancey, "Health and Disease on the Plantations of Cameroon, 1884–1939," in Patterson and Hartwig, *Disease in African History*, 153, 160, 174.

206. Kuczynski, *Demographic Survey*, 761.

207. Shelford, "Ten Years' Progress," 347; Percy Girourd, "The Devel-

opment of Northern Nigeria," *Journal of the African Society* VII no. 28 (July 1908), 334–37. Overview of "economic dislocation" in northern Nigeria in 1900–1908 followed by resettlement and adjustment 1909–16 in Lovejoy and Hogendorn, *Slow Death for Slavery*, 216–20.

208. Baillaud, "Problem of Agricultural Development," 120. On forest clearance and malaria: Feierman and Janzen, *Social Basis of Health*, 1.

209. Davidson, *The Black Man's Burden*.

210. Anon., "Colonial Medical Report, Southern Nigeria, for 1905," *Journal of Tropical Medicine* IX (1906), 55 (my italics). *See also*: *P.P.* 1912–13 LXII [Cd 6538], 12, 67, 69; *P.P.* 1914 LXIII [Cd 7519], 7; Cohen, "Malaria and French Imperialism," 29.

211. Hoffmann, "Yellow Fever," 920 (my italics); Manson, "The Malaria Parasite," 226; Curtin, "End of the 'White Man's Grave'?" 88.

212. On parliamentary legislation, July 1926, barring alienation of Nigerian land to non-Africans: Crowder, *Under Colonial Rule*, 319; on Italian Fascist government mass colonization in Libya; French colonization in Morocco, Tunisia, Ivory Coast; German colonization in Duoala and Cameroon see: J. D. Fage and Roland Oliver, eds, *Cambridge History of Africa*, VII: *From 1905 to 1940* (Cambridge, Cambridge University Press, 1986), 297, 344, 410–11.

213. Baillaud, "Problem of Agricultural Development," 127–28.

7 *Afterword: To the Epidemiologic Transition?*

1. *The World Health Report 1995, Bridging the Gaps* (Geneva, WHO, 1995), v. The five "Giant Evils" listed by William Beveridge in his *Report* of 1 December 1942 were Want, Disease, Ignorance, Squalor and Idleness.

2. Anon., "Benelovence" (*sic*), *Maadi Messenger* of the Maadi Community Church (Cairo, Egypt) XVIII no. 15 (15 May 1994), 5; BBC World Service program 17 April 1994, "Hymns of Praise," discussion of the dark hidden meanings of the problems troubling Lazarus alternating with dramatic choral music by Verdi and Berlioz; Reuters report, "Russians Try to Come to Terms with Leprosy," *Egyptian Gazette*, 13 November 1996, 8 containing Orientalist statements such as "the disease which stalked Europe after it was brought to the region after the Crusades."

3. See Chapter 6, note 52. Party slogan "Ignorance is Strength," George Orwell, *Nineteen Eighty-Four: A Novel* (New York, Signet, 1950), 15. According to Vitebsky, "The very essence of 'Development' is to declare an essence in someone else, in order to end their previous state of knowledge by transmuting it into ignorance—a sort of reverse alchemy": Piers Vitebsky, "Is Death the Same Everywhere? Contexts of Knowing and Doubting," in Mark Hobart, ed., *An Anthropological Critique of Development: The Growth of Ignorance* (London, Routledge, 1993), 108.

4. Abdel R. Omran, "The Epidemiologic Transition: A Theory of the Epidemiology of Population Change," *Milbank Memorial Fund Quarterly* XLIX no. 4 part I (October 1971), 509–38. See also Abdel R. Omran, "The Epidemiologic Transition Theory: A Preliminary Update," *Journal of Tropical Pediatrics* XXIX (1983), 305–16. As a

medical man, Omran was especially concerned with mortality rates; however, in any population growth equation *fertility* rates are another important factor. Here old-style Demographic Transition Theory does not have equal relevance in all parts of the world and specifically in sub-Saharan Africa; for an early breakthrough to this insight: Gavin Kitching, "Proto-industrialization and Demographic Change," *Journal of African History* XXIV (1983), 221–40.

5. David R. Phillips and Yola Verhasselt, "Health and Development: Retrospect and Prospect," in Phillips and Verhasselt, eds, *Health and Development* (London, Routledge, 1994), 307: "Table Four, Trends in Human Development," *Human Development Report 1993*: published for the United Nations Development Programme (Oxford, Oxford University Press, 1993), 142–43; Steven Feierman and John M. Janzen, "The Decline and Rise of African Population: The Social Context of Health and Disease," in Feierman and Janzen, eds, *The Social Basis of Health and Healing in Africa* (Berkeley, University of California Press, 1992), 25ff.

6. Omran, "Epidemiologic Transition (1991)," 536; Thomas McKeown, *The Modern Rise of Population* (London, Edward Arnold, 1976), 152–63; Thomas McKeown, *The Origins of Human Disease* (Oxford, Basil Blackwell, 1988), 9–10, 60–61, 84–87. For an assessment see Massimo Livi-Bacci, "The Nutrition–Mortality Link in Past Times: A Comment," in Robert I. Rotberg and Theodore K. Rabb, eds, *Hunger and History: The Impact of Changing Food Production and Consumption Patterns on Society* (Cambridge, Cambridge University Press, 1985), 95–100; Alex Mercer, *Disease Mortality and Population in Transition* (Leicester, Leicester University Press, 1990), 4–6. For an economist's firm support for the "rising standard of living argument" when paired with "social equality" (as in Sweden, as opposed to the USA), see: Richard G. Wilkinson, *Unhealthy Societies: The Afflictions of Inequality* (London, Routledge, 1996).

7. Anne Hardy, *The Epidemic Streets: Infectious Disease and the Rise of Preventive Medicine, 1856–1900* (Oxford, Clarendon Press, 1993); Simon Szreter, "The Importance of Social Intervention in Britain's Mortality Decline *c.* 1850–1914: A Reinterpretation of the Role of Public Health," *Social History of Medicine* I (1988), 1–37.

8. Paul Ewald, *Evolution of Infectious Disease* (New York, Oxford University Press, 1994).

9. Ian Scott and David Seemungal, "A Growing Problem: Human Population Growth and the Population Studies Programme," *TRP3: Research and Funding News from the Wellcome Trust* V (1995), 7–9. However, not all western-educated people in the world's South accept that runaway population growth is a pressing problem.

10. For a pioneering model: David Levine, *Reproducing Families: The Political Economy of English Population History* (Cambridge, Cambridge University Press, 1988); Kitching, "Proto-industrialization," 221, 239–40. For application to sub-Saharan Africa: Jay O'Brien, "Differential High Fertility and Demographic Transition: Peripheral Capitalism in Sudan," in Dennis D. Cordell and Joel W. Gregory, eds, *African Population and Capitalism: Historical Perspectives* (Boulder, CO, Westview Press, 1987), 185;

Meredeth Turshen, "Population Growth and the Deterioration of Health: Mainland Tanzania, 1920–1960," in Cordell and Gregory, *African Population and Capitalism*, 195–99; Marc Dawson, "Health, Nutrition, and Population in Central Kenya, 1890–1945," ibid, 202–203, 212–17; Bogumil Jewsiewicki, "Towards a Historical Sociology of Population in Zaire: Proposals for the Analysis of the Demographic Regime," ibid., 272–74.

11. Michael Walzer, *Thick and Thin: Moral Arguments at Home and Abroad* (Notre Dame, IN, Notre Dame University Press, 1994), 64, 93.

12. Basil Davidson, *Black Man's Burden: The Curse of the Nation State* (London, James Currey, 1992), 46–51, 197–242, 290–322; Michael Geyer and Charles Bright, "World History in a Global Age," *American Historical Review* C no. 4 (October 1995), 1049; Yasmin Alibhai-Brown, "For Africa, the Only Answer Lies Within," *The Independent*, 15 October 1994, 14.

13. WHO, *Bridging the Gaps*, 4; Omran, "Epidemiologic Transition (1971)," 530.

14. Patrick A. Twumasi, "Colonial Rule, International Agency, and Health: The Experience of Ghana," in Toyin Falola and Dennis Ityavyar, eds, *The Political Economy of Health in Africa* (Athens, OH, Ohio, University Monographs in International Studies, 1992), 114–15; F. M. Mburu, "The Impact of Colonial Rule on Health Development: The Case of Kenya," ibid., 100–4; Dennis A. Ityavyar, "The Colonial Origins of Health Care Services: The Nigeria Example," ibid., 83–85; John Farley, *Bilharzia: A History of Imperial Tropical Medicine* (Cambridge, Cambridge University Press, 1991), 292; B. Hyma and A. Ramesh, "Traditional Medicine: Its Extent and Potential for Incorporation into Modern National Health Systems," in Phillips and Verhasselt, *Health and Development*, 65–82; U. A. Igun, "The Underdevelopment of Traditional Medicine in Africa," in Falola and Ityavyar, *Political Economy of Health in Africa*, 143–83; and the six chapters in the section "Twentieth-Century African Medicine," in Feierman and Janzen, *Social Basis of Health*, 285–406; Mark Hobart, "Introduction: The Growth of Ignorance?" in Hobart, *An Anthropological Critique*, 1–30. To counter this problem the medical school at the University of Ilorin, Nigeria (my own sub-Saharan university) used community-based health concerns as the starting point for medical education and research.

15. Farley, *Bilharzia*, 72–75; E. Richard Brown, *Rockefeller Medicine Men: Capitalism and Medical Care in America* (Berkeley, University of California Press, 1979): criticized by Ronald Numbers in *American Historical Review* LXXXV no. 3 (June 1980), 727–28.

16. Armando Solórzano, "Sowing the Seeds of Neo-Imperialism: The Rockefeller Foundation's Yellow Fever Campaign in Mexico," *International Journal of Health Services* XXII no. 3 (1992), 529–54; Marcos Cueto, "'Sanitation from Above': Yellow Fever and Foreign Intervention in Peru, 1919–1922," *Hispanic American Historical Review* LXXII no. 1 (1992), 1–22.

17. Solórzano, "Neo-Imperialism," 550.

18. Maurice King, *Medical Care in Developing Countries: A Primer on the Medicine of Poverty and A Symposium from Makerere*

(Nairobi, Oxford University Press, 1966), 1:4, 1:8–9.

19. Fang Ru-Kang, "Health, Environment and Health Care in the People's Republic of China," in Phillips and Verhasselt, *Health and Development*, 259, 262; Frank Dikötter, "The Discourse of Race and the Medicalization of Public and Private Space in Modern China (1895–1949)," *History of Science* XXIX part 4 no. 86 (December 1991), 410–14, 419; Joshua S. Horn, *"Away With All Pests": An English Surgeon in People's China*, (London, Paul Hamlyn, 1960); Noshir H. Antia, "Leprosy Control by People's Program: 'A New Concept in Technology Transfer'," *International Journal of Health Services* XVII no. 2 (1987), 327–31; Teresa Poole, "Chinese Peasants Encouraged to Heal Themselves," *The Independent* 19 April 1995, 10; Griffith Feeney and Yuan Jianhau, "Below Replacement Fertility in China? A Close Look at Recent Evidence," *Population Studies* XLVIII (1994), 381–94.

20. Andrew Spielman, Uriel Kitron and Richard J. Pollack, "Time Limitation and the Rise of Research in the Worldwide Attempt to Eradicate Malaria," *Journal of Medical Entomology* XXX no. 1 (1993), 10.

21. Toyin Falola, "The Crisis of African Health Care Services," in Falola and Ityavyar, *Political Economy of Health in Africa*, 21–23.

22. Gill Walt, "WHO under Stress: Implications for Health Policy," *Health Policy* XXIV, (1993), 138–40. Falola lists the problems associated with the scientific medical "curative approach" inherited from the colonial period: "(a) the *inability* to accept the fact that good health is associated with good food, hygienic environments, and the provisions of basic amenities such as clean water; (b) modern medical facilities . . . have increased the cost of health care services beyond what the majority of the population can afford. Policy based on spending the bulk of the budget on medical technology ends up catering for an affluent few": Falola, "Crisis," 19–20 (my italics).

23. John C. Caldwell and Pat Caldwell, "What Have We Learned about the Cultural, Social and Behavioral Determinants of Health? From Selected Readings to the First Health Transition Workshop," *Health Transition Review* I no. 1 (1991), 13.

24. Tim Beardsley, "Trends in Preventative Medicine: Better Than a Cure," *Scientific American*, January 1995, 88–95; M. King, "Health is a Sustainable State," *The Lancet* CCCXXXI (1990), 664–67; Axel Kroeger, "Past and Present Trends of Community Health in Tropical Countries", *Transactions of the Royal Society of Tropical Medicine and Hygiene* LXXXVIII (1994), 497. Faiza Rady, "Health in the Market," ed. Gamal Nkrumah, *Al Ahram Weekly*, 27 July–2 August 1995, 5; Wil Gesler, "The Global Pharmaceutical Industry: Health, Development and Business," in Phillips and Verhasselt, *Health and Development*, 97–108, and the editors' wrap-up comments, ibid., 311–12.

25. *Human Development Report* 1993, 205.

26. World Bank figures show that the debt of the less developed countries (LDC) increased between 1980 and 1989 from $580 billion to $1,341 billion, and that the LDC were paying more in interest and debt repayment than they were receiving in new loans; between 1983 and 1989, "a net total of $223 billion was transferred from the poorer countries

of the Southern hemisphere to the financial institutions of the North": Sheena Asthana, "Economic Crisis, Adjustment and the Impact on Health," in Phillips and Verhasselt, *Health and Development*, 52; Davidson, *Black Man's Burden*, 218–22; David Orr, "Aid May Dry Up as Donors Lose Patience with Kenya," *The Independent*, 27 May 1995, 8.

27. Asthana, "Economic Crisis," 55–63; Rady, "Health in the Market," 5. Reporting on the 13–15 November 1996 World Food Summit held in Rome, Tariz Tadros noted that sub-Saharan African countries were now producing substantially less food than they were thirty years ago when they had half their current population. "Food for All?", *Al-Ahram Weekly* (14–20 November 1996), 7.

28. Penny Price, "Maternal and Child Health Care Strategies," in Phillips and Verhasselt, *Health and Development*, 145. On recent cutbacks in resources for female education in Nigeria: Asthana, "Economic Crisis," 61–62. On World Bank awareness of the importance of primary education for teaching girls about child care: Julio Frenk *et al.*, "Elements for a Theory of Health Transition," *Health Transition Review* I no. 1 (1991), 28. See also John C. Caldwell, "'Health Transition' The Cultural, Social and Behavioral Determinants of Health in the Third World," *Social Science and Medicine* XXXVI no. 2 (1993), 125–35, esp. 131–34. The *idea* that the education of girls in basic principles of hygiene would have important local health benefits was hardly new. In 1887 T. G. Hewlett, provincial sanitary inspector for Bombay, reminded higher authority that he had strongly recommended that girls be educated in hygiene in village schools ten years earlier; in the interval, nothing had been done: *Parliamentary Papers* 1887 LXIII [Cd 5209], 128.

29. Carol Vlassoff cites the following recent articles which attest that "epidemiological data" do not as yet demonstrate any clear link: J. Leslie, M. Lycette and M. Buvinic, "Weathering Economic Crisis: The Crucial Role of Women in Health," in D. Bell and M. Reich, eds, *Health, Nutrition and the Economic Crisis: Approaches to Policy in the Third World* (Dover, MA, Auburn House, 1988); L. M. Whiteford, "Maternal Health in the Dominican Republic," *Social Science and Medicine* XXXVII (1993); Carol Vlassoff, "Gender Inequalities in Health in the Third World: Uncharted Ground," *Social Science and Medicine* XXXIX no. 9 (1994), 1256.

30. Christopher Lasch, *The Revolt of the Elites & the Betrayal of Democracy* (New York, Norton, 1995), 3–4, 25–49. Maurice King had pointed out that to mention that humanitarian principles exist "is now hardly even respectable," King, *Medical Care*, 1:8.

31. Walt, "WHO under Stress", 136–37; Price, "Maternal and Child," 145. Reviewing Rima D. Apple's *Mothers and Medicine: A Social History of Infant Feeding 1890–1950* (Madison, University of Wisconsin Press, 1987), Janet Golden ignored the issue of infant formula manufacturers as contributors to death and instead was impressed by the way that the author had probed "the connections between the medical profession, and the manufacturers and with her ability to demonstrate how medical theories were translated into medical practice"; *Isis* LXXX no. 1 (1989), 109–10.

32. Director-General of WHO,

Hiroshi Nakajima, marked "No Tobacco Day, 1995" by revealing that tobacco was responsible for the death of 3 million people each year. It was also stated that advertising in the Third World especially targeted young people and women: Reuters Report, *Egyptian Gazette*, 31 May 1995, 4. A few days earlier it was revealed that former British Prime Minister Margaret Thatcher's appointment "as a non-executive director of the tobacco firm Philip Morris reportedly brings [her] an annual £550,000": "Iron Lady with the Midas Touch," *The Independent* 27 May 1995, 25. Following a full-page Philip Morris ad advocating freedom of choice in smoking was the following article: "Philip Morris Memo Likens Nicotine's Effect to Drugs: Tobacco Component 'Alters' Smoker's State; Firm Plays Down Draft [Memo]," *Wall Street Journal Europe* 11 December 1995, 5–6.

33. Mercer, *Disease Mortality*, 165–66. For an update on the fast changing legal situation see the array of articles in the *Independent* 22 March 1997, 4; "All companies now under siege in US," "Tories accused of tobacco industry pay off," "'This is the start of the facade cracking.'"

34. Charles Glass has reminded the literary world that the Anglo-French Sykes-Picot agreement and Treaty of Lausanne (1922) which carved up the old Ottoman Empire was carefully designed by Sykes, W. S. Churchill and others to give the UK full control of the oil fields of Mosul: "How the Kurds Were Betrayed," *Times Literary Supplement* 6 September 1996, 14.

35. *The Lancet* CCCXLVIII (19 October 1996), 1071.

36. John W. Peabody, "An Organizational Analysis of the World Health Organization: Narrowing the Gap between Promise and Performance," *Social Science and Medicine* LX no. 6 (1995), 737–40; Editorial, "Fortress WHO," *The Lancet* CCCXLV (28 January 1995), 204; WHO, *Bridging the Gaps*, 9. See also: Randy Shilts, *And the Band Played On: Politics, People & the AIDS Epidemic* (New York, Viking Penguin, 1993); Paul Farmer, *AIDS & Accusation: Haiti and the Geography of Blame* (Berkeley, University of California Press, 1993); Allan Brandt, "The Syphilis Epidemic and its Relation to AIDS," *Science* CCXXXIX (1988), 63; Karen A. Stanecki and Peter O. Way, "Negative Population Growth: Is it Likely for Africa?" *AIDS & Society: International Research and Policy Bulletin* IV no. 1 (October/November 1992), 4–5; James N. Gribble and Samuel H. Preston, eds, *The Epidemiological Transition: Policy and Planning Implications for Developing Countries: Workshop Proceedings* (Washington, DC, National Academy Press, 1993), 39–40; Susan Watts, Sheldon Watts and Rose Okello, "Medical Geography and AIDS," *Annals of the Association of American Geographers* LXXX no. 2 (June 1990), 301–304.

37. "Koch," *Dictionary of Scientific Biography*, 425–27. See also Linda Bryder, *Below the Magic Mountain: A Social History of Tuberculosis in Twentieth Century Britain* (Oxford, Oxford University Press, 1988); Allan Mitchell, "Obsessive Questions and Faint Answers: The French Response to Tuberculosis in the Belle Epoque," *Bulletin of Medical History* LXII (1988), 215–35.

38. WHO "estimates that the annual number of new cases of tuberculosis will increase from 7.5 million in 1990 to 10.2 million in 2000": "The Global Challenge

of Tuberculosis," *The Lancet* CCCXLIV (30 July 1994), 277.

39. Spielman *et al.*, "Attempt to Eradicate Malaria," 116–17; Ewald, *Evolution of Infectious Disease*, 207–12. "According to WHO estimates, nearly half of the world population is at risk in more than 100 countries (with an estimated 110 million cases and 270 million people carrying the malaria parasites). . . . It remains a major cause of death (with 1–1.5 million deaths annually, particularly among young children": Phillips and Verhasselt, "Introduction," in *Health and Development*, 8; Anon., *Implementation of the Global Malaria Control Strategy* (Geneva, WHO, 1993), 16. See also: "Time to put *malaria control* on the global agenda," *Nature CCCLXXXVI* (10 April 1997), 535, 535–41: notes: [talks are underway with] "the pharmaceutical industry to find ways to reverse its unprecedented withdrawal from vaccine research and development of antimalarial drugs."

40. According to Hunter "The principle has to be established [i.e. *has not yet been established*] that economic development should not create sickness and disease": J. M. Hunter *et al.*, *Water Resource Development: The Need for Intersectoral Negotiation* (Geneva, WHO, 1993), 100.

Select Bibliography

Abu-Lughod, Janet, *Before European Hegemony: The World System* AD *1250–1350* (Oxford 1989)

Acworth, H. A., "Leprosy in India," *Journal of Tropical Medicine* II (1899)

Adas, Michael, *Machines as the Measure of Men: Science, Technology and Ideologies of Western Dominance* (Ithaca, NY 1989)

Ajayi, J. F. A and Michael Crowder, eds, *History of West Africa* (New York 1976)

Alchon, Suzanne Austin, *Native Society and Disease in Colonial Ecuador* (Cambridge 1991)

Anderson, Roy M. and Robert M. May, *Infectious Diseases in Humans* (Oxford 1991)

Annett, H. E., J. E. Dutton and J. H. Elliott, *Report on the Malaria Expedition to Nigeria of the Liverpool School of Tropical Medicine and Medical Parasitology* (Liverpool 1901)

Anon., "Cholera at Sunderland," *Edinburgh Medical and Surgical Journal* XXXVII (1832)

Anon., "Professor Koch's Investigations on Malaria," *British Medical Journal* (1900)

Anon., "The Depreciation of the Attractions of the Indian Medical Service and Its Remedies," *Journal of Tropical Medicine* IX (1906)

Armstrong, H. C., "Account of Visit to Leprosy Institutions in Nigeria," *Leprosy Review* IV (1935)

Arnold, David, "Cholera and Colonialism in British India," *Past and Present* CXIII (1986)

Arnold, David, "Cholera Mortality in British India, 1817–1947," in Tim Dyson, ed., *India's Historical Demography: Studies in Famine, Disease and Society* (London 1989)

Arnold, David, ed., *Imperial Medicine and Indigenous Societies* (Manchester 1988)

Asthana, Sheena, "Economic Crisis, Adjustment and the Impact on Health," in D. R. Phillips and Y. Verhasselt, eds, *Health and Development* (London 1994)

Austen, Ralph, *Africa in Economic History* (London 1987)

Austen, Ralph and Woodruff D. Smith, "Private Tooth Decay and Public Economic Virtues: The Slave-Sugar Triangle, Consumerism, and European Industrialization," in J. E. Inikori and S. L. Engerman, eds, *The Atlantic Slave Trade* (Durham, NC 1992)

Ayandele, E. A., *The Missionary Impact on Modern Nigeria 1842–1914: A Political and Social Analysis.* (London 1966)
Baillaud, Emile, "The Problem of Agricultural Development in West Africa," *Journal of the African Society* XVIII (1906)
Baker, Brenda J. and George J. Armelagos, "The Origin and Antiquity of Syphilis: Paleopathological Diagnosis and Interpretation," *Current Anthropology* XXIX no. 5 (1988)
Barber, Malcolm, "Lepers, Jews and Moslems: The Plot to Overthrow Christendom in 1321," *History* LXVI (1981)
Bardet, Jean-Pierre *et al.*, *Peurs et terreurs face à la contagion* (Paris 1988)
Basset, André, "Épidémiologie des tréponématoses: vrais et faux-semblants de la syphilis," in Bardet, *Peurs et terreurs* (Paris 1988)
Bayly, C. A., *Indian Society and the Making of the British Empire* (Cambridge 1988)
Bayly, C. A., *Imperial Meridian: The British Empire and the World, 1780–1830* (London 1989)
Beier, Lucinda McCray, *Sufferers & Healers: The Experience of Illness in Seventeenth Century England* (London 1987)
Bercé, Yves-Marie, *Le Chaudron et la lancette: croyances populaires et médecins préventive (1798–1830)* (Paris 1984)
Bériac, Françoise, *Histoire des lépreaux au Moyen Age: Une société d'exclus* (Paris 1983)
Berlin, Isaiah, *The Crooked Timber of Humanity* (New York 1991)
Bernal, Martin, *Black Athena: The African Roots of Classical Civilization* (New Brunswick, NJ 1987)
Biraben, Jean-Noël, *Les Hommes et la peste en France et dans les pays Europeéns et Méditerranéens*, I: *La Peste dans l'histoire* (Paris 1975); II: *Les Hommes face à la peste* (Paris 1976)
Bisson, T. N., "The 'Feudal Revolution'," *Past and Present* CXLII (1994)
Blackburn, Robin, *The Overthrow of Colonial Slavery 1776–1848* (London 1988)
Bloom, Khaled, *The Mississippi Valley's Great Yellow Fever Epidemic of 1878* (Baton Rouge 1993)
Boahen, Adu, ed., *UNESCO General History of Africa VII: Africa under Colonial Domination 1880–1935* (London 1985)
Bourdelais, Patrice, "Cholera: A Victory for Medicine?" in R. Schofield, ed., *The Decline of Mortality in Europe* (Oxford 1991)
Bourgeois, Albert, *Lépreux et maladreriers du Pas-du-Calais (X–XVIIIe siècles)* (Arras 1972)
Boyajian, James C., *Portuguese Trade in Asia under the Hapsburgs, 1580–1640* (Baltimore 1993)
Boyce, Rubert, "The Colonization of Africa," *Journal of the African Society* X (1911)
Boyce, Rubert, "The Distribution and Prevalence of Yellow Fever in West Africa," *Journal of Tropical Medicine and Hygiene* XIII (1910)
Boyce, Rubert, *Mosquito or Man? The Conquest of the Tropical World* (London 1910)
Braudel, Fernand, *Civilization & Capitalism: 15th–18th Century, III: The Perspective of the World* (London 1985)

Bristow, Edward, *Vice and Vigilance: Purity Movements in Britain since 1700* (Dublin 1977)

Brown, Richard E., *Rockefeller Medicine Men: Capitalism and Medical Care in America* (Berkeley 1979)

Browne, Stanley G., "Leprosy," in E. E. Sabben-Clare, D. J. Bradley and K. Kirkwood, eds, *Health in Tropical Africa during the Colonial Period* (Oxford 1980)

Brundage, Anthony, *England's "Prussian Minister": Edwin Chadwick and the Politics of Government Growth, 1832–1854* (University Park, PA 1988)

Brunton, Deborah, "Smallpox Inoculation and Demographic Trends in Eighteenth Century Scotland," *Medical History* XXXVI (1992)

Bull, Marcus, *Knightly Piety and the Lay Response to the First Crusade: The Limousin and Gascony,* c. *970–1130* (Oxford 1993)

Bulst, Neithard and Robert Delort, eds, *Maladie et société (XIIe XIIIe siècles)* (Paris 1989)

Burkholder, Mark A. and Lyman L. Johnson, *Colonial Latin America* (Oxford 1990)

Bynum, W. F., "Treating the Wages of Sin: Venereal Disease and Specialism in Eighteenth Century Britain," in W. F. Bynum and Roy Porter, eds, *Medical Fringe and Medical Orthodoxy 1750–1850* (London 1987)

Cain, P. J. and A. G. Hopkins, *British Imperialism: Innovation and Expansion, 1688–1914* (London 1993)

Calvi, Giulia, *Histories of a Plague Year: the Social and Imaginary in Baroque Florence* (Berkeley 1989)

Cameron, Euan, *The European Reformation* (Oxford 1991)

Campbell, Ann Montgomery, *The Black Death and Men of Learning* (New York 1966)

Campbell, Sheila, Bert Hall and David Klausner, eds, *Health, Disease and Healing in Medieval Culture* (New York 1992)

Cantlie, James, *Report on the Conditions under which Leprosy Occurs in China, Indo-China, Malaya, the Archipelago, and Oceania, Compiled Chiefly during 1894* (London 1897)

Carmichael, Ann G., *Plague and the Poor in Renaissance Florence* (Cambridge 1986)

Carmichael, Ann G., and Arthur M. Silverstein, "Smallpox in Europe before the Seventeenth Century: Virulent Killer or Benign Disease?," *Journal of the History of Medicine* XLII (1987)

Carrigan, Jo An, "Yellow Fever: Scourge of the South," in Savitt and Young, *Disease and Distinctiveness* (Knoxville 1988)

Carter, Henry Rose, *Yellow Fever: An Epidemiological and Historical Study of its Place of Origin* (Baltimore 1931)

Cartwright, F. F., *A Social History of Medicine* (New York 1977)

Cartwright, Samuel A., "Report on the Diseases and Physical Peculiarities of the Negro Race," in Arthur L. Caplan, H. Engelhardt and J. McCartney, eds, *Concepts of Health and Disease: Interdisciplinary Perspectives* (Reading, MA 1981)

Casamieva, Fernando, "Smallpox and War in Southern Chile in the Late

Eighteenth Century," in Cook and Lovell, eds, *"Secret Judgment of God"* (Norman, OK 1991)

Cell, John W., "Anglo-Indian Medical Theory and the Origins of Segregation in West Africa," *American Historical Review* XCI, no. 2 (1986)

Chatterji, K. R., "Survey Reports: Report on Leprosy Survey Work Done at Salbani Police Station, Midnapore, Bengal," *Leprosy in India* III no. 2 (1932)

Chauliac, Guy de, *La Grande Chirurgie* (Paris 1890)

Choksy, Khan Bahadur, "Leprosy Legislation in India," *Lepra* X (1910)

Cipolla, Carlo M., *Cristofano and the Plague: A Study in the History of Public Health in the Age of Galileo* (London 1973)

Cipolla, C. M., *Public Health and the Medical Profession in the Renaissance* (Cambridge 1976)

Clot-Bey, A. B., *Mémoires de A. B. Clot Bey* (Cairo 1949)

Cochrane, Robert G., *Leprosy in India: A Survey* (London 1927)

Cohen, William B., "Malaria and French Imperialism," *Journal of African History* XXIV (1983)

Coleman, William, *Yellow Fever in the North: The Methods of Early Epidemiology* (Madison, WI 1987)

Colley, Linda, *Britons: Forging the Nation 1770–1837* (London 1992)

Conrad, Lawrence I., "Epidemic Disease in Formal and Popular Thought in Early Islamic Society," in T. Ranger and P. Slack, eds, *Epidemics and Ideas* (Cambridge 1992)

Conrad, Lawrence I., "The Social Structure of Medicine in Early Islam," *Social History of Medicine* XXXVII (1985)

Conrad, Lawrence I, Michael Neve, Vivian Nutton, Roy Porter and Andrew Wear, *The Western Medical Tradition: 800 BC to AD 1800* (Cambridge 1995)

Cook, Harold J., "The New Philosophy and Medicine in Seventeenth Century England," in D. C. Lindberg and R. S. Westman, eds, *Reappraisals of the Scientific Revolution* (Cambridge 1990)

Cook, Noble David, *Demographic Collapse: Indian Peru, 1520–1620* (Cambridge 1981)

Cook, Noble David and W. George Lovell, eds, *"Secret Judgments of God": Old World Disease in Colonial Spanish America* (Norman, OK 1991)

Cooter, Roger, "Anticontagionism and History's Medical Record," in P. Wright and A. Trencher, eds, *The Problem of Medical Knowledge* (Edinburgh 1982)

Corbin, Alain, "La Grande Peur de la syphilis," in Bardet *et al.*, *Peurs et terreurs* (Paris 1988)

Corbin, Alain, *Les Filles de noce: misère sexualle et prostitution (19e et 20e siècles)* (Paris 1978)

Cordell, Dennis D. and Joel W. Gregory, *African Population & Capitalism: Historical Perspectives* (Boulder, CO 1987)

Couto, G. and C. de Rezende, "Control of Infectious Diseases in Brazil and Especially in Rio de Janeiro," *Yellow Fever Bureau Bulletin* II (1913)

Craigie, David, "An Account of the Epidemic Cholera at Newburn in

January and February 1832," *Edinburgh Medical and Surgical Journal* XXXVII (1832)

Creighton, Charles, *A History of Epidemics in Britain from A.D. 664 to the Extinction of Plague* (Cambridge 1891)

Crosby, Alfred W., *The Columbian Exchange: Biological Consequences of 1492* (Westport, CT 1972)

Crosby, Alfred W., "Hawaiian Depopulation as a Model for the Amerindian Experience," in T. Ranger and P. Slack, eds, *Epidemics and Ideas* (Cambridge 1992)

Cueto, Marcos, "Sanitation from Above: Yellow Fever and Foreign Intervention in Peru, 1919–1922," *Hispanic American Historical Review* LXXII, no. 1 (1992)

Curtin, Philip D., *Death by Migration: Europe's Encounter with the Tropical World in the Nineteenth Century* (Cambridge 1989)

Curtin, P. D., "The End of the 'White Man's Grave'?: Nineteenth-Century Mortality in West Africa," *Journal of Interdisciplinary History* XXI no. 1 (1990)

Curtin, P. D., "Medical Knowledge and Urban Planing in Tropical Africa," *American Historical Review* XC no. 3 (1985)

Davidson, Basil, *The Black Man's Burden: Africa and the Curse of the Nation State* (New York 1992)

Dawson, Marc H., "Socioeconomic Change and Disease: Smallpox in Colonial Kenya, 1880–1920," in S. Feierman and J. M. Janzen, eds, *The Social Basis of Health and Healing in Africa* (Berkeley 1992)

De Cock, K. M. *et al.*, "Epidemic Yellow Fever in Eastern Nigeria, 1986," *The Lancet* 19 March 1988

Delaporte, François, *Disease and Civilization: The Cholera in Paris, 1832* (Cambridge, MA 1986)

Delumeau, Jean, *La Peur en Occident: XIV–XVIIIe siècles: une cité assiégée* (Paris 1978)

Digby, Anne, *Making a Medical Living: Doctors and Patients in the English Market for Medicine 1720–1911* (Cambridge 1994)

Dikötter, Frank, "The Discourse of Race and the Medicalization of Public and Private Space in Modern China (1895–1949)," *History of Science* XXIX (1986)

Dobyns, Henry F., *Their Number Became Thinned: Native American Population Dynamics in Eastern North America* (Knoxville, TN 1983)

Dols, Michael W., *The Black Death in the Middle East* (Princeton, NJ 1977)

Dols, M., "Leprosy in Medieval Arabic Medicine," *Journal of the History of Medicine* XXXIV (1979)

Douglas, Mary, "Witchcraft and Leprosy: Two Strategies of Exclusion," *Man* new series, XXVI (1991)

Drescher, Seymour, "The Ending of the Slave Trade and the Evolution of European Scientific Racism," in J. E. Inikori and S. Engerman, eds, *The Atlantic Slave Trade* (Durham, NC 1992)

Duffy, John, "The Impact of Malaria on the South," in Savitt and Young, eds, *Disease and Distinctiveness* (Knoxville, TN 1988)

Dumett, Raymond, "Disease and Mortality among Gold Miners of Ghana:

Colonial Government and Mining Company Attitudes and Policies, 1900–1938," *Social Science and Medicine* XXXVII (1993)

Durey, Michael, *The Return of the Plague: British Society and the Cholera 1831–2* (Dublin 1979)

Elliott, J. H., *Spain and its World 1500–1700* (New Haven 1989)

Emch-Dériaz, Antoinette, *Tissot: Physician of the Enlightenment* (Berne 1992)

Engelhardt, H. Tristram, Jr., "The Disease of Masturbation: Values and the Concepts of Disease," in Arthur Caplan and H. Engelhardt Jr, *Concepts of Health and Disease: Interdisciplinary Perspectives* (Reading, MA 1981)

Enthoven, R. E., *The Folklore of Bombay* (Oxford 1924)

Evans, David, "Tackling the 'Hideous Scourge': The Creation of Venereal Disease Centres in Early Twentieth Century Britain," *Social History of Medicine* V, no. 3 (1992)

Evans, Richard, "Epidemics and Revolutions: Cholera in Nineteenth Century Europe," *Past and Present* CXX (1988)

Ewald, Paul E., *Evolution of Infectious Diseases* (Oxford 1994)

Falola, Toyin and Dennis Ityavyar, *The Political Economy of Health in Africa* (Athens, OH 1992)

Farley, John, *Bilharzia: A History of Imperial Tropical Medicine* (Cambridge 1991)

Farmer, Paul, *AIDS and Accusation: Haiti and the Geography of Blame* (Berkeley 1992)

Feierman, Steven and John M. Janzen, eds, *The Social Basis of Health & Healing in Africa* (Berkeley 1992)

Fenner, Frank, *Smallpox and its Eradication* (Geneva 1988)

Flinn, M. W., "Plague in Europe and the Mediterranean Countries," *Journal of European Economic History* VIII, no. 1 (1979)

Floud, Roderick, K. Wachter and A. Gregory *Height, Health and History: Nutritional Status in the United Kingdom, 1750–1980* (Cambridge 1989)

Foa, Anne, "The New and the Old: The Spread of Syphilis (1494–1530)," in Edward Muir and Guido Ruggiero, eds, *Sex and Gender in Historical Perspective* (Baltimore 1990)

Fogel, Robert William, *Without Consent or Contract: The Rise and Fall of American Slavery* (New York 1991)

Foucault, Michel, *The Birth of the Clinic: An Archaeology of Medical Perception* (London 1989)

Foucault, M., *Madness and Civilization: A History of Insanity in the Age of Reason* (London 1967)

Foucault, M., *Power/Knowledge: Selected Interviews and Other Writings, 1972–1977* (New York 1980)

French, Roger, "The Arrival of the French Disease in Leipzig," in Bulst and Delort, *Maladie et société* (Paris 1989)

Frenkel, Stephen and John Western, "Pretext or Prophylaxis? Racial Segregation and Malarial Mosquitoes in a British Tropical Colony: Sierra Leone," *Annals of the Association of American Geographers* LXXVII, no. 2 (1988)

Frost, Richard H., "The Pueblo Indian Smallpox Epidemic in New Mexico, 1898–1899," *Bulletin of the History of Medicine* (1990)

Gale, Thomas S., "Segregation in British West Africa," *Cahiers d' Études Africaines* XX no. 4 (1980)

Garcia-Ballester, Luis, "Changes in the *Regimina Sanitatis*: The Role of the Jewish Physicians," in Campbell *et al.*, eds, *Health, Disease and Healing in Medieval Culture* (New York 1992)

Geggus, David, "Yellow Fever in the 1790s: The British Army in Occupied Saint Domingue," *Medical History* XXIII (1979)

Germond, R. C., "A Study of the Last Six Years of the Leprosy Campaign in Basutoland," *International Journal of Leprosy* IV (1936)

Gilman, Carolyn, *The Grand Portage Story* (St Paul, MN 1992)

Ginzburg, Carlo, *Ecstasies: Deciphering the Witches' Sabbath* (New York 1991)

Goodyear, James D., "The Sugar Connection: A New Perspective on the History of Yellow Fever," *Bulletin of the History of Medicine* LII (1978)

Gorgas, W. C., "Recent Experiences of the United States Army with Regard to Sanitation of Yellow Fever in the Tropics," *Journal of Tropical Medicine* VI (1903)

Greene, Jack P., *Imperatives, Behaviors, and Identities: Essays in Early American Cultural History* (Charlottesville, VA 1992)

Grmek, Mirko, *Diseases in the Ancient Greek World* (Baltimore 1989)

Gruzinski, Serge, *The Conquest of Mexico: The Incorporation of Indian Societies into the Western World, 16th–18th Centuries* (Cambridge 1993)

Guerra, Francisco, "The Dispute over Syphilis: Europe versus America," *Cleo Medica* XII no. 1 (1978)

Guiteras, J., "Endemicity of Yellow Fever," *Yellow Fever Bulletin* II (1913)

Gupta, Ashin Das, *Indian Merchants and the Decline of Surat* c. *1700–1750* (Wiesbaden 1979)

Gussow, Zachary and George S. Tracy, "Stigma and the Leprosy Phenomenon: The Social History of a Disease in the Nineteenth and Twentieth Centuries," *Bulletin of the History of Medicine* XLIV (1970)

Hall, Leslie A., "Forbidden by God, Despised by Men: Masturbation, Medical Warnings, Moral Panic and Manhood in Great Britain, 1850–1950," *Journal of the History of Sexuality* II no. 3 (1992)

Hall, Leslie A., *Hidden Anxieties: Male Sexuality, 1900–1950* (Cambridge 1992)

Hamlin, Christopher, "Muddling in Bumbledom: On the Enormity of Large Sanitary Improvements in Four British Towns, 1855–1885," *Victorian Studies* XXXII, no. 1 (1988)

Hamlin, C., "Predisposing Causes and Public Health in Early Nineteenth Century Medical Thought," *Social History of Medicine* V, no. 1 (1992)

Hardy, Anne, "Parish Pump to Private Pipes: London's Water Supply in the 19th Century," in W. F. Bynum and Roy Porter, eds, *Living and Dying in London* (London, 1991)

Harrison, Mark, *Public Health in British India: Anglo-Indian Preventive Medicine 1859–1914* (Cambridge 1994)

Hartwig, Gerard and K. Patterson, *Disease in African History: An Introduction and Case Studies* (Durham, NC 1975)

Hasan, Khwaja Arif, *The Cultural Frontier of Health in Village India: Case Study of an Indian Village* (Bombay 1967)

Henderson, Donald A., "The History of Smallpox Eradication," in Abraham M. Lilienfeld, ed., *Times, Places, and Persons: Aspects of the History of Epidemiology* (Baltimore 1978)

Henige, David, "When Did Smallpox Reach the New World (And Why Does It Matter?)," in Paul Lovejoy, ed., *Africans in Bondage: Studies in Slavery and the Slave Trade: Essays in Honor of Philip D. Curtin* (Madison, WI 1986)

Henriot, Christian, "Medicine, V.D. and Prostitution in Pre-Revolutionary China," *Social History of Medicine* V, no. 1 (1992)

Henriot, C., "Prostitution et 'Police des Moeurs' à Shanghai aux XIXe–XX siècles," in his *La Femme en Asie Orientale* (Lyon 1988)

Herbert, Eugenia W., "Smallpox Inoculation in Africa," *Journal of African History* XVI no. 4 (1975)

Heyningen, E. B. van, "Agents of Empire: The Medical Profession in the Cape Colony 1880–1910," *Medical History* XXXIII (1989)

Higman, B. W., *Slave Populations of the British Caribbean 1807–1834* (Baltimore 1988)

Hilton, Boyd, *Age of Atonement: The Influence of Evangelicalism on Social and Economic Thought, 1795–1865* (Oxford 1988)

Hobson, John, *Imperialism: A Study* (London 1902)

Hoffmann, W. H., "Yellow Fever in Africa from the Epidemiological Standpoint," in Mohamed Bay Khalil, ed., *Proceedings: International Congress on Tropical Medicine in Cairo, December 1928* V (Cairo 1932)

Hopkins, Donald R., *Princes and Peasants: Smallpox in History* (Chicago 1983)

Horn, Joshua S., *"Away with all Pests . . ." An English Surgeon in People's China* (London 1960)

Howard, A. C., "Leprosy in Nigeria," *International Journal of Leprosy* IV (1936)

Hrbek, Ivan, "Egypt, Nubia and the Eastern Deserts," in Roland Oliver, ed., *The Cambridge History of Africa. III From* c. *1050*–c. *1600* (Cambridge 1977)

Hume, John Chandler Jr, "Colonialism and Sanitary Medicine: The Development of Preventive Health Policy in the Punjab, 1860–1900," *Modern Asian Studies* XX no. 4 (1986)

Humphreys, Margaret, *Yellow Fever and the South* (New Brunswick, NJ 1992)

Hunter, W. W., *Orissa, Or the Vicissitudes of an Indian Province Under Native and British Rule* (London 1872)

Hutchinson, Jonathan, "On Circumcision as Preventive of Masturbation," *Archives of Surgery* II (1890–1)

Hutchinson, Jonathan, *On Leprosy and Fish-Eating: A Statement of Facts and Explanation* (London 1906)

Hyam, Ronald, *Empire and Sexuality: The British Experience* (Manchester 1990)

Iliffe, John, *The African Poor: A History* (Cambridge 1987)

Inikori, Joseph E., "Underpopulation in Nineteenth Century West Africa: The Role of the Export Slave Trade," in *African Historical Demography* (Edinburgh 1981)

Inikori, Joseph E. and Stanley L. Engerman, eds, *The Atlantic Slave Trade: Effects on Economies, Societies, and Peoples in Africa, the Americas, and Europe* (Durham, NC 1992)

Irvine, W. C., "Christian Teaching and Spiritual Work in the Asylums," in *Report on a Conference of Leper Asylum Superintendents and Others* (Cuttack 1920)

Irwin, Robert, *The Middle East in the Middle Ages: The Early Mamluk Sultanate 1250–1382* (Carbondale, IL 1986)

Israel, Jonathan I., *European Jewry in the Age of Mercantilism 1550–1750* (Berkeley 1991)

Jacob, Margaret C., *The Cultural Meaning of the Scientific Revolution* (New York 1988).

Jacquart, Danielle and Claude Thomasset, *Sexuality and Medicine in the Middle Ages* (Cambridge 1988)

Jaggi, O. P., *Epidemics and Other Tropical Diseases* (Delhi 1979)

Joesting, Edward, *Kauai: The Separate Kingdom* (Honolulu 1984)

Joralemon, Donald, "New World Depopulation and the Case of Disease," *Journal of Anthropological Research* XXXVIII (1982)

Joshua-Raghavar, A., *Leprosy in Malaysia, Past, Present and Future* (Selangor 1983)

Joyce, Patrick, "Work," in F. M. L. Thompson, ed., *The Cambridge Social History of Britain* II (Cambridge 1990)

Kamel, Ahmed, "On the Epidemiology and Treatment of Plague in Egypt: The 1940 Epidemic," *Journal of the Egyptian Public Health Association* XVI, no. 2 (1941)

Kamen, Henry, *Inquisition and Society in Spain in the Sixteenth and Seventeenth Century* (Bloomington, IN 1985)

Kamen, H., *Spain 1469–1714: A Society of Conflict* (London 1991)

Karant-Nunn, Susan C., "Continuity and Change: Some Effects of the Reformation on the Women of Zwickau," *Sixteenth Century Journal* XII, no. 2 (1982)

Kearns, Gerry, "Environmental Management in Islington 1830–55," in W. F. Bynum and Roy Porter, eds, *Living and Dying in London* (London, 1991)

Kearns, Gerry, "Private Property and Public Health Reform in England 1830–70," *Social Science and Medicine* XXVI, no. 1 (1988)

Kidwell, Clara Sue, "Aztec and European Medicine in the New World, 1521–1600," in Lola Romanucci-Ross, D. Moerman and L. Tancredi, eds, *The Anthropology of Medicine: From Culture to Method* (New York 1982)

King, Maurice, *Medical Care in Developing Countries: A Primer on the Medicine of Poverty and A Symposium from Makerere* (Nairobi 1966)

Kingsley, Mary, *West African Studies* (London 1901)

Kiple, Kenneth F. and Brian T. Higgins, "Yellow Fever and the Africanization of the Caribbean," in Verano and Ubelaker, *Disease and Demography in the Americas* (Washington, DC 1992)

Klein, Ira, "Cholera, Theory and Treatment in Nineteenth Century India," *Journal of Indian History* LVIII (1980)

Kuczinski, R. R., *Demographic Survey of the British Colonial Empire*, I: *West Africa* (Oxford 1949)

Kuhnke, LaVerne, *Lives at Risk: Public Health in Nineteenth Century Egypt* (Berkeley 1990)

Kuykendall, Ralph S., *The Hawaiian Kingdom, 1854–1874: Twenty Critical Years* (Honolulu 1953)

Lasch, Christopher, *The Revolt of the Elites & the Betrayal of Democracy* (New York 1995)

Lawrence, C. J., "Medicine as Culture: Edinburgh and the Scottish Enlightenment." Unpublished PhD thesis, University College London 1984

Leavitt, Judith Walzer and Ronald L. Numbers, *Sickness and Health in America: Readings in the History of Medicine and Public Health* (Madison, WI 1985)

Le Roy Ladurie, Emmanuel, *Montaillou: The Promised Land of Error* (New York 1978)

Lindberg, David C. and Robert S. Westman, eds, *Reappraisals of the Scientific Revolution* (Cambridge 1990)

Little, L. K., *Religious Poverty and the Profit Economy in Medieval Europe* (Ithaca, NY 1978)

Livingstone, Frank B., "The Duffy Blood Groups, Vivax Malaria, and Malaria Selection in Human Populations: A Review," *Human Biology* LVI, no. 3 (1984)

Livingstone, Frank B., "On the Origin of Syphilis: An Alternative Hypothesis," *Current Anthropology* XXXII, no. 5 (1991)

Lockhart, James, *The Nahaus after the Conquest: A Social and Cultural History of the Indians of Central Mexico, Sixteenth through Eighteenth Centuries* (Stanford, CA 1992)

Lovell, W. George, "'Heavy Shadows and Black Night': Disease and Depopulation in Colonial Spanish America," *Annals of the Association of American Geographers* LXXXII, no. 3 (1992)

Luckin, Bill, "States and Epidemic Threats," *Bulletin of the Social History of Medicine* XXXIV (1984)

McCuster, John J. and Russell R. Menard, *The Economy of British America 1697–1789* (Chapel Hill, NC 1985)

MacDonald, Robert H., "The Frightful Consequences of Onanism: Notes on the History of a Delusion," *Journal of the History of Ideas* XXVIII (1967)

MacLaren, A. A., "Bourgeois Ideology and Victorian Philanthropy: The Contradictions of Cholera," in his *Social Class in Scotland: Past and Present* (Edinburgh 1976)

McLaren, Angus, *A History of Contraception from Antiquity to the Present Day* (Oxford 1990)

MacLeod, D. Peter, "Microbes and Muskets: Smallpox and the Participation of the Amerindian Allies of New France in the Seven Years War," *Ethnohistory* XXX, no. 1 (1992)

MacLeod, Roy and Milton Lewis, eds, *Disease, Medicine, and Empire: Perspectives on Western Medicine and the Experience of European Expansion* (London 1988)

McNeill, William, *Plagues and Peoples* (Garden City, NY 1976)

MacPherson, C. B., *The Political Theory of Possessive Individualism* (Oxford 1962)

McVaugh, Michael R., *Medicine before the Plague: Practitioners and their Patients in the Crown of Aragon, 1285–1345* (Cambridge 1994)

Madden, Frank, *The Surgery of Egypt* (Cairo 1922)

Madden, Frank, "Thirty Years of Surgery in Qasr el Aini Hospital, 1898–1928," in Mohamed Bey Khalil, ed., *Comptes Rendus* (Congrès International de Médecine Tropicale et d'Hygiène, Le Caire, Egypt, Décembre 1928) (Cairo 1931)

Maier, D., "Nineteenth Century Ashante Medical Practices," *Comparative Studies in Society and History* XXI (1979)

Majeed, J., "James Mill's 'The History of British India' and Utilitarianism as a Rhetoric of Reform," *Modern Asian Studies* XXIV, no. 2 (1990)

Malthus, Thomas, *Essay on Population* (first published 1798) (Cambridge 1989)

Mambrini, P. du Toit de, *De l'Onanisme: ou Discours philosophique et moral sur la luxure artificielle et sur tous les crimes relatifs* (Lausanne 1760)

Manchester, Keith, "Leprosy: The Origin and Development of the Disease in Antiquity," in D. Gourevitch, ed., *Maladie et maladies, histoire et conceptualisation* (Geneva 1992)

Manchester, Keith and Charlotte Roberts, "The Palaeopathology of Leprosy in Britain: A Review," *World Archaeology* XII, no. 2 (1989)

Manson, Patrick, "The Malaria Parasite," *Journal of the African Society* VI, no. 23 (1907)

Marland, Hilary, ed., *The Art of Midwifery: Early Modern Midwives in Europe* (London 1993)

Mason, Michael, *The Making of Victorian Sexuality* (Oxford 1994)

Mayer, T. F. G., "Leprosy in Nigeria," *Leprosy in India* II, no. 4 (1930)

Meade, Teresa, "Cultural Imperialism in Old Republic Rio de Janeiro: The Urban Renewal and Public Health Project," in T. Meade and M. Walker, eds, *Science, Medicine and Cultural Imperialism* (London 1991)

Meade, Teresa and Mark Walker, eds, *Science, Medicine and Cultural Imperialism* (London 1991)

Mérab, J., *Impression d'Éthiopie: L'Abyssinie sous Ménéluk II* (Paris 1921)

Mercer, Alex, *Disease Mortality and Population in Transition: Epidemiological-Demographic Change in England since the Eighteenth Century as Part of a Global Phenomenon* (Leicester 1990)

Merrens, H. Roy and George D. Terry, "Dying in Paradise: Malaria, Mortality and the Personal Environment in Colonial South Carolina," *Journal of Southern History*, no. 4 (1984)

Meyer, Gregg S., "Criminal Punishment for the Transmission of Sexually Transmitted Diseases: Lessons from Syphilis," *Bulletin of the History of Medicine* LXV, no. 4 (1991)

Miller, Genevieve, "Putting Lady Mary in her Place: A Discussion of Historical Causation," *Bulletin of the History of Medicine* LV (1981)

Miller, Joseph C., *Way of Death: Merchant Capitalism and the Angolan Slave Trade 1730–1830* (London 1988)

Mintz, Sidney W., *Sweetness and Power: The Place of Sugar in Modern World History* (New York 1985)

Mollaret, Henri H., "Le Cas de la peste," *Annales de Démographie Historique* (1989)

Monath, Thomas P., "Yellow Fever: Victor, Victoria? Conqueror, Conquest? Epidemics and Research in the Last Forty Years and the Prospects for the Future," *American Journal of Tropical Medicine and Hygiene* XLV, no. 1 (1991)

Moore, R. I., *The Formation of a Persecuting Society* (Oxford 1987)

Moreau-Neret, A., "L'Isolement des lepreaux au Moyen-Age et la problème de 'lepreux errants'," *Fédération des Sociétés d'Histoire et d'Archélogie de l'Aisne: Memoires* XVI (1970)

Morris, R. J., *Cholera 1832: The Social Response to an Epidemic* (London 1979)

Morris, R. J., "Clubs, Societies and Associations," in F. M. L. Thompson, ed., *The Cambridge Social History of Britain 1750–1950* II (Cambridge 1990)

Mortimer, Richard, "The Priory of Butley and the Lepers of West Somerton," *Bulletin of the Institute of Historical Research* LIII, no. 127 (1980)

Muir, Ernest, "The Leprosy Situation in Africa," *Journal of the Royal African Society* XXXIV (1940)

Muir, Ernest, "Methods of Campaign against Leprosy in India," *Leprosy Review* III, no. 2 (1931)

Muir, Ernest, "Native Ideas and Practices Regarding Leprosy," *Leprosy Review* VII, no. 4 (1936)

Moulin, Anne Marie, "L'Ancien et le Nouveau: la réponse médicale à l'épidémie de 1493," in N. Bulst and R. Delort, eds, *Maladie et société* (Paris 1989)

Murrin, John M., "Beneficiaries of Catastrophe: The English Colonies in America," in Eric Foner, ed., *The New American History* (Philadelphia 1990)

Needham, Joseph, "Medicine and Chinese Culture," in his *Clerks and Craftsmen in China* (Cambridge 1970)

Neuman, R. P., "Masturbation, Madness, and the Modern Concepts of Childhood and Adolescence," *Journal of Social History* VIII, no. 1 (1975)

Nicholas, Ralph W., "The Goddess Sitala and Epidemic Smallpox in Bengal," *Journal of Asian Studies* XLI, no. 1 (1981)

Nicholls, G. Heaton, "Empire Settlement in Africa in Relation to Trade and the Native Races," *Journal of the African Society* XXV (1926)

Noordeen, S. K., "Estimated Number of Leprosy Cases in the World," *Leprosy Review* LXIII, no. 3 (1992)

Nutton, Vivian, "The Seeds of Disease: An Explanation of Contagion and Infection from the Greeks to the Renaissance," *Medical History* XXVII (1983)

Oldrieve, Frank, *India's Lepers: How to Rid India of Leprosy* (London 1924)

Omran, Abdel R., "The Epidemiologic Transition: A Theory of the Epidemiology of Population Change," *Milbank Memorial Fund Quarterly* XLIX, no. 4 part I (1971)

Orwell, George, *Nineteen-Eighty Four: A Novel* (New York 1949; Signet edn 1950)

Osterwald, Jean Frédéric, *The Nature of Uncleanness Considered* (London 1708)

Ottosson, Per-Gunnar, "Fear of the Plague and the Burial of Plague Victims in Sweden 1710–1711," in N. Bulst and R. Delort, eds, *Maladie et société* (Paris 1989)

Pagden, Anthony, *European Encounters with the New World: From Renaissance to Romanticism* (New Haven 1993)

Palmer, Richard, "The Church, Leprosy and Plague in Medieval and Early Modern Europe," in W. J. Shiels, *The Church and Healing* (Oxford 1982)

Pankhurst, Richard, "The History of Leprosy in Ethiopia to 1935," *Medical History* XXVIII (1984)

Panzac, Daniel, *La Peste dans l'Empire Ottoman* (Paris 1985)

Park, Katharine, "Medicine and Society in Medieval Europe, 500–1500," in A. Wear, ed., *Medicine in Society* (Cambridge 1992)

Patterson, K. David, "Yellow Fever Epidemics and Mortality in the United States, 1693–1905," *Social Science and Medicine* XXXIV (1992)

Patterson, K. David and Gerald W. Hartwig, *Disease in African History* (Durham, NC 1978)

Payenneville, Dr, "Rapport sur l'organisation de la lutte anti vénerienne en France," in M. A. Khalil, ed., *Comptes Rendus* V (Cairo 1932)

Pelling, Margaret, "Appearance and Reality: Barber-Surgeons, the Body and Disease," in A. L. Beier and Roger Finlay, eds, *London 1500–1700: The Making of a Metropolis* (London 1986)

Pelling, Margaret, *Cholera, Fever and English Medicine 1825–1865* (Oxford 1978)

Phillips, David R. and Yola Verhasselt, eds, *Health and Development* (London 1994)

Pickstone, John V., "Ferriar's Fever to Kay's Cholera: Disease and Social Structure in Cottonopolis," *History of Science* XXII (1984)

Pollitzer, R., *Cholera* (Geneva 1959)

Porter, H. C., *The Inconstant Savage: England and the North American Indian, 1500–1660* (London 1979)

Porter, Dorothy and Roy Porter, "The Politics of Prevention: Anti-Vaccinationism and Public Health in Nineteenth Century England," *Medical History* XXXII (1988)

Porter, Roy, "Love, Sex and Madness in Eighteenth Century England," *Social Research* LIII (1986)

Porter, Roy, "Love, Sex and Medicine: Nicolas Venette and his Tableau de l'Amour Conjugal," in Peter Wagner, ed., *Erotica and the Enlightenment* (Frankfurt am Main 1990)

Porter, Roy, "The Patient in England, *c.* 1660–*c.* 1800," in A. Wear, ed., *Medicine in Society* (Cambridge 1992)

Porter, Roy, ed., *The Popularization of Medicine 1650–1850* (London 1992)

Porter, Roy, "Quacks and Sex: Pioneering or Anxiety Making?," in his *Health for Sale: Quackery in England 1660–1850* (Manchester 1989)

Postma, Johannes Menna, *The Dutch in the Atlantic Slave Trade* (Cambridge 1990)

Prem, Hanns J., "Disease Outbreaks in Central Mexico During the Sixteenth

Century," in N. D. Cook and W. G. Lovell, eds, *"Secret Judgments of God"* (Norman, OK 1991)

Prothero, R. Mansell, *Migrants and Malaria* (London 1965)

Quétel, Claude, *History of Syphilis* (Cambridge 1990)

Raj, Kapil, "Knowledge, Power and Modern Science: The Brahmins Strike Back," in Deepak Kumar, ed., *Science and Empire: Essays in Indian Context (1700–1947)* (Anamika Prakashan 1991)

Rake, Beaven *et al.*, *Leprosy in India: Report on the Leprosy Commission in India 1890–91* (Calcutta 1892)

Ramenofsky, Ann, *Vectors of Death: The Archaeology of European Contact* (Albuquerque 1987)

Ramsey, Matthew, *Professional and Popular Medicine in France, 1770–1830* (Cambridge 1988)

Ranger, Terence, "Godly Medicine: The Ambiguities of Medical Mission in Southeast Tanzania, 1900–1945," in S. Feierman and J. M. Janzen, eds, *Social Basis of Health and Healing* (Berkeley 1992)

Ranger, Terence and Paul Slack, eds, *Epidemics and Ideas: Essays on the Historical Perception of Pestilence* (Cambridge 1992)

Raychaudhuri, Tapan, "Europe in India's Xenology: The Nineteenth Century Record," *Past and Present* CXXXVII (1992)

Razzell, Peter, *Edward Jenner's Cowpox Vaccine: The History of a Medical Myth* (Firle, Sussex 1977)

Reff, Daniel T., "Contact Shock in Northwestern New Spain, 1518–1764," in J. W. Verano and D. H. Ubelaker, eds, *Disease and Demography in the Americas* (Washington, DC 1992)

Richardson, Ruth, *Death, Dissection and the Destitute* (London 1987)

Riddle, John M., *Contraception and Abortion from the Ancient World to the Renaissance* (Cambridge, MA 1992)

Rigau-Pérez, José G., "Smallpox Epidemics in Puerto Rico during the Prevaccine Era (1518–1803)," *Journal of the History of Medicine* XXXVII, no. 4 (1982)

Risse, Guenter, "Medicine in the Age of Enlightenment," in A. Wear, ed., *Medicine in Society* (Cambridge 1992)

Robisheaux, Thomas, "Peasants and Pastors: Rural Youth Control and the Reformation in Hohenlohe, 1540–1680," *Social History* VI, no. 3 (1981)

Roper, Lyndal, "Discipline and Respectability: Prostitution and the Reformation in Augsburg," *History Workshop Journal* XIX (1985)

Rosenberg, Charles, "Cholera in Nineteenth Century Europe: A Tool for Social and Economic Analysis," *Comparative Studies in Society and History* XIII (1966)

Rosenberg, Charles, *Explaining Epidemics and Other Studies in the History of Medicine* (Cambridge 1992)

Ross, Ronald, *Memoirs: With a Full Account of the Great Malaria Problem and Its Solution* (London 1923)

Ross, Ronald, "Missionaries and the Campaign against Malaria," *Journal of Tropical Medicine* XIII (1910)

Ross, W. Felton, "Leprosy Control: Past, Present and Future," *Proceedings of the 3rd International Workshop of Leprosy Control in Asia* (T'ai-pei 1986)

Rossiaud, Jacques, *Medieval Prostitution* (Oxford 1988)
Rossiaud, Jacques, "Prostitution, Sex and Society in French Towns in the Fifteenth Century," in Philippe Ariès and André Béjin, eds, *Western Sexuality: Practice and Precept in Past and Present Times* (Oxford 1985)
Rothenberg, Gunther E., "The Austrian Sanitary Cordon and the Control of Bubonic Plague: 1710–1871," *Journal of the History of Medicine* XXVIII (1973)
Rouse, Irving, *The Tainoes: Rise and Decline of the People Who Greeted Columbus* (New Haven 1993)
Rousseau, Jean Jacques, *Emile, or Education* (first published 1762) (London 1911)
Sahagún, Bernardion de, *Florentine Codex: General History of the Things of New Spain* (Salt Lake City 1955)
Said, Edward, *Culture and Imperialism* (London 1993)
Said, Edward, *Orientalism* (London 1978)
Santra, I., "Survey Reports: Leprosy Survey in the Punjab," *Leprosy in India* III, no. 2 (1931)
Savitt, Todd L., *Medicine and Slavery: The Diseases and Health Care of Blacks in Antebellum Virginia* (Urbana, IL 1978)
Savitt, Todd L. and James H. Young, *Disease and Distinctiveness in the American South* (Knoxville, TN 1988)
Sellelink, J., *Geschiedenis der Cholera in Oose-Indië vóór 1817* (Utrecht 1885)
Sen, A. K., *Poverty and Famines: An Essay on Entitlement and Deprivation* (Oxford 1981)
Shahar, Shulamith, "Des Lépreux pas comme les autres: l'ordre de Saint-Lazare dans le Royaume Latin de Jérusalem," *Revue Historique* CCLXVII (1982)
Shelford, Frederick, "Ten Years" Progress in West Africa," *Journal of the African Society* VI (1906–7)
Siraisi, Nancy G., *Medieval & Early Renaissance Medicine: An Introduction to Knowledge and Practice* (Chicago 1990)
Skidmore, Thomas, "Racial Ideas and Social Policy in Brazil, 1870–1940," in Richard Graham, ed., *The Idea of Race in Latin America* (Austin, TX 1990)
Slack, Paul, *The Impact of Plague in Tudor and Stuart England* (London 1995)
Smith, Adam, *Theory of Moral Sentiment* (first published 1759) (Oxford 1976)
Smith, C. Stanley, "Leprosy in Kigezi, Uganda Protectorate," *Leprosy Review* II, no. 4 (1931)
Smith, J. R., *The Speckled Monster: Smallpox in England 1670–1970, with Particular Reference to Essex* (Chelmsford 1987)
Snell, K. D. M., *Annals of the Labouring Poor: Social Change and Agrarian England, 1660–1900* (Cambridge 1987)
Snowden, Frank M., *Naples in the Time of Cholera, 1884–1911* (Cambridge 1995)
Solórzano, Armando, "Sowing the Seeds of Neo-Imperialism: The

Rockefeller Foundation's Yellow Fever Campaign in Mexico," *International Journal of Health Services* XXII, no. 3 (1992)
Sonbol, Amira, *The Creation of a Medical Profession in Egypt, 1800–1922* (Syracuse, NY 1992)
Spitzer, Leo, "The Mosquito and Segregation in Sierra Leone," *Canadian Journal of African Studies* II, no. 1 (1968)
Stannard, David E., *American Holocaust: Columbus and the Conquest of the New World* (Oxford 1992)
Stengers, Jean, and Anne Van Neck, *Histoire d'une grande peur: la masturbation* (Brussels 1984)
Stepan, Nancy, *Beginnings of Brazilian Science: Oswaldo Cruz, Medical Research and Policy, 1890–1920* (New York 1976)
Stepan, Nancy, *The Idea of Race in Science: Great Britain 1800–1960* (London 1982)
Stopes, Marie Carmichael, *Married Love: A New Contribution to the Solution of Sex Difficulties* (London 1918)
Strachey, John, *India* (London 1888)
Strahan, S. A. K., *Marriage and Disease: A Study of Hereditary and the More Important Family Degenerations* (London 1892)
Strayer, Robert, *The Making of Mission Communities in East Africa: Anglicans and Africans in Colonial Kenya, 1875–1935* (London 1978)
Ten Have, Henk A. M. J., G. Kimsma and S. Spicker, *The Growth of Medical Knowledge* (Dordrecht 1990)
Thapar, Romila, "Imagined Religious Communities? Ancient History and the Modern Search for a Hindu Identity," *Modern Asian Studies* XXIII, no. 2 (1989)
Thin, George, *Leprosy* (London 1891)
Thompson, F. M. L., *The Rise of Respectable Society: A Social History of Victorian Britain 1830–1900* (Cambridge, MA 1988)
Thornton, John, *Africa and Africans in the Making of the Atlantic World, 1400–1680* (Cambridge 1992)
Tissot, S. A. A. D., *Onanism or, A Treatise upon the Disorders Produced by Masturbation or, The Dangerous Effects of Secret and Excessive Venery* (London 1756)
Todorov, Tzvetan, *The Conquest of America* (New York 1992)
Touati, François-Olivier, "Une Approche de la maladie et du phénomène hospitalier aux XIIe et XIIIe siècles: la léproserie du Grand-Beaulieu à Chartres," *Histoire des Sciences Médicales* XIV, no. 1 (1980)
Trudgill, Eric, "Prostitution and Paterfamilias," in H. J. Dyos and M. Wolff, eds, *The Victorian City: Images and Realities* (London 1973)
United Nations, *Human Development Report for 1993* (Oxford 1993)
Unschald, Paul U., "Epistemological Issues and Changing Legitimation: Traditional Chinese Medicine in the Twentieth Century," in Charles Leslie and Allan Young, eds, *Paths to Asian Medical Knowledge* (Berkeley 1992)
Upadhyay, V. S., *Socio-Cultural Implications of Leprosy: An Essay in Medical Anthropology* (Calcutta 1988)
Vaughan, Megan, *Curing Their Ills: Colonial Power and African Illness* (Cambridge 1991)

Vaughan, Megan, "Syphilis in Colonial East and Central Africa: The Social Construction of an Epidemic," in T. Ranger and S. Slack, eds, *Epidemics and Ideas* (Cambridge 1992)

Verano, John W. and Douglas H. Ubelaker, eds, *Disease and Demography in the Americas* (Washington, DC 1992)

Vigarello, Georges, *Concepts of Cleanliness: Changing Attitudes in France since the Middle Ages* (Cambridge 1988)

Walkowitz, Judith, *City of Dreadful Delight: Narratives of Sexual Danger in Late Victorian London* (Chicago 1992)

Walter, John and Roger Schofield, eds, *Famine, Disease and the Social Order in Early Modern Society* (Cambridge 1991)

Walzer, Michael, *Thick and Thin: Moral Arguments at Home and Abroad* (Notre Dame, IN 1994)

Washbrook, D. A., "Progress and Problems: South Asian Economic and Social History *c.* 1720–1860," *Modern Asian Studies* XXII, no. 1 (1988)

Watts, S. J., *A Social History of Western Europe 1450–1720: Tensions and Solidarities among Rural People* (London 1984)

Wayson, N. E., "Leprosy in Hawaii," *Leprosy Review* III, no. 1 (1932)

Wear, Andrew, ed., *Medicine in Society: Historical Essays* (Cambridge 1992)

Weber, Eugene, *From Peasants into Frenchmen: The Modernization of Rural France* (Stanford, CA 1976)

Webster, Charles, *The Great Instauration: Science, Medicine and Reform, 1626–1669* (London 1975)

Willis, Justin, "The Nature of a Mission Community: The Universities' Mission to Central Africa in Bonde," *Past and Present* CXL (1993)

Wills, John E. Jr., "European Consumption and Asian Production in the Seventeenth and Eighteenth Centuries," in John Brewer and Roy Porter, eds, *Consumption and the World of Goods* (London 1993)

Wilson, Samuel M., *Hispaniola: Caribbean Chiefdoms in the Age of Columbus* (Tuscaloosa, AL 1990)

Worboys, Michael, "The Discovery of Colonial Malnutrition between the Wars," in D. Arnold, ed., *Imperial Medicine and Indigenous Societies* (Manchester 1988)

Worboys, Michael, "Manson, Ross and Colonial Medical Policy: Tropical Medicine in London and Liverpool, 1899–1914," in R. MacLeod and L. Lewis, eds, *Disease, Medicine and Empire* (London 1988)

World Health Organization, *Prevention and Control of Yellow Fever in Africa* (Geneva 1986)

World Health Organization, *The World Health Report 1995: Bridging the Gaps* (Geneva 1995)

Wright, Henry, *Leprosy and its Story: Segregation and its Remedy* (London 1885)

Wright, Ronald, *Stolen Continents: The American Indian Story* (London 1993)

Zier, Mark, "The Healing Power of the Hebrew Tongue: An Example from Late Thirteenth Century England," in S. Campbell *et al.*, eds, *Health, Disease and Healing in Medieval Culture* (New York 1992)

Index